International
Diabetes Center

Learning to Live *Well* with Diabetes

Editorial Committee:
Donnell D. Etzwiler, M.D.
Marion J. Franz, R.D., M.S.
Priscilla Hollander, M.D.
Judy Ostrom Joynes, R.N., M.A.

Editors:

Neysa C. M. Jensen
Michael P. Moore

Diabetes Center, Inc.
Minnetonka, Minnesota

Acknowledgements

The Editorial Committee members and the International Diabetes Center gratefully acknowledge and extend our sincere thanks to the following people, whose skills and efforts helped to make this book possible:

Production Manager
Neysa C. M. Jensen

Preparation of Manuscripts and Typesetting
Carol Hargarten, B.A.

Illustrations
Andrew Grivas, M.A.
Medical Illustrator,
Biomedical Graphic Communications
University of Minnesota

Cover and Intro Art Chapters 1-7
Michael Pearson Advertising
Minneapolis, Minnesota

Illustrations Chapters 6, 28, 29
Tom Foty Advertising Art
Minneapolis, Minnesota

© 1985 All Rights Reserved
Revised, 1987.
International Diabetes Center
Park Nicollet Medical Foundation
5000 West 39th Street
Minneapolis, Minnesota 55416
Phone: 612/927-3393

Library of Congress Cataloging-in-Publication Data

Learning to live well with diabetes.

Includes index
1. Diabetes — popular works.   I. Etzwiler, Donnell D.
II. Jensen, Neysa C. M.
RC660.L338 1987   616.4'62   87-5369
ISBN 0-937721-23-9

About the
International Diabetes Center

The International Diabetes Center (IDC) believes that excellence in diabetes management can be achieved only when informed individuals with the disease work with concerned health professionals in planned systems of care and using the most modern techniques. Through its education, clinical research, team management, and outreach programs, the IDC is working to ensure that this goal is reached and the quality of life improved for all people with diabetes.

A division of the Park Nicollet Medical Foundation, the IDC translates the latest research knowledge and advanced medical technology into practical systems of diabetes management. The IDC is on the leading edge of major changes in the health care system, developing education and treatment models that set an example in cost containment and are applicable to other chronic conditions.

Education
The IDC evolved from the Diabetes Education Center, founded in 1967 by IDC Director Dr. Donnell D. Etzwiler. Nearly 6,000 individuals with diabetes and their family members and more than 6,000 health professionals from the United States and other nations have come to the IDC to learn more about diabetes.

Care
The IDC, in conjunction with Park Nicollet Medical Center (PNMC), offers ongoing treatment through large pediatric and adult diabetes clinics. Specialized outpatient services are offered at IDC/PNMC, including an ambulatory (outpatient) insulin start program, diabetes and pregnancy program, and eye, foot, neurology, urology, and renal clinics.

IDC nutrition and nurse educators and family counselors offer consultative services in areas such as meal planning, weight loss, blood glucose monitoring and insulin injection skills, emotional adjustment to diabetes, and family problem solving. All focus on maximizing the individual's and family's ability to achieve good diabetes control while living fully. Feedback and suggestions for future management are provided to the person's physician.

Clinical Research
IDC research evaluates the latest discoveries and technological advances and translates them into the most effective health care delivery systems possible. The IDC was part of some of the first clinical testing of human insulins, and continues to assess the effectiveness of new insulins, oral agents, and other diabetes medications. The IDC/PNMC is one of the centers taking part in the Diabetes Control and Complications Trial, a nationwide study of the practicality and effects of strict blood glucose control.

Outreach
The IDC is actively spreading its mission in cooperation with health professionals in communities throughout Minnesota, in many other states, and in several other nations. IDC staff hold leadership positions in the American Diabetes Association and its Minnesota Affiliate, American Association of Diabetes Educators, American Dietetic Association, and International Diabetes Federation. IDC staff members speak throughout the world on topics related to diabetes, with the common theme being the importance of involving people with chronic health problems and their families in a close team working relationship with their health care providers.

Learning to Live *Well* with Diabetes
Table of Contents

Section IV—Special Topics on Diabetes

Section V—Diabetes and Youth

The Authors

Barbara Balik, R.N., M.S.
Pediatric Nurse Practitioner,
International Diabetes Center

Jose Barbosa, M.D.
Associate Professor,
Division of Endocrinology and Metabolism,
University of Minnesota School of Medicine,
Minneapolis, Minnesota

Richard M. Bergenstal, M.D.
Assistant Director for Adult Diabetes,
International Diabetes Center
Adult Endocrinologist,
Park Nicollet Medical Center

Randi Birk, M.A., L.P.
Family Counselor,
International Diabetes Center

Helen R. Bowlin, R.N., B.S.N.Ed.
Health Professional Coordinator
International Diabetes Center

Nancy Cooper, R.D., B.S.
Nutrition Educator,
International Diabetes Center

Donald A. Duncan, M.D.
Consultant, International Diabetes Center
Nephrologist, Park Nicollet Medical Center

Donnell D. Etzwiler, M.D.
Director, International Diabetes Center
Pediatric Diabetologist,
Park Nicollet Medical Center

Catherine Feste
Motivation Specialist
Minneapolis, Minnesota

Marion J. Franz, R.D., M.S.
Director of Nutrition,
International Diabetes Center

Broatch Haig, R.D., B.S.
Nutrition Coordinator, Outreach Services,
International Diabetes Center

Priscilla Hollander, M.D.
Assistant Director for Diabetes Studies,
International Diabetes Center
Adult Endocrinologist,
Park Nicollet Medical Center

Judy Ostrom Joynes, R.N., M.A.
Director of Education,
International Diabetes Center

Ron Kitzman, R.Ph.
Consultant, International Diabetes Center
Director of Pharmacy, Methodist Hospital
Minneapolis, Minnesota

Wayne Leebaw, M.D.
Consultant, International Diabetes Center
Endocrinologist, Meadowbrook Endocrinology Clinic
Minneapolis, Minnesota

LeAnn McNeil, R.N., M.S.
Director of Research
International Diabetes Center

William J. Mestrezat, M.D.
Consultant, International Diabetes Center
Director of Retina/Vitreous Services
Park Nicollet Medical Center

Arlene Monk, R.D., B.S.
Nutrition Educator,
International Diabetes Center

Patricia M. Moynihan, R.N., M.P.H.
Director, Outreach Services,
International Diabetes Center

Lucy Mullen, R.N., B.S.
Diabetes Nurse Educator,
International Diabetes Center

Leonard A. Nordstrom, M.D.
Cardiologist,
Park Nicollet Medical Center

Beth Olson, R.N., B.A.
Foot Care Specialist
International Diabetes Center
Nurse Clinician, Foot Clinic,
Park Nicollet Medical Center

Leslie Pratt, M.D.
Obstetrics/Gynecology,
Park Nicollet Medical Center

Martha L. Spencer, M.D.
Assistant Director for Diabetes in Youth,
International Diabetes Center
Pediatric Endocrinologist,
Park Nicollet Medical Center

Introduction

Before You Read This Book . . . .

. . . take a moment to think about your current needs for information on diabetes. **Learning to Live *Well* with Diabetes** was written to be used by people with many different needs related to diabetes and to continue to be useful for many years.

The key word is "used." There is a great deal of information presented, but this information will be relatively useless if it is just read and then put on your bookshelf. It can be most useful if you set a fairly specific objective each time you begin reading. Within the overall goal of living well with diabetes there are many specific objectives; for example to lose weight, improve blood glucose (sugar) control, adjust emotionally, do everything possible to avoid complications, or help someone else do these things.

To help you discover the best way **Learning to Live *Well* with Diabetes** can be used to meet your needs, I would like to present a brief guide to what it contains.

As you can see from the Table of Contents, there are five sections, each containing chapters that discuss specific areas of diabetes and written for either a general or specific audience. Some of the main concepts of diabetes, especially those related to prevention of health problems, are explained and discussed in several different sections. This will allow you to read some of the later chapters without having to go back to refresh your memory about concepts discussed earlier.

The first section is a general overview of diabetes information. It covers all the basic areas we at the International Diabetes Center feel are necessary to get started toward living well. Especially important are the two topics that are seldom addressed when diabetes information is presented: emotional adjustment to the disease, and motivation to do what is necessary to control it and live well. No amount of information will improve a person's life unless you are ready and willing to put it to good use. Much of the information in the first section will also be very helpful for those who do not have diabetes, but who want to know what it is and how it can be controlled. And anyone may benefit from the chapters on nutrition and exercise, which are vital parts of a healthy lifestyle with or without diabetes.

Section two will help people on insulin therapy take the steps necessary to work with their health care providers to improve diabetes control. It is important to know what to expect in the way of good diabetes care and then make sure you receive it. Of course, it is equally important to be able and willing to work as part of your health care team to follow through with the daily practices that are the main ingredients of your health care plan. A chapter on possible complications outlines how these daily practices help a person avoid health problems—today and in the future.

Section three looks at aspects of diabetes care for people with Type II (non-insulin-dependent) diabetes. It is important for these people, who usually develop diabetes after the age of 40, to realize that their form of the disease is just as serious as Type I (insulin-dependent) diabetes, which usually develops at an earlier age. The key here is to work closely with a health care team that can help make lifestyle changes needed to control diabetes and prevent or reduce the severity of health complications.

Section four covers in more detail some of the concepts that have been mentioned or discussed briefly in earlier sections. The chapter titles will help you decide when you are ready to use the information discussed. The chapter on diabetes research may provide the motivation you need to control your diabetes as well as possible. Exciting things are being done to not only find a cure but improve our ability to control diabetes!

Section five contains a fun chapter to be read with a child who has diabetes (and brothers, sisters and friends too) to help establish a basic understanding of diabetes. There are also two chapters for parents or other relatives of children with diabetes. Parents need not only information but also much support from others to help with a very important challenge.

Learning to Live *Well* with Diabetes has been designed to be easy to use. The wide margins are meant to be written in, and many chapters end with a place for note-taking. As you read, please highlight especially useful information and jot down questions for your health care providers, notes to yourself, ideas that occur to you, anything that will help you or a loved one live well. If you are so inclined, please take the time to write to me to let us know how we might improve this book. Use it in good health!

Section I

General Information to Get You Started:

Diabetes
Nutrition
Exercise
Testing
Skills
Emotional Adjustment
Motivation

For Individuals and Families with
Insulin-Dependent (Type I) Diabetes
OR
Non-Insulin-Dependent (Type II) Diabetes

Diabetes?

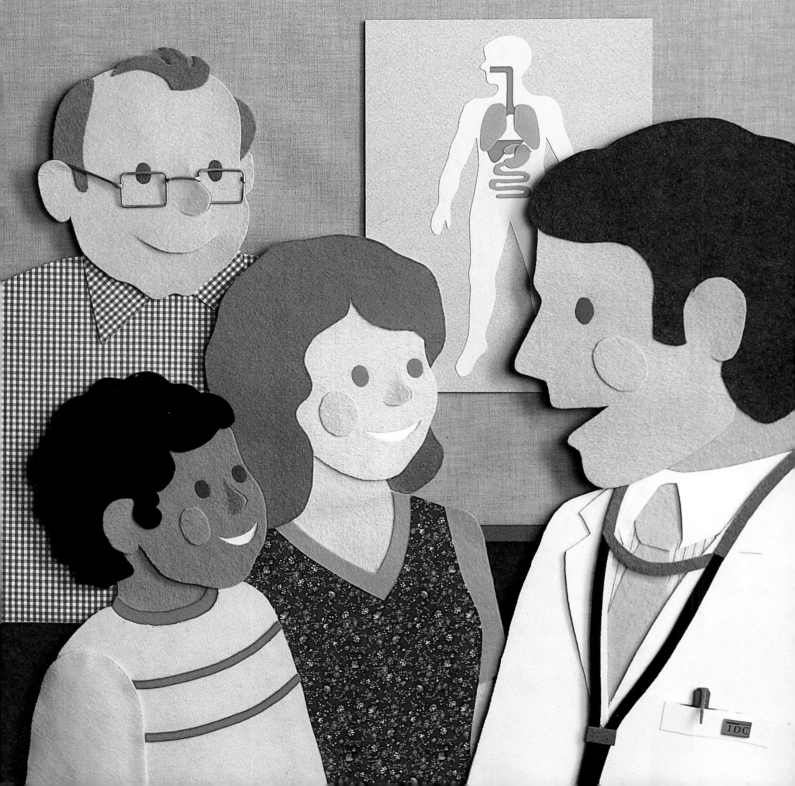

Chapter 1
Diabetes: What Is It?

Donnell D. Etzwiler, M.D.

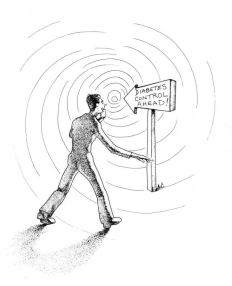

If you, a member of your family, or a friend had to develop diabetes, there has never been a better time. Although there is still no cure for this disease, there is a tremendous amount of research being conducted. And, yes, there does appear to be a "light at the end of the tunnel." This thought should not be used as an excuse to ignore your diabetes. It is meant to encourage you to achieve the best possible physical condition so you can take full advantage of the breakthroughs of the future. It is now more important than ever to control your diabetes.

Diabetes is a serious disease that has been known for thousands of years and was described in the earliest medical writings. But it has not been until relatively recently that the seriousness of the disease and its accompanying complications have been understood and fully appreciated. In the mid-1960s the American Diabetes Association (ADA) was considering becoming a voluntary health agency. In 18 communities throughout the United States, a sampling of the public along with health professionals, community leaders, and heads of health agencies were asked, "Would the American Diabetes Association receive public support if it became a voluntary health agency?"

When the results were analyzed, the ADA was informed that such an effort would fail because there was little public interest in diabetes! The public's perception of diabetes was that it is a relatively innocent disease and of concern only to older overweight people. Treatment of the disease was considered by the public to consist mostly of dietary management and weight loss. If this were unsuccessful, the public thought that a diabetes pill could be taken. It was recognized that a few people with diabetes might require insulin, but otherwise they were thought to need little medical help and could live a normal life.

In the years since this survey the true nature of diabetes and its many associated complications have been recognized, and the American Diabetes Association has become an important national voluntary health agency and a major benefactor to research, education, and care.

In 1974, Congress established a National Diabetes Commission, which was responsible for determining how many Americans have diabetes, what problems exist, and what are its financial costs. The Commission was also asked to identify all research being conducted in the field and what plan was needed for the future. On the basis of this data, a five-year action plan was submitted to Congress. The results of the National Commission Report on Diabetes startled even those familiar with the field of diabetes. It was found that:

- At least eleven million Americans have diabetes.
- 500,000 to 600,000 new cases of diabetes are diagnosed each year.
- Diabetes is the fifth leading cause of death by disease.
- Diabetes is the leading cause of new cases of blindness among people between 20 and 74 years old.
- People with diabetes are twice as likely as others to develop heart disease and suffer a heart attack or stroke.
- People with diabetes are 17 times more prone to kidney disease.
- People with diabetes are 40 times more likely to have amputations.
- The estimated cost of diabetes to this nation in 1985 was more than 14 billion dollars.

How long has diabetes been known?

We now know that diabetes is indeed a serious disease and that it can be controlled, but this has not always been so. A brief history of diabetes will help you understand the changes that have occurred through the years.

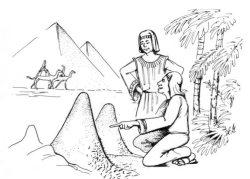

Diabetes was described in the earliest known medical literature, an Egyptian manuscript known as the Ebers Papyrus, which was written about 1500 B.C. Later in Arabic and Chinese literature, people who drank large amounts of water and voided huge amounts of urine were described and recognized as suffering from the disease. The early literature even describes diagnostic tests in which urine from the patient was poured near ant hills. If the ants were attracted to the urine, it was known that sugar was present, and the diagnosis was made. The Greek physician Aretaeus (120-200 A.D.) first called the disease "diabetes," which means to syphon or to flow through. The Latin word "mellitus," which means honeyed, is often added (diabetes mellitus) to indicate the presence of sugar in the urine.

In the 1860s, a German doctor named Paul Langerhans examined under the microscope pieces of the pancreas, a pistol-shaped gland located behind the stomach. He noticed that certain cells took up different colored dyes. These cells seemed to appear together as groups or islands scattered throughout the pancreas. They made up only about 1 percent of the entire gland, and because of their scattered appearance they were referred to as the "islets of Langerhans." But their function was a mystery.

Today, we know that these islets contain the beta cells, which make, store, and release the body's supply of insulin, a substance that lowers blood sugar (glucose). They also contain alpha cells, which produce and release glucagon, a substance which raises blood sugar. Glucagon is described in Chapter 8.

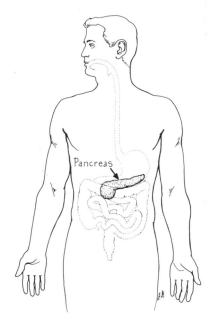

One of the first really significant diabetes experiments occurred in the 1880s when Oscar Minkowski and Joseph von Mering discovered that the pancreas is closely involved with the disease. These scientists were not interested specifically in diabetes, but they did want to know what effect various organs of the body had on the digestion and use of food. They found that when the pancreas of a dog was removed, the animal began urinating more frequently, sugar appeared in the urine, and the animal ultimately died. This experiment drew the scientific world's attention to the pancreas and its possible relationship to diabetes.

A major breakthrough in the treatment of diabetes occurred in 1921. Two researchers chose to spend a summer trying to isolate a substance from the pancreas that they thought might be helpful in treating the disease. The senior researcher was a surgeon named Dr. Frederick Banting, who had no special training or experience in diabetes. Dr. Banting was assisted by a young medical student named Charles Best. They were quite an unlikely pair of diabetes researchers. But together they succeeded in isolating an extract from the pancreas of dogs that when injected into diabetic dogs, caused the blood sugar (glucose) to decrease. The extract came from the islet cells of the pancreas and was first referred to as isletin, but later became known as insulin. Dr. Banting received the Nobel prize for medicine in 1923 for the discovery of insulin.

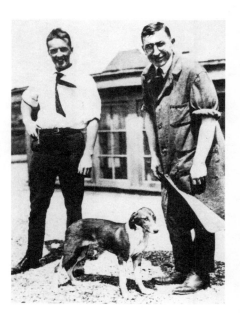

Charles Best (left) and Dr. Frederick Banting with the first dog to be kept alive by insulin.

Before the discovery of insulin, young people who developed diabetes lived for only a few weeks or months.

Before the discovery of insulin, young people who developed diabetes lived for only a few weeks or months. Daily injections of insulin reversed that pattern, and the world rejoiced in the belief that indeed a cure for diabetes had been found. It was thought that if people with diabetes took their insulin regularly and ate properly, they would live a normal life.

In the 1930s, however, information began to appear in the literature about problems that were occurring in people who had been treated with insulin since the onset of their disease. These problems included loss of eyesight, poor blood supply to the lower legs and feet, and increased numbers of heart attacks.

Despite these alarming findings, it was not until after World War II, in the late 1940s and early 1950s, that extensive research work in the field of diabetes was resumed. At that time, Dr. Saul Berson and Dr. Rosalyn Yalow, two researchers in New York, tried to measure the amount of insulin present in the blood. Since the amount of insulin in the blood is very small—about one part per billion—this was obviously a difficult task. They devised an ingenious method of measuring this tiny amount of insulin, and to their surprise found that there was not an absence of insulin in all people with diabetes. They found that in some people there was little or no insulin in the blood, but in others there were normal amounts. And in many overweight people with diabetes, they found more insulin in the blood than in that of people who did not have diabetes. These amazing discoveries stimulated increasing amounts of diabetes research. Dr. Yalow received the Nobel prize for medicine in 1977.

In the early 1950s, a researcher in England, Dr. Frederick Sanger, was conducting studies unrelated to diabetes, but which resulted in some interesting new information. Sanger, a molecular scientist, was trying to determine the structure of protein molecules. He needed a readily available source of small protein molecules, and chose insulin. Insulin is a protein that is relatively pure, readily available, and inexpensive. Sanger found that the insulin molecule resembles two lengths of chain bound together by sulfa atoms. He also found that the individual links of the insulin chains varied in different animals. Insulin from pigs differed from human insulin in only one of the 51 tiny links that make up the two chains, while beef insulin differed in three sites. Whale insulin and insulin from other animals had other variations, so it became apparent that not all insulin was exactly the same.

Sanger's work caused some scientists to question the accepted cause of diabetes. For a long time it had been thought that diabetes was a result of the pancreas not producing a sufficient quantity of insulin. Researchers now began to wonder if some people have diabetes because they are not able to produce a good quality of insulin.

In the late 1960s, Dr. Donald Steiner of the University of Chicago found a substance that apparently is first made in the islets of the pancreas and is then changed into insulin. This substance, **proinsulin** ("pro" means "before"), was found to be about one twentieth as effective in lowering blood glucose as was insulin. The discovery of proinsulin helped researchers understand how insulin is formed in the pancreas.

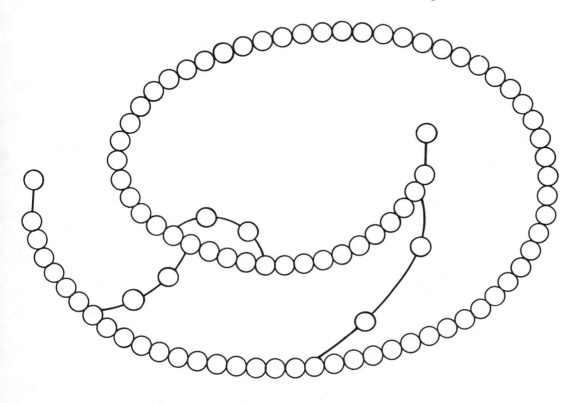

Proinsulin

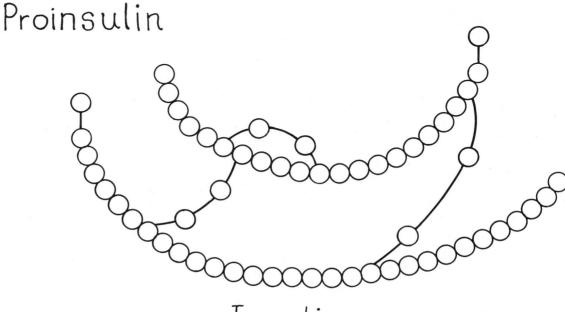

Insulin

Carbohydrates

Fats

Protein

P

What does insulin do in the body?

When diabetes occurs in a young person and some lean adults, there is usually a shortage or complete lack of insulin. The insulin cells in the pancreas are scarred or destroyed, so they cannot make enough insulin. To understand how the lack of insulin affects a person's health, it is necessary to understand how insulin normally functions in the body.

If one thinks of the body as a complex machine, it is apparent that like any machine, it has to have sources of energy to perform its work. Three sources of energy are found in foods—carbohydrate (sugars and starches), fat (oils and fats), and protein (meat, fish, etc.).

After chewing and swallowing, foods are digested in the stomach and intestines. Then they are absorbed through the walls of the intestines and go into the bloodstream, where they are carried to the millions of cells which make up all parts of the body. The fuel most readily available for use by all the body's cells immediately after eating is a carbohydrate called glucose. Glucose is a simple form of sugar that can be used by body cells.

As the amount of glucose in the blood rises after we eat, the pancreas detects this and sends out a "message" in the blood to all of the individual cells in the body. The message says "There is a lot of glucose available, use it." This "message" is insulin. Insulin attaches itself to specific places on the wall of each cell in the body. These places are called insulin receptor sites. They allow insulin to signal the wall of the cell to open up and take in the glucose circulating in the blood. Insulin at the same time signals the rest of the cell that glucose is being taken in and should be used as the main source of energy.

When the amount of glucose in the blood is low, the pancreas stops sending out insulin. Without insulin, body cells can't take in glucose, so they switch to using fat and protein as their main source of energy. It is in this sophisticated manner that the body is able to determine which energy fuel is available and properly use the foods we eat. When diabetes develops, either the pancreas is unable to produce insulin or the cells are unable to receive the insulin message. The result is that the body can no longer use foods correctly.

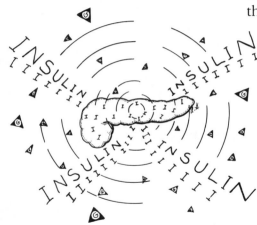

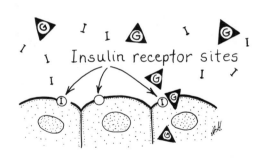

Insulin receptor sites

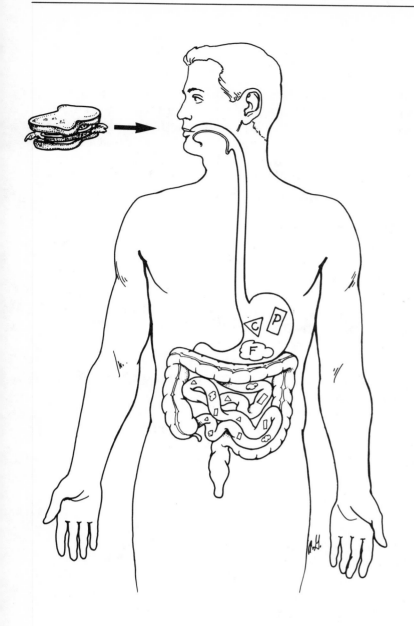

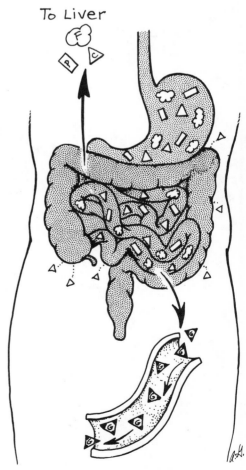

To Liver

Glucose △
enters bloodstream

9

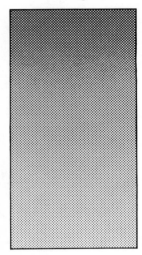

160 mg/dl

60 mg/dl

Normal blood
glucose range

In people who do not have diabetes, the amount of glucose in the blood is closely controlled at all times. When people without diabetes do not eat for several hours, the amount of glucose in the blood rarely falls below 60 mg/dl, and even after gorging themselves on sweets, these individuals are able to keep the blood glucose below 160 mg/dl. [Blood glucose is measured in milligrams (thousandths of a gram) of glucose in each deciliter, or approximately 1 1/2 ounces of blood.]

This very fine control is exceedingly important because we know that if blood glucose gets too high, it can become dangerous. The kidneys must then filter the glucose from the blood and wash it out of the body in the urine. When this occurs the person must drink large amounts of fluids to provide enough water to "wash" out the excess glucose. It is difficult to replace all of the water that is lost, and the body may quickly become dehydrated, or literally dried out. This can be a serious threat to life.

When there is no insulin to allow the body cells to use glucose for energy, they demand another source of energy to carry out their work. Fat and protein are the only other sources of energy available, so the cells switch to using fat and protein. These fuels are harder for the cells to use, which is why they prefer to use glucose. The cells can't burn fat and protein completely, and some of the unused material, or by-products, begin to build up in the body. These by-products are called **ketones**.

As the ketones increase, a condition called **ketoacidosis** appears. ("Osis" means "a condition of," so ketoacidosis means an acid condition resulting from ketones.) As this occurs the person's mouth becomes dry, and he or she experiences abdominal pain. If ketoacidosis is not recognized and treated promptly with insulin and fluids, the person may begin vomiting, breathing heavily, lose consciousness, and eventually may die because of severe ketoacidosis.

Ketoacidosis is a serious threat to a person with diabetes whose body does not produce insulin. It is a preventable condition, but you must understand what it is, how to detect it, and what to do. Despite this it is estimated that 40,000 individuals are hospitalized with ketoacidosis each year and 4,000 die. More information about how to prevent, detect, and treat ketoacidosis can be found in Chapters 8 and 10.

It is also dangerous if blood glucose gets too low. The brain can use only glucose for its source of energy, so when there is little glucose available it begins sending out emergency signals to the rest of the body. The person then experiences hunger, headaches, confusion, loss of consciousness, and may even have convulsions. If the blood glucose is very low over many hours, brain damage may result. It is therefore vitally important that the body closely control the amount of glucose in the blood, not allowing it to become too high or low.

Although diabetes is sometimes referred to as "sugar diabetes," it is important to realize that whenever the way we use carbohydrate is changed, there is also a change in the use of both fat and protein. The inability to use carbohydrate properly immediately results in large amounts of fats being emptied into the bloodstream and sent to the cells as an alternate source of energy. Abnormally high levels of fats (cholesterol and triglycerides) are thought to be harmful to the blood vessel walls over the years. Proper management of diabetes is an attempt to restore the normal pattern of food usage and energy production.

When the body can't use carbohydrate properly, there is also a change in the use of fat and protein.

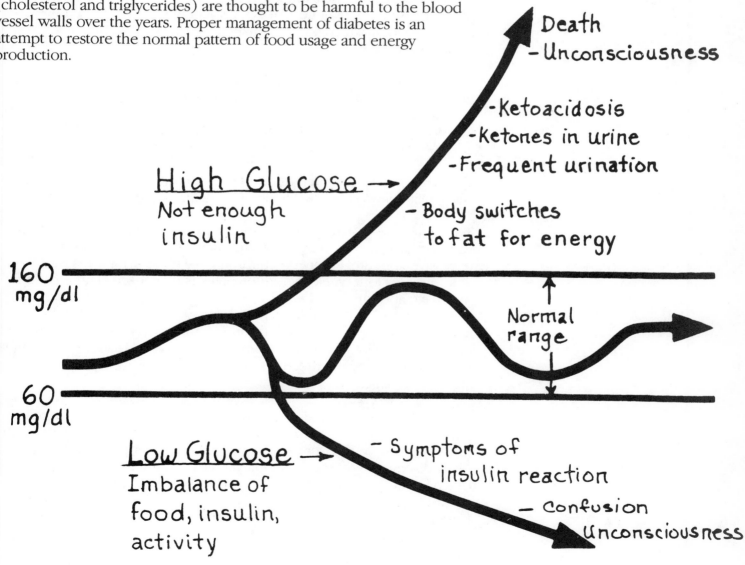

Is there more than one kind of diabetes?

There are different types of diabetes, and they may be treated quite differently. We mentioned earlier that when young people and some lean adults develop diabetes, it is usually because they have lost their ability to produce insulin. Older people, however, may have normal or high levels of insulin in the blood yet have high blood glucose levels and diabetes. This indicates that there is more than one kind of diabetes. It should help you understand why people with diabetes may be treated differently. It is also important to remember that each individual with the disease has different medical needs, different likes and dislikes, a different lifestyle, etc., so every diabetes treatment plan must be adapted to the individual being treated.

Both types of diabetes mentioned above have long been recognized, and basically share the same problem—the inability of the body to properly use carbohydrate. They have been given separate names as the differences in the causes of diabetes have become better understood.

The type of diabetes that usually occurs in children and young adults has traditionally been called "juvenile diabetes." Since all of these people require daily insulin injections to survive, the term used for this form of the disease is **insulin-dependent diabetes mellitus (IDDM)**, or abbreviated more simply as **Type I** (one) diabetes.

The type of diabetes often referred to as "adult diabetes" is now called **non-insulin-dependent diabetes mellitus (NIDDM)** or **Type II** (two) diabetes.

Type I diabetes usually appears abruptly in children or young adults, with symptoms of extreme thirst, frequent urination, tiredness, and excessive appetite. Rarely do children have these symptoms for more than three or four weeks before diabetes is diagnosed. These patients may have abdominal pain and vomiting at the time they first come to the doctor and are sometimes mistakenly thought to have the flu or appendicitis. If we could look through a microscope at the pancreas of one of these people with early symptoms of Type I diabetes, we might find that the islets are already decreased in number and show other signs of damage.

Type II diabetes differs significantly in its onset. Many times there is a past medical history of glucose in the urine or a gradual increase in the blood glucose level over months or years. In older people, diabetes is often discovered during a routine physical examination or at the time of a hospital admission for some other reason. The onset of the disease in this group is frequently not associated with any symptoms. Under a microscope, the pancreas of one of these people would probably appear normal.

Types of Diabetes

	Type I Insulin-Dependent	Type II Non-Insulin Dependent	Gestational
Onset	Usually in children or young adults.	Usually in obese adults over age 40.	Occurs in 3-5% of pregnant women.
Cause	Heredity and other factors lead to failure of pancreas' ability to produce insulin.	Inherited tendency plus obesity leads to resistance of body cells to action of insulin.	Hormonal changes lead to high blood glucose.
Symptoms	Extreme thirst and excessive appetite, tiredness, and frequent urination. May progress to ketoacidosis.	May be no obvious symptoms, or just slight fatigue and frequent thirst and urination.	Usually none; may be fatigue.
Diagnosis	Fasting blood glucose test.	Fasting blood glucose test.	Oral glucose tolerance test.
Treatment	Meal planning, exercise, and insulin injections.	Meal planning, exercise, and sometimes pills or insulin injections.	Meal planning, exercise and sometimes insulin injections.
Acute Complications	Insulin reactions and ketoacidosis.	Usually none.	Usually none.
Intermediate Complications	Failure of growth and development; problems during pregnancy.	Problems during pregnancy.	Problems during pregnancy.
Long-Term Complications	Small blood vessel problems in eyes, kidneys, nerves; large blood vessel problems in heart, brain, and extremities.	Large blood vessel problems in heart, brain, extremities; small blood vessel problems in eyes, feet, nerves, and kidneys.	Usually none; high blood glucose usually goes away after delivery. Woman is more likely to develop diabetes later in life.
Prevention of Problems	Diabetes education and blood glucose control aid ability to work with health care team to control diabetes.	Diabetes education, weight loss, and blood glucose control.	Blood glucose monitoring to allow strict control during pregnancy.

The daily problems confronting people with Type I diabetes are quite different from those of people with Type II diabetes. People with Type I diabetes are likely to develop sudden problems resulting from the blood glucose being too low (insulin reactions) or too high (which can lead to ketoacidosis). These serious disorders must be treated immediately and will be discussed in Chapter 8. These two problems seldom occur in Type II diabetes.

Even the problems which slowly arise over the years in Type I and Type II diabetes are different. People with Type I diabetes more frequently develop destruction of the small blood vessels in the eyes and kidneys. People with Type II diabetes are more prone to damage in the large blood vessels, which causes blood circulation problems, stroke, and heart disease.

Pregnant women sometimes develop a form of diabetes that is considered separate from Type I and Type II diabetes. It is called **gestational diabetes**, and it is usually discovered when the woman has urine tests and/or a blood test for glucose done during routine visits for supervision of her pregnancy. These women may or may not require insulin, but their blood glucose must be controlled very carefully during the remainder of the pregnancy if problems are to be avoided. The symptoms of gestational diabetes often go away at the end of the pregnancy. See Chapter 17 for more information about diabetes and pregnancy.

How do doctors know if a person has diabetes?

The diagnosis of diabetes in children (Type I) is relatively easy. The symptoms of thirst, frequent urination, and tiredness mentioned earlier should prompt the doctor to test the patient's blood glucose level immediately. A blood glucose test when Type I diabetes is present is usually quite high, and the diagnosis can be made immediately. It is important to start treatment as soon as possible. The young person should be seen the same day by a physician, and insulin and nutritional therapy are usually started immediately. Almost all young people with diabetes are dependent on daily injections of insulin. The kinds of insulins used in treating diabetes will be discussed in Chapters 8 and 9.

In Type II diabetes, the diagnosis may be more difficult, because there is usually no obvious illness. The blood glucose levels are not always higher than normal, and blood glucose measurements taken after eating may not be unusually high. Sometimes a test called a **glucose tolerance test** is used to identify Type II diabetes. The concept behind this test is to give the person a large amount of a sugar drink and then test the blood glucose level at ½, 1 and 2 hours later.

In people with newly diagnosed Type II diabetes, starting treatment is usually not an emergency, and diabetes management may start with meal planning and weight reduction. Some adults may take diabetes pills in addition to meal planning. These medications have been available since the mid1950s. There appear to be two ways in which the diabetes pills lower the glucose in the blood. Some stimulate the pancreas to make more insulin, while others are thought to increase the sensitivity of body cells to insulin in the blood. (These pills are not useful in Type I diabetes because the islet cells have been destroyed, so there is nothing for the pill to stimulate.) See Chapter 14 for more information about pills for Type II diabetes.

Why control?

The primary goal of treatment of diabetes is to restore the body's ability to properly use carbohydrates, which in turn results in normal fat and protein usage. All experts now agree that with good control the sudden or acute complications of diabetes (insulin reactions and ketoacidosis), may be minimized or even eliminated.

If diabetes is not controlled over periods of weeks or months, intermediate problems may develop. Young people in poor control may experience a failure of growth and development. Poor control of diabetes in women who become pregnant can result in an increased number of stillbirths and birth defects. It is important that women with diabetes make certain their diabetes is in very good control before becoming pregnant and throughout the pregnancy. Some studies have shown that the risk of birth defects is eight times higher when the mother's diabetes is poorly controlled. Again, see Chapter 17 for more details.

Most experts agree that good diabetes control reduces the risk of complications.

In the past all diabetes experts did not agree that good control of diabetes reduces the risks of long-term complications such as heart attacks, strokes, and eye and kidney problems. There are now increasing numbers of reports, however, which suggest that good control does minimize the risk of blindness, kidney disease, and nerve damage. There are not yet any good long-term studies that show whether disease of the large blood vessels, which can cause heart disease and stroke, occurs less often in people with good diabetes control, although most experts believe this is true.

Summary

Diabetes is a severe disease that affects almost eleven million Americans and cannot be cured at the present time. Control of the disease requires keeping blood glucose at or near normal levels (60-160 mg/dl), which restores the body's ability to correctly use carbohydrate, fat, and protein. To achieve such control requires informed people with diabetes who cooperate closely with knowledgeable and concerned health professionals in a planned system of care.

It is the purpose of this book to help people with diabetes and their family members understand the disease and discover how important it is to work as a part of the health care team in an individualized program of diabetes care. Indeed, there is a light at the end of the tunnel, and it is growing brighter every day!

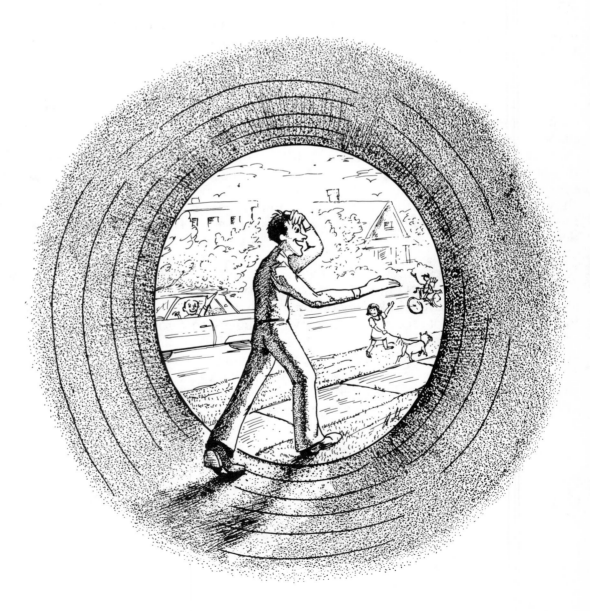

NOTES

Nutrition

Chapter 2
Nutrition: The Cornerstone of Diabetes Management

Marion Franz, R.D., M.S.

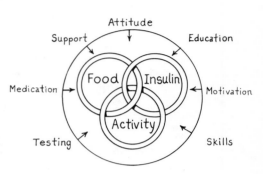

From the information in Chapter 1, you now know that controlling diabetes means keeping your blood glucose (sugar) as close to the normal range for as much of the time as possible. And because diabetes is basically a disease in which the body has problems using food, it is easy to understand why good nutrition and close control of the food you eat are so important. Exercise, and if necessary, proper medication, such as taking insulin or diabetes pills, are also important parts of diabetes management. But control of food intake has been called the "cornerstone of diabetes management."

What can good nutrition do for the person with diabetes?

Good nutrition can do the same thing for people with diabetes that it can for everyone else—and more! People who do not have diabetes often pay little attention to what or how much they eat. They can do this because their body appropriately uses the food they eat. It uses what it needs for energy and maintenance and then stores the remainder as fat. It also keeps blood glucose levels in a normal range. The result, of course, is that if a person overeats, he or she becomes fat or "obese," and may also have dangerously high levels of fat in the bloodstream.

Because you have diabetes, your body will no longer appropriately adjust when you eat food. It is up to you to control the quantity and quality of food you put into your body. Insulin or diabetes pills, and exercise can help to control your blood glucose, but these things can only lower blood glucose so much. If you ignore your responsibility to eat sensibly, then you are missing the chance to control your diabetes and live a healthier and more energetic life.

The word diet has no place in healthy meal planning for diabetes.

To eat sensibly you must first understand some basic things about nutrition, such as how much food you need and how to plan meals and snacks accordingly. This chapter will not only help you do those things, but it will also change any negative ideas you might have about going on a "diabetic diet." The word "diet" often has a negative meaning of drastic caloric reduction and boring meals and has no place in healthy meal planning for diabetes. This chapter will teach you how to sensibly eat foods you like and how to plan meals with more variety and good nutrition than those eaten by most people in our society.

How does good nutrition help control diabetes?

The first and major goal of nutritional management is to help maintain a normal blood glucose level. To keep the blood glucose normal, we need to first determine a meal plan that you feel you can follow and that meets your nutritional needs. Once you are satisfied with your meal plan, your insulin needs can be adjusted to your food intake.

If you have insulin-dependent (Type I) diabetes, that will be the insulin you need to inject daily. If you have non-insulin-dependent (Type II) diabetes, you may be able to keep blood glucose in the normal range by controlling the amount and kinds of food you eat and by losing weight, or you may be given insulin or diabetes pills to supplement your natural insulin or to help it work more effectively.

The amount of physical activity you normally get will affect your food needs and blood glucose levels, whether you have Type I or Type II diabetes. The best way to achieve a balance of all these factors is by working with a team of qualified health care professionals, including a doctor, dietitian, and nurse. The more knowledge you have, the better you can work with health care providers and become a part of this team.

It is important to maintain normal blood glucose levels to prevent the acute complications of diabetes (complications that happen in a relatively short period of time). These are hypoglycemia (too low a blood glucose level), which can lead to an insulin reaction; and hyperglycemia (too high a blood glucose level), which can lead to ketoacidosis. Research also suggests that it is important to maintain normal blood glucose to prevent and/or delay the onset of the chronic (happens over a long period of time) complications of diabetes. These acute and chronic complications are discussed in Chapters 8, 11, and 16, and also in Chapters 19-23. In order to achieve normal blood glucose levels, however, you will need to be willing to watch your food intake.

The second goal of nutritional management is to provide a meal plan that is nutritionally adequate. The nutritional recommendations for people with diabetes would benefit everyone. The **Dietary Guidelines for Americans** suggest that everyone should: 1) attain and maintain a desirable body weight; 2) eat more complex carbohydrates (starch), with an emphasis on fiber; 3) limit refined and simple sugars; 4) cut back on fats, especially saturated fats and cholesterol; 5) use alcohol only in moderation, if at all; and 6) eat a variety of foods. These guidelines are identical to those recommended for people with diabetes, so your entire family will benefit from following the nutritional guidelines for diabetes. Perhaps it is more important for you to watch your food intake, but it is important for everyone!

The third goal of nutritional management is to provide a daily number of calories that will help you attain or maintain a desirable body weight. For children, it is important to ensure that there are enough calories to provide for normal growth. Adults with Type I diabetes who are lean will also require adequate calories to maintain body weight. During pregnancy it is especially important that women who have diabetes also have adequate caloric intake to meet their needs and the needs of the growing baby.

People with Type II diabetes who are obese will find it important to try and reach a desirable body weight. With obesity, the body becomes resistant to the action of insulin. The body is composed of millions of cells that require the energy from blood glucose that comes from the food we eat. On the outside of each cell there are places called **insulin receptor sites**, where insulin attaches and allows blood glucose to enter the cell. With obesity, there appears to be a decrease in the number of insulin receptor sites, which causes the cells to become resistant to the action of insulin. As an individual loses weight, the number of receptor sites increases, allowing the body to use insulin better. It is also thought that something happens inside the cells of some individuals with Type II diabetes to cause the body to become resistant to the action of insulin. Therefore, you will use insulin most effectively when you are at a desirable body weight.

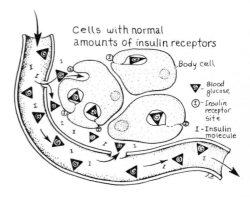

Cells with normal amounts of insulin receptors

Body cell

Blood glucose

Ⓘ - Insulin receptor site

I - Insulin molecule

Finally, the fourth goal of nutritional management is to attain and maintain healthy levels of blood fats (lipids). The two lipids most commonly tested for are cholesterol and triglycerides. High levels of these lipids are associated with development of heart and blood vessel disease. Healthy goals are to keep cholesterol below 180-200 milligrams and triglycerides below 150 milligrams.

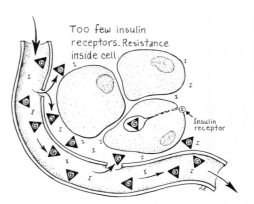

Too few insulin receptors. Resistance inside cell.

Insulin receptor

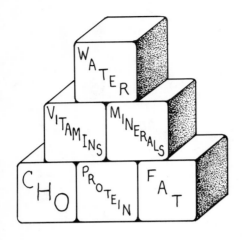

What are the nutrients in food?

We all eat and need food for a variety of reasons: for energy; for growth and maintenance and repair of the body; for the regulation of body processes that keep our bodies running smoothly; and, very importantly, for enjoyment—food is a large part of our social lives!

The six basic nutrients in food are **carbohydrates, proteins, fats, vitamins, minerals, and water.** The last three do not add calories to the diet and do not require insulin in order to be used by the body.

Carbohydrates are absorbed through the intestinal wall as glucose and then are carried by the blood to the liver. Some of the blood glucose will be stored in the liver and muscle in the form of **glycogen.** Glycogen can be converted back to glucose to be used later and during exercise. Some of the glucose will be carried through the bloodstream and used by the cells for an immediate source of energy. Carbohydrate not needed for glycogen storage or as an immediate energy source is changed by the liver to fat, which is stored in fat cells for future fuel needs. Insulin is required to allow this whole process to take place.

Carbohydrates

Fats

Protein

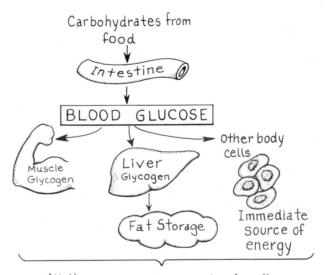

Protein from food is broken down to **amino acids** in the intestines and absorbed through the intestinal walls into the bloodstream. Amino acids are used in forming new body tissue for growth or for repair of body tissue. They can also be used as a backup source of energy. If not enough carbohydrate is available for energy, the liver will change amino acids into glucose. Amino acids can also be changed to fat and stored for future energy needs.

Insulin allows the body to build amino acids into new body tissue for growth and to repair body tissue for healing. This is why children in poor control of their diabetes do not grow well, and why adults in poor control of their diabetes may not heal as rapidly as they should. Insulin is also needed for amino acids to be used as a secondary source of energy or to be stored as fat.

22

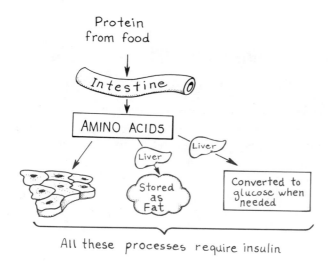

Protein
from food

Intestine

AMINO ACIDS

Liver

Stored
as
Fat

Liver

Converted to
glucose when
needed

All these processes require insulin

Most fat is found in foods in the form of **triglycerides** and is absorbed through the intestinal wall and taken to the fat cells to be stored and used when necessary as a source of body fuel. Insulin allows triglycerides to enter the fat cells for storage. However, if there is too much insulin available, it prevents stored fat from leaving the fat cells. Too much insulin also may increase your appetite.

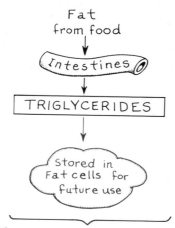

Fat
from food

Intestines

TRIGLYCERIDES

Stored in
Fat cells for
future use

This process requires insulin

If a person does not have enough insulin, glucose will not be used properly, and the body switches over to burning fat as its main source of fuel. When fat is burned more rapidly than the body can handle, large quantities of ketones are the result. This causes diabetic ketoacidosis.

Insulin, therefore, is important not only in the body's use of carbohydrate, but in the use of protein and fat as well. If there is not enough insulin available the levels of cholesterol and triglycerides will often be high. The goal of diabetes management is to have enough insulin available to keep blood glucose and fat levels normal, but not too much, since too much insulin can promote obesity and make it difficult to lose weight.

What percentage of calories should come from carbohydrate, protein, and fat?

Calorie values are determined by burning pure nutrients and measuring the heat they produce. One gram of carbohydrate and one gram of protein each supplies 4 calories, whereas one gram of fat supplies 9 calories and one gram of alcohol supplies 7 calories (approximately 30 grams equal one ounce). The average American diet contains approximately 35 to 40 percent of the calories from carbohydrate, 15 to 20 percent from protein, and 40 to 50 percent from fat.

It has been recommended that all Americans shift calories from fat sources to carbohydrate sources. *The American Diabetes Association Nutrition Recommendations and Principles for Persons with Diabetes Mellitus: 1986* suggests that for people with diabetes, up to 55 to 60 percent of the calories should come from carbohydrate. However, this needs to be individualized depending on blood glucose and lipid (fat) control, as well as lifestyle. Starches and "naturally occurring" sugars with fiber should be emphasized. However, moderate amounts of refined sugars can be eaten, depending on weight and blood glucose control. The recommended percentage of calories from protein is 15 to 20 percent. It is unknown whether a high protein diet contributes to the development of kidney problems in persons with diabetes, but caution is recommended in its use. Ideally, less than 30 percent of the calories will come from fat, but again, this must be individualized.

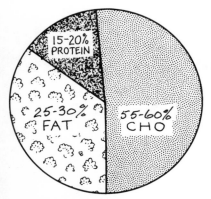

Average American diet

Recommended diet for everyone including people with diabetes

General Nutritional Recommendations for People with Diabetes

Nutrient	Recommended Percent of Calories	Calories Per Gram	Effect on Blood Glucose	Emphasis
Carbohydrate	55-60%	4	Main source	Complex CHO, Fiber
Protein	15-20%	4	Secondary source	Adequate for growth and maintenance
Fat	25-30%	9	Very little	Reduced saturated Fats and Cholesterol

24

What types of carbohydrate foods are best to include in the meal plan?

There are three different types of carbohydrates found in foods: sugar, starch, and fiber. Sugar is found in foods as either refined sugars or as "naturally occurring" sugars. Foods containing refined sugar include soft drinks, jams, jellies, honey, syrup, candies, desserts, etc. Foods containing naturally occurring sugar include fruits, vegetables, and milk. Starches are found in breads, cereals, pastas, and starchy vegetables. Fiber gives structure to some foods and cannot be digested by our bodies. Fiber is found in whole grain breads and cereals, fruits, vegetables, nuts, and in legumes such as dried peas, beans and lentils.

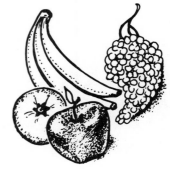

"Naturally occurring" Sugars

Recent research suggests that different carbohydrate-containing foods affect the blood glucose level differently. This difference may not be related to the type of carbohydrate (sugar, starch or fiber) as much as to what is called the glycemic index of foods. The glycemic index suggests which carbohydrate foods will raise blood glucose quickly and which will cause a more gradual rise in blood glucose. We are just beginning to learn which foods fall into which categories, as well as differences that occur when foods are eaten separately or as part of a meal.

Phyllis Crapo, R.D., from the University of California, was the first investigator to challenge the commonly held view that simple carbohydrates (sugar) always raise blood glucose levels faster and higher than complex carbohydrates (starches). Recent scientific reports have raised additional questions about the effects of carbohydrates on blood glucose levels because there are many other factors that may affect how the body responds to food.

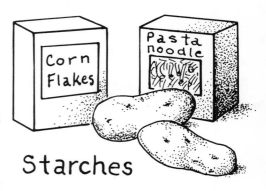

Starches

However, it is now possible to begin to predict how carbohydrate foods will be absorbed and affect blood glucose levels. Studies have shown that diets containing higher amounts of fiber and carbohydrate are associated with lower blood glucose and fat levels. Additional studies have shown that it may not be the fiber that is important, but rather the higher amount of carbohydrate. Higher carbohydrate diets seem to improve the body's ability to use carbohydrate.

This does not mean that fiber in foods is not important. Fiber helps lower blood fats, aids bowel function, and is associated with a lower incidence of certain types of cancer. (How to increase the fiber content of your diet is discussed in the next section.)

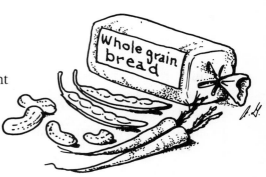

Fibers

The form in which food is eaten may also play a role in blood glucose response. Whole foods, which have a smaller surface area exposed to digestive enzymes, may be absorbed slower than foods that have been ground up. Cooking also has an effect; if foods are eaten raw, blood glucose level does not rise as high as when they have been cooked.

The meal in which the carbohydrate food is eaten may also be important. Slowly digested carbohydrates eaten in one meal not only cause less blood glucose response after that meal but also less glucose response after the next meal. And carbohydrates taken in smaller amounts over several hours will cause a smaller blood glucose response than if the same amount of carbohydrate were eaten all at once.

The above is general information. Carbohydrate foods may affect each individual a little differently. Blood glucose monitoring (which will be discussed in Chapters 4 and 5) can help you test your response to foods and help you and your dietitian determine the meal plan most effective for you.

Fiber

As mentioned above, fiber seems to help slow the absorption of nutrients, especially certain types of fiber. Fibers most helpful in slowing digestion are pectin (from fruits and vegetables), guar (from legumes, such as dried peas, beans and lentils), and oat fibers. You are encouraged to use as many food sources of fiber in your diet as you can. The average American diet contains 10-15 grams of dietary fiber per day; 30-40 grams would be better for everyone, including people with diabetes. The following table summarizes approximate information on dietary fiber:

Food Containing Dietary Fiber

Food	Portion	Fiber in grams (Approximate Averages)
Vegetables	1/2 cup to 3/4 cup cooked 1 cup to 2 cups raw	2
Fruits: fresh or canned	1/2 cup, 1 small fresh	2
Breads: whole wheat breads and crackers	1 slice or 1 ounce	2
Cereals: dry or cooked cereals Bran cereals	Varies 1/3 to 1/2 cup	3 8
Starchy vegetables: potatoes, brown rice, bulgur, green peas	1/2 cup	3
Legumes: peas, beans, lentils	1/3 cup	5 to 8
Nuts, seeds, peanut butter	1 oz. (1/4 cup) or 2 Tbsp.	3

Fat

It is recommended that calories from fat in the diet be reduced. Foods that contain fat are usually higher in calories than other foods. Diets that are high in most fats have been shown to be related to a higher blood cholesterol level, which increases the risk of heart disease.

Cholesterol is a type of fat found in animal foods and is also made in the human body. Fats, especially saturated fats, stimulate the liver to make cholesterol. This is why it is recommended that all Americans (especially those with diabetes) cut back on the amount of fat they consume. Countries in which the people consume a high percentage of their calories from fat have a higher incidence of heart disease in comparison to countries where the people consume a lower percentage of their calories from fat.

Here are some terms you need to understand when we discuss fat:

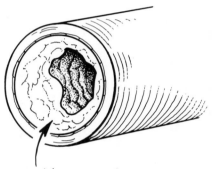

Fatty deposit in an artery

Atherosclerosis—An accumulation of a fatty-like deposit in arteries. This deposit appears to be composed primarily of cholesterol. When the deposit builds up to the point where blood can no longer flow through the artery, a heart attack may occur. If the blockage occurs in arteries going to the brain, a stroke may occur.

Cholesterol—A wax-like substance produced by the body in the liver. In foods, cholesterol is only found in animal foods. Cholesterol is an important first step in the production of some body hormones as well as bile salts and acids. However, elevated cholesterol levels have been associated with an increased incidence of heart disease. Average cholesterol levels in the United States are 200-250 mg/dl. A more ideal level would be 180-200 mg/dl. Your doctor can measure your cholesterol level with a laboratory blood test.

Lipids—Another term for fat. Two types of lipids are cholesterol and triglycerides.

Triglycerides—The form in which fat is found in most foods. Also, the form in which fat is carried in the bloodstream and stored in fat cells for future use.

Lipoproteins—Since lipids cannot dissolve in the blood, they require a carrier in order to be transported in the body. Lipo means fat, and protein is the carrier. There are three main types of lipoproteins:

Low density lipoprotein (LDL)—carrier of cholesterol to tissues. It is affected by the total amount of fat and amount of saturated fat in your diet.

Very low density lipoprotein (VLDL)—carrier of triglycerides to the fat cells for storage.

High density lipoprotein (HDL)—carrier of cholesterol back to the liver where it can be disposed of. It is known as "good" cholesterol since an elevated level appears to help protect against heart disease. It is not affected as much by diet as it is by exercise. Individuals who exercise regularly have higher levels of HDL.

Saturated fats increase blood cholesterol levels.

Saturated fat—The type of fat generally found in animal foods. It is usually solid at room temperature. Saturated fats have the effect of increasing blood cholesterol levels. Food sources include: animal fats, palm and coconut oil, solid shortenings, chocolate, and products containing dairy fat.

Unsaturated fat or poly-unsaturated fat—The type of fat generally found in vegetable oil. It is liquid at room temperature. Food sources include: safflower, sunflower, corn, soybean, and cottonseed oils; soft margarines; and walnuts. The general effect of these fats is to lower blood cholesterol levels.

Mono-unsaturated fat—Fats that do not affect blood cholesterol levels. Food sources are: olive and peanut oil, nuts (except walnuts), and olives. It is not known for certain today if these fats are neutral and do not affect blood cholesterol levels or if their effect is similar to the polyunsaturated fats in lowering blood cholesterol level.

Omega-three fatty acids—This is the type of fat found in fish oils, especially from cold-water and fatty fish. This type of fat lowers blood cholesterol and triglyceride levels and prevents blood platelets from clotting, so it appears to be an especially beneficial type of oil. It is not currently recommended that it be taken as a supplement; instead persons are encouraged to eat fish three to four times a week. Ocean fish that are found in cold, deep water are the sources of this oil: salmon, sardines, mackerel, albacore tuna, sablefish, and herring. Other good sources are rainbow trout, cod, flounder, haddock, crab, and shrimp.

To reduce total fat in your meal plan:

- Limit meat portion sizes. Try to limit yourself to six meat exchanges or 6 ounces of meat per day.
- Use lean meats, such as fish and poultry, as often as possible.
- Avoid high fat meats, such as sausage, frankfurters, prime cuts of meats, and luncheon meats (cold cuts).
- Cook to get rid of as much fat as possible—broil, bake, boil, etc. Remove fat before making gravies and sauces.
- Use skim milk. If you now drink whole milk, move down gradually from 2% to 1% and then to skim milk.
- Use a margarine with a liquid vegetable oil as the first ingredient. A tub margarine will be more unsaturated than a stick margarine.
- Use liquid vegetable oils whenever possible. In recipes calling for 1 cup of solid shortening, substitute 3/4 cup of liquid vegetable oil; replace 1/2 cup shortening with 1/3 cup vegetable oil.
- Use low fat dairy products. Low fat yogurt can be substituted for sour cream and mayonnaise. Try some of the skim milk cheeses.
- Limit intake of eggs to three per week.

Salt

All Americans are also encouraged to cut back on their salt intake. Obesity, inherited tendency (genetics), and high salt intake increase the risk of developing high blood pressure. People with diabetes have a greater risk of developing high blood pressure, so it is important to reduce any of the other risk factors if possible. The average American daily diet contains 8 to 12 grams of salt; much more than the 5 grams that is recommended. Salt is approximately 40 percent sodium and 60 percent chloride. One teaspoon of salt is 5 grams (5,000 milligrams) and contains 2,300 milligrams of sodium. It is the sodium that contributes to the development of high blood pressure.

To reduce salt in your meal plan:

- Taste foods before salting.
- Use only a small amount of salt in cooking.
- Avoid foods containing obvious amounts of salt, such as crackers and snack foods, pickles, olives, etc.
- Limit use of processed foods such as high salt meat products (ham, bacon, sausage, cold cuts).
- Limit use of "fast foods."

Is there an easy way to plan meals?

Some amount of thought must always go into planning meals, and this is especially true for people with diabetes. To make this easier for you, the American Diabetes Association and the American Dietetic Association have divided foods into six groups called "exchange lists." Each list is based on the amounts of carbohydrate, protein, and fat contained in foods. These nutrients are used in the calculations because they supply calories and because they require insulin for the body to use them correctly. There are six exchange lists: starch/bread, meat, vegetables, fruit, milk, and fat.

Each list contains foods in specific portions that are approximately equal in the amount of carbohydrate, protein, and fat—and therefore calories—they contain. It is important to use the correct portion sizes. For example:

1 slice bread = 3/4 cup dry cereal = 1 small potato
1 apple = 1/2 banana = 1-1/4 cup strawberries

Specific portions of foods are approximately equal in nutritional value and can therefore be substituted or "exchanged" for one another. *Exchange Lists for Meal Planning*, the standard publication for meal planning, received a new look in 1986. The updated version reflects nutritional principles of the '80s. A symbol was added for fiber so you can easily identify good sources of fiber. A different symbol was added next to foods containing more than 400 mg. of sodium, so you can see which foods contain large amounts of sodium. The following table summarizes the carbohydrate, protein, and fat content of the exchange lists.

Nutrient Content of Exchanges

One Exchange	Portion	Calories	CHO	Protein	Fat
Starch/Bread	Varies	80	15	3	trace
Meat, Lean	1 oz.	55	—	7	3
Medium Fat	1 oz.	75	—	7	5
High Fat	1 oz.	100	—	7	8
Vegetable	1/2 c. cooked 1 c. raw	25	5	2	—
Fruit	Varies	60	15	—	—
Milk, Skim	1 cup	90	12	8	trace
Fat	Varies	45	—	—	5

How can the exchange lists be used effectively?

Foods are listed on the exchange lists in portion sizes. In order to follow your meal plan, it will be important to judge portion sizes correctly. When you begin, it may be a good idea to weigh and measure the correct portion sizes. However, you will soon learn to "eyeball" the portion sizes quite accurately. Periodically (once or twice a year) it is a good idea to again weigh and measure portion sizes to be sure you are still using correct portion sizes. This is especially important if you are gaining unwanted weight and are not sure why. Foods are listed in portion size by tablespoon or measuring cup amount. However, meat is listed by ounces. One ounce of cooked meat, with the bone and fat removed, is one exchange. An average size serving will be 3 ounces of cooked meat. This will be approximately the size of the palm of a woman's hand and 1/2 inch thick. The exchange lists are described below and printed at the end of this chapter.

What's in an exchange?

One: The Starch/Bread list is first because it contains foods higher in carbohydrate as well as fiber, which should form the basis of a sound meal plan. Each food item in this list contains approximately 15 grams of carbohydrate, 3 grams of protein, a trace of fat, and 80 calories. Whole grain products on the list average 2 grams of dietary fiber per serving. Some foods are higher in fiber and have a fiber symbol next to them. This list includes cereal, grains, pasta, dried beans and peas, starchy vegetables, breads, crackers, snacks, and some starch foods prepared with fat. If in doubt about the correct portion of a starch food not on this list, a general rule is that 1/2 cup cereal, grain, or pasta or 1 ounce of a bread product is one serving.

$$\text{Breads, crackers, etc.} = 15g \boxed{C}_{\text{CHO}} + 3g \boxed{P}_{\text{Proteins}} = 80 \text{ calories}$$

Two: The Meat and Meat Substitutes list is next for convenience in planning meals. Meats are divided into one of three lists depending on the amount of fat they contain. One ounce of a lean meat contains approximately 7 grams of protein, 3 grams of fat, and 55 calories. One ounce of a medium-fat meat contains approximately 7 grams of protein, 5 grams of fat, and 75 calories. One ounce of a high-fat meat contains approximately 7 grams of protein, 8 grams of fat, and 100 calories. These are cooked meats with the bone and fat removed and with no fat or flour added in the preparation. You are encouraged to use more lean and medium-fat meat, poultry, and fish in your meal plan and to limit your choices from the high-fat group to three servings per week.

1oz. Lean meats $= 7g \boxed{P} + 3g \text{ F} = 55 \text{ calories}$
Protein   Fat

Medium-fat meats $= 7g \boxed{P} + 5g \text{ F} + 75 \text{ calories}$
Protein   Fat

1oz. High-fat meats $= 7g \boxed{P} + 8g \text{ F} = 100 \text{ Calories}$
Protein   Fat

Three: Vegetable exchanges contain about 5 grams of carbohydrate, 2 grams of protein, and 25 calories. Vegetables contain 2 to 3 grams of dietary fiber per serving. The serving size is 1/2 cup cooked vegetables or vegetable juice or 1 cup raw vegetables. Starchy vegetables such as corn, peas, and potatoes are on the starch/bread list, and vegetables having less than 20 calories per serving are on the Free Food List.

$\frac{1}{2}$ Many cooked vegetables $= 5g \text{ C} + 2g \boxed{P} = 25 \text{ calories}$
CHO   Proteins

Four: Fruit exchanges are based on the amount of fruit or fruit juice contributing 15 grams of carbohydrate and 60 calories. Fresh, frozen, and dried fruits have about 2 grams of fiber per serving. Fruit juices contain very little dietary fiber. Fruits vary in portion sizes because they differ in the amount of water they contain. The serving size for one fruit serving is generally 1/2 cup or 1 small fresh fruit, 1/2 cup fruit juice, or 1/4 cup of dried fruit.

$$\bigcirc = 15g\ \nabla\kern-0.8em C = 60\ \text{calories}$$

½ cup or Small fruit   CHO

Five: Milk exchanges are based on foods containing 12 grams of carbohydrate and 8 grams of protein. The amount of fat in milk is measured in percent of butterfat, and the calories vary depending on what kind of milk you choose. Skim or very low fat milk is recommended for use and contains a trace of fat and 90 calories.

$$1\ \bigsqcup = 12g\ \nabla\kern-0.8em C + 8g\ \boxed{P} + \text{trace}\ \text{F} = 90$$

Milk   CHO   Proteins   fat   Calories

Six: Fat exchanges are based on the amount of food contributing 5 grams of fat and 45 calories. Portion sizes vary and in general are small.

$$= 5g\ \text{F} = 45\ \text{Calories}$$

Corn Oil butter
Fats   Fat

Free Foods: Free foods contain less than 20 calories per serving. You can eat as much as you want of items that have no serving size specified. Free foods with a serving size specified should be limited to two or three servings per day; one at each meal or snack time, or a total of approximately 50 to 60 extra calories per day.

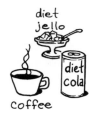

diet jello
diet cola
coffee

< 20 Calories per serving

Combination Foods: Combination foods do not fit into only one exchange list, but are combinations of several exchanges. This list helps to fit some common combination foods into your meal plan. For additional foods see *Exchanges for All Occasions.*

Foods for Occasional Use: Moderate amounts of some foods can be used in your meal plan in spite of their sugar or fat content, depending on maintaining blood glucose control. Because they are concentrated sources of carbohydrate and fats, the portion sizes are very small. The more careful everyone can be of these foods the better.

An individualized meal plan is essential!

It is important that each person with diabetes have a meal plan that is designed specifically for his or her caloric and nutritional needs, as well as to suit his or her lifestyle. A meal plan tells you how many exchanges you can select for each meal and at snack times. A sample meal planning card is shown below:

My Meal Plan

Meal Plan for: Jane Smith   Date: Jan. 6, 1987

Dietitian: M. Franz   Phone: 555-1234

	Grams	Percent
Carbohydrate	230	53%
Protein	80	18%
Fat	60	29%
Calories 1800		

Time	Meal Plan	Menu Ideas	Menu Ideas
7:30 a.m.	3 Starch — Meat — Vegetable 1 Fruit 1 skim Milk 1 Fat	1 cup oatmeal 1 slice whole wheat toast ½ grapefruit 1 cup skim milk 1 tsp. margarine	
	___ ___		
12:30 p.m.	2 Starch 2 Meat 0-1 Vegetable 1 Fruit 1 skim Milk 1 Fat	2 slices w.w. bread 2 oz. sliced turkey lettuce & tomato slices 1 apple 1 cup skim milk 1 tsp. margarine	
3:00	1 Fruit or Starch	3 graham cracker squares	
6:30	2 Starch 3 Meat 2 Vegetable 1 Fruit — Milk 2 Fat	1 baked potato with 1 tsp. margarine 1 small roll with 1 tsp. margarine 3 oz. broiled chicken breast ½ cup green beans dinner salad with low calorie salad dressing 15 grapes	
10:00	1 Fruit 1 Starch 0-1 Fat	1 orange 3 cups popcorn	

Copyright © 1986 by the American Diabetes Association,® Inc./The American Dietetic Association

As you can see, this meal plan card tells you how many calories are planned for you; how many grams and percentages of carbohydrate, protein and fat; times for your meals and snacks; and number of servings to select from each exchange list at each meal and at snack times.

Using the exchange lists to plan your meals will allow you more flexibility while helping to keep your diabetes in good control. However, different foods from the same exchange list may affect your blood glucose differently than they affect another person's blood glucose. By doing self blood glucose monitoring (a form of testing described in Chapters 4 and 5) you can determine for yourself the effect each food has on you. You can then avoid those foods that cause an excessive rise in blood glucose levels. It will be approximately one to two hours after eating before you can see the maximum effect of your food intake reflected in blood glucose levels.

1. Your caloric and nutrient requirements.
2. Your lifestyle—what you feel will be convenient for you to do on a consistent basis. The meal plan is worthless if you will not or cannot follow it.
3. Your diabetes therapy:
Insulin—Food needs to be coordinated with the predictable time action of various insulins. In people who do not have diabetes, the body will release the amount of insulin needed to metabolize the amount of food eaten at that time. Unfortunately, injected insulin cannot do this. It is important to take insulin injections at approximately the same time each day, making it also essential to eat meals and snacks of approximately consistent values at scheduled times.
Type II Diabetes Pills—Some people require a diabetes pill to help control their blood glucose levels. Food must then be matched to the time action of these diabetes pills.
Diet Alone—If your diabetes is being controlled by diet only, exact timing of your meals is not as important. What will be important is the amount eaten. Eating three small meals and a few snacks to spread your food intake over the day, however, will help you control blood glucose levels.
4. Activity level—Your normal level of physical activity will be reflected in your caloric requirements. If you take insulin, unusually large amounts of exercise will cause your body to use the insulin more effectively, and depending on your blood glucose level before exercise and how well conditioned you are, may lower blood glucose levels. Therefore, based on your blood glucose level prior to and after exercise, extra food may need to be added. Routine exercise times will be planned for in the meal pattern.

However, what is most important is your acceptance of the meal plan. You must feel you can follow it and live with it. If this is the case, you can learn to adjust your insulin dose (or your health care provider can advise you) based on your blood glucose levels prior to and after meals.

The following are two sample meal plans and menus:

Plan A.
1500 calories
190 grams carbohydrate (52%)
75 grams protein (20%)
45 grams fat (28%)

	Exchanges	Food
Breakfast:		
Starch/Bread	2	1 slice whole wheat toast
		1/2 cup Raisin Bran
Fruit	1	1/2 grapefruit
Skim Milk	1/2	1/2 cup skim milk
Fat	1	1 tsp. margarine
Lunch:		
Starch/Bread	2	2 slices whole wheat bread
Meat	2	2 oz. turkey
Vegetable	0-1	carrot sticks
Fruit	1	1 apple
Milk	1	1 cup skim milk
Fat	1	1 tsp. margarine
Snack:		
Fruit	1	15 grapes
Dinner:		
Starch/Bread	1	1 small baked potato
Meat	3	3 oz. lean roast beef
Vegetable	2	1/2 cup green beans
		dinner salad
Fruit	1	1/3 cup pineapple chunks
Fat	1	1 tsp. margarine
		low calorie salad dressing
Evening Snack:		
Starch/Bread	1	5 snack crackers
Milk	1/2	1/2 cup skim milk
Fat	0-1	(in crackers)

Plan B.
2100 calories
280 grams carbohydrate (54%)
90 grams protein (18%)
65 grams fat (28%)

	Exchanges	Food
Breakfast:		
Starch/Bread	3	1 English muffin 3/4 cup Cherrios
Fruit	1	1 orange
Skim Milk	1	1 cup skim milk
Fat	1	1 tsp. margarine sugar-free jelly
Snack:		
Fruit or Bread	1	1 apple
Lunch:		
Starch/Bread	3	1 cup veg. beef soup 2 slices whole wheat bread
Meat	2	2 oz. lean beef
Vegetable	0-1	2 tomato slices lettuce
Fruit	1	12 cherries
Milk	1	1 cup skim milk
Fat	1	1 tsp. mayonnaise
Snack:		
Starch/Bread	1	3 graham cracker squares
Fruit	1	1 fruit roll-up
Dinner:		
Starch/Bread	2	1 large potato 1 roll
Meat	3	3 oz. broiled fish
Vegetable	2	1/2 cup carrots dinner salad
Fruit	1	1-1/4 cup strawberries
Fat	3	1 Tbsp. salad dressing 1 tsp. margarine 2 Tbsp. sour cream
Evening Snack:		
Starch/Bread	1	1 oz. small bagel
Fruit	1	1/3 cantaloupe
Fat	0-1	1 tsp. margarine

What effect does alcohol have on diabetes?

The decision to use or not use alcoholic beverages must be made by each individual. To make this decision, you need to be aware of the effects of alcohol on blood glucose levels and the rest of your body.

Alcohol is broken down in the liver, but the liver can process only about one ounce of alcohol per hour. The overall effect of alcohol is to lower the blood glucose level, especially if you have not eaten for several hours. Alcohol cannot be converted to blood glucose. If the calories from alcohol are not used as an immediate source of energy, they are stored as fat. The body's use of alcohol does not require insulin; alcohol seems to increase the effects of insulin.

When you have not eaten for several hours, your liver uses its stored carbohydrate (glycogen). Normally, the liver then changes other sources, such as protein, into glucose to maintain the blood glucose level. When the liver is processing alcohol, the formation of glucose from other sources is blocked. People in poor control of their diabetes usually have lower glycogen stores, so they are at greater risk of hypoglycemia.

Hypoglycemia can occur even before a person is aware of being mildly intoxicated. Two ounces of alcohol is enough to produce hypoglycemia in a person who hasn't eaten for several hours.

Alcohol is also a concentrated source of calories, providing seven calories per gram. Alcohol provides energy but has no other nutritional value. One ounce of 86 proof liquor contains 70 calories. Sweet wines and beers contain carbohydrates in addition to alcohol, so they have even more calories.

Large doses of alcohol sometimes cause a small but short-term rise in blood glucose, but this is followed a couple of hours later by a fall in blood glucose to below normal blood glucose levels.

When diabetes is well controlled, the blood glucose level is not affected by the moderate use of alcohol if it is consumed shortly before, during, or immediately after eating. Alcohol should not be used if you have: high triglyceride levels, gastritis, pancreatitis, or certain types of kidney and heart diseases. Alcohol also interacts with certain drugs such as barbituates and tranquilizers. If you choose to drink alcohol, discuss your use of alcohol with your health care provider.

Guidelines for use of alcohol

Individuals with diabetes can use alcohol in their meal plan by following some simple guidelines. These guidelines refer to the occasional use of alcoholic beverages; approximately 2 ounces of alcohol not more than once or twice a week.

Limit yourself to two ounces of alcohol per day. Occasional use of carbohydrate-free alcohol by normal weight people whose insulin-dependent diabetes is well controlled may be regarded as an "extra." No food should be omitted, though, because of the possibility of alcohol-induced hypoglycemia. If used daily, the energy value of alcohol should be included in your daily meal plan. One ounce of alcohol is contained in each of the following amounts of alcoholic beverages:

- 1.5 ounces of a distilled beverage—whiskey, scotch, rye, vodka, gin, cognac, rum, dry brandy
- 4 ounces of dry wine; 2 ounces of a dry sherry
- 12 ounces of beer, preferably "light."

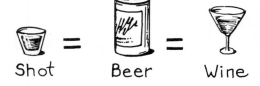

Shot = Beer = Wine

Never drink on an empty stomach. Take precautions to avoid hypoglycemia, especially when drinking before meals or during times when your insulin is most effective. Two ounces of alcohol taken shortly before a meal, or directly after, should be safe.

Count the calories. People with Type II diabetes, for whom weight is a concern, must count the calories from alcohol in their meal plan. Alcohol calories are best substituted for fat exchanges, because alcohol is metabolized in a manner similar to fat. (Each of the above equivalents containing one ounce of alcohol is equal to two fat exchanges.) However, people with Type I diabetes should not subtract any food from their meal plan.

Use alcohol only in moderation. Sip slowly and make a drink last a long time. Since symptoms of alcohol intoxication and hypoglycemia are similar, it is easy to mistake the low blood glucose for intoxication and delay necessary treatment. Even one drink is enough to give your breath the smell of alcohol. If you lose consciousness due to hypoglycemia, people might think you have had too much to drink and be reluctant to help you.

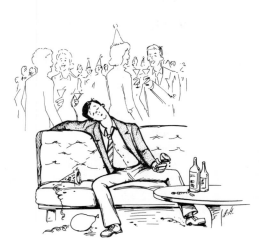

Avoid drinks containing large amounts of sugar. Liqueurs, sweet wines, and sweet mixes (such as tonic, soda pop or fruit juices) are examples of drinks containing sugar. Drink mixes, if used, should be sugar-free. Beer and ale contain malt sugar, which should be substituted for carbohydrate in the meal plan. Light beer is recommended because it has approximately 3 to 6 grams of carbohydrate per can in contrast to regular beer, which has 15 grams of carbohydrate per can. Dry wines are also better choices than a sweet wine.

Don't let a drink make you careless. Alcohol can have a relaxing effect and may dull judgment. Be sure meals and snacks are taken on time and selected with the usual care.

Carry or wear identification. Visible medical emergency identification should be carried or worn especially when drinking.

If you are taking diabetes pills, be aware of the possible effect of alcohol with these pills. In some people with non-insulin-dependent diabetes (10-30 percent), the diabetes pills (the sulfonylurea group) interact with alcohol to produce deep flushing, nausea, quickened heart beat and impaired speech.

Nutrition Information for Alcoholic Beverages

Beverage	Serving	Alcohol (gms)	Carbohydrate (gms)	Calories	Exchanges for Non-Insulin Dependent Diabetics
Beer:	12 oz.	13.0	13.7	151	1 bread, 2 fat
Light Beer	12 oz.	10.1	6	90	2 fat
Extra Light Beer	12 oz.	8.1	3.3	70	1½ fat
Near Beer	12 oz.	1.5	12.3	60	1 bread
Distilled Spirits:					
86 proof (gin, rum, vodka, whiskey, scotch)	1½ oz.	15.3	Trace	107	2 fat
Dry brandy or cognac	1 oz.	10.7	Trace	75	1½ fat
Table wines:					
Red or Rose	4 oz.	11.6	1.0	85	2 fat
Dry white	4 oz.	11.3	.4	80	2 fat
Sweet wine	4 oz.	11.8	4.9	102	1/3 bread, 2 fat
Light wine	4 oz.	6.4	1.3	48-58	1 fat
Sparkling wines:					
Champagne	4 oz.	11.9	3.6	98	2 fat
Sweet Kosher wine	4 oz.	11.9	12.0	132	1 bread, 2 fat
Appetizer/dessert wines:					
Sherry	2 oz.	9.4	1.5	73	1½ fat
Sweet sherry, port, muscatel	2 oz.	9.4	7.0	94	½ bread, 1½ fat
Vermouths, dry	3 oz.	12.6	4.2	105	2 fat
Sweet	3 oz.	12.2	13.9	141	2 fat, 1 bread

Summary

The field of nutrition is changing rapidly. As facts emerge and concepts change, nutritional recommendations will also undergo evaluation and change. However, with the information available to us today, it is possible to make meal planning for persons with diabetes more flexible and enjoyable while controlling blood glucose and blood fat levels as well. More nutritious eating habits can lead to improved health and a longer life for all family members who share the changes being made by the person with diabetes.

NOTES

Exchange Lists for Meal Planning

List 1 — Starch/Bread Exchanges

Each item in this list contains approximately 15 grams of carbohydrate, 3 grams of protein, a trace of fat, and 80 calories. Whole grain products average about 2 grams of fiber per serving. Some foods are higher in fiber. Those foods that contain 3 or more grams of fiber per serving are identified with the fiber symbol. ✇

You can choose your starch exchanges from any of the items on this list. If you want to eat a starch food that is not on this list, the general rule is that:

- ■ 1/2 cup of cereal, grain or pasta is one serving
- ■ 1 ounce of a bread product is one serving.

Your dietitian can help you be more exact.

Cereals/Grains/Pasta

✇Bran cereals, concentrated	1/3 cup
✇Bran cereals, flaked	1/2 cup
(such as Bran Buds®, All Bran®)	
Bulgur (cooked)	1/2 cup
Cooked cereals	1/2 cup
Cornmeal (dry)	2-1/2 Tbsp.
Grapenuts	3 Tbsp.
Grits (cooked)	1/2 cup
Other ready-to-eat	
unsweetened cereals	3/4 cup
Pasta (cooked)	1/2 cup
Puffed cereal	1-1/2 cup
Rice, white or brown (cooked)	1/3 cup
Shredded wheat	1/2 cup
✇Wheat germ	3 Tbsp.

Dried Beans/Peas/Lentils

✇Beans and peas (cooked)	
(such as kidney, white,	
split, blackeye)	1/3 cup
✇Lentils (cooked)	1/3 cup
✇Baked beans	1/4 cup

Starchy Vegetables

✇Corn	1/2 cup
✇Corn on cob, 6 in. long	1
✇Lima beans	1/2 cup
✇Peas, green (canned or frozen)	1/2 cup
✇Plantain	1/2 cup
Potato, baked	1 small (3 oz.)
Potato, mashed	1/2 cup
Squash, winter (acorn, butternut)	3/4 cup
Yam, sweet potato, plain	1/3 cup

Bread

Bagel	1/2 (1 oz.)
Bread sticks, crisp,	
4 in. long x 1/2 in.	2 (2/3 oz.)
Croutons, low fat	1 cup
English muffin	1/2
Frankfurter or	
hamburger bun	1/2 (1 oz.)

Pita, 6 in. across	1/2
Plain roll, small	1 (1 oz.)
Raisin, unfrosted	1 slice (1 oz.)
✇Rye, pumpernickel	1 slice (1 oz.)
Tortilla, 6 in. across	1
White (including	
French, Italian)	1 slice (1 oz.)
Whole wheat	1 slice (1 oz.)

Crackers/Snacks

Animal crackers	8
Graham crackers, 2½ in. square	3
Matzoth	3/4 oz.
Melba toast	5 slices
Oyster crackers	24
Popcorn	
(popped, no fat added)	3 cups
Pretzels	3/4 oz.
Rye crisp, 2 in. x 3½ in.	4
Saltine-type crackers	6
Whole wheat crackers,	
no fat added	
(crisp breads, such as Finn®,	
Kavli®, Wasa®)	2-4 slices (3/4 oz.)

Starch Foods Prepared with Fat

(Count as 1 starch/bread serving, plus 1 fat serving.)

Biscuit, 2-1/2 in. across	1
Chow mein noodles	1/2 cup
Corn bread, 2 in. cube	1 (2 oz.)
Cracker, round butter type	6
French fried potatoes,	
2 in. to 3½ in. long	10 (1½ oz.)
Muffin, plain, small	1
Pancake, 4 in. across	2
Stuffing, bread (prepared)	1/4 cup
Taco shell, 6 in. across	2
Waffle, 4½ in. square	1
Whole wheat crackers, fat added	
(such as Triscuits®)	4-6 (1 oz.)

✇ *3 grams or more of fiber per serving*

42

List 2 — Meat Exchanges

Each serving of meat and substitutes on this list contains about 7 grams of protein. The amount of fat and number of calories varies, depending on what kind of meat or substitute you choose. The list is divided into three parts based on the amount of fat and calories: lean meat, medium-fat meat, and high-fat meat. One ounce (one meat exchange) of each of these includes:

	Carbohydrate (grams)	Protein (grams)	Fat (grams)	Calories
Lean	0	7	3	55
Medium-Fat	0	7	5	75
High-Fat	0	7	8	100

You are encouraged to use more lean and medium-fat meat, poultry, and fish in your meal plan. This will help decrease your fat intake, which may help decrease your risk for heart disease. The items from the high-fat group are high in saturated fat, cholesterol, and calories. You should limit your choices from the high-fat group to three (3) times per week. Meat and substitutes do not contribute any fiber to your meal plan.

 Meats and meat substitutes that have 400 milligrams or more of sodium per exchange are indicated with this symbol.

Tips

1. Bake, roast, broil, grill, or boil these foods rather than frying them with added fat.

2. Use a nonstick pan spray or a nonstick pan to brown or fry these foods.

3. Trim off visible fat before and after cooking.

4. Do not add flour, bread crumbs, coating mixes, or fat to these foods when preparing them.

5. Weigh meat after removing bones and fat, and after cooking. Three ounces of cooked meat is about equal to 4 ounces of raw meat. Some examples of meat portions are:

   2 ounces meat (2 meat exchanges) =
   1 small chicken leg or thigh
   1/2 cup cottage cheese or tuna

   3 ounces meat (3 meat exchanges) =
   1 medium pork chop
   1 small hamburger
   1/2 of a whole chicken breast
   1 unbreaded fish fillet
   cooked meat, about the size of a deck of cards

6. Restaurants usually serve prime cuts of meat, which are high in fat and calories.

Lean Meat and Substitutes
(One exchange is equal to any one of the following items.)

Beef: USDA Good or Choice grades of lean beef, such as round, sirloin, and flank steak; tenderloin; and chipped beef 🖊 ....1 oz.

Pork: Lean pork, such as fresh ham; canned, cured or boiled ham 🖊 ; Canadian bacon 🖊 , tenderloin ....1 oz.

Veal: All cuts are lean except for veal cutlets (ground or cubed) ....1 oz. Examples of lean veal are chops and roasts.

Poultry: Chicken, turkey, Cornish hen (without skin) ....1 oz.

Fish: All fresh and frozen fish ....1 oz.
Crab, lobster, scallops, shrimp, clams (fresh or canned in water 🖊) ....2 oz.
Oysters ....6 medium
Tuna 🖊 (canned in water) ....1/4 cup
Herring (uncreamed or smoked) ....1 oz.
Sardines (canned) ....2 medium

Wild Game: Venison, rabbit, squirrel ....1 oz.
Pheasant, duck, goose (without skin) ....1 oz.

Cheese: Any cottage cheese ....1/4 cup
Grated parmesan ....2 Tbsp.
Diet cheeses 🖊 (with less than 55 calories per ounce) ....1 oz.

Other: 95% fat-free luncheon meat ....1 oz.
Egg whites ....3 whites
Egg substitutes with less than 55 calories per 1/4 cup ....1/4 cup

Medium-Fat Meat and Substitutes
(One exchange is equal to any one of the following items.)

Beef: Most beef products fall into this category.
Examples are: all ground beef, roast (rib, chuck, rump),
steak (cubed, Porterhouse, T-bone), and meatloaf...........................1 oz.

Pork: Most pork products fall into this category.
Examples are: chops, loin roast, Boston butt, cutlets.........................1 oz.

Lamb: Most lamb products fall into this category.
Examples are: chops, leg, and roast ....1 oz.

Veal: Cutlet (ground or cubed, unbreaded) ....1 oz.

Poultry: Chicken (with skin), domestic duck or goose (well-drained of fat),
ground turkey ....1 oz.

Fish: Tuna 🖊 (canned in oil and drained) ....1/4 cup
Salmon 🖊 (canned) ....1/4 cup

Cheese: Skim or part-skim milk cheeses, such as:
Ricotta ....1/4 cup
Mozzarella ....1 oz.
Diet cheeses 🖊 (with 56-80 calories per ounce)........................1 oz.

Other: 86% fat-free luncheon meat 🖊 ....1 oz.
Egg (high in cholesterol, limit to 3 per week) 1
Egg substitutes with 56-80 calories per 1/4 cup ....1/4 cup
Tofu (2½ in. x 2¾ in. x 1 in.)...4 oz.
Liver, heart, kidney, sweetbreads (high in cholesterol) ....1 oz.

High-Fat Meat and Substitutes

Remember, these items are high in saturated fat, cholesterol, and calories,
and should be used only three (3) times per week.

(One exchange is equal to any one of the following items.)

Beef: Most USDA Prime cuts of beef, such as ribs, corned beef 🥓 ....1 oz.

Pork: Spareribs, ground pork, pork sausage 🥓 (patty or link) ....1 oz.

Lamb: Patties (ground lamb) ....1 oz.

Fish: Any fried fish product ....1 oz.

Cheese: All regular cheeses 🥓 , such as American, Blue, Cheddar,
Monterey, Swiss...1 oz.

Other: Luncheon meat 🥓 , such as bologna, salami, pimento loaf ....1 oz.
Sausage 🥓 , such as Polish, Italian...1 oz.
Knockwurst, smoked ....1 oz.
Bratwurst 🥓 ....1 oz.
Frankfurter 🥓 (turkey or chicken) ....1 frank (10/lb.)
Peanut butter (contains unsaturated fat) ....1 Tbsp.

Count as one high-fat meat plus one fat exchange:

Frankfurter 🥓 (beef, pork, or combination).........................1 frank (10/lb.)

🥓 *400 mg or more of sodium per exchange*

List 3 — Vegetable Exchanges

Each vegetable serving on this list contains about 5 grams of carbohydrate, 2 grams of protein, and 25 calories. Vegetables contain 2-3 grams of dietary fiber. Vegetables which contain 400 mg of sodium per serving are identified with a 🥓 symbol.

Vegetables are a good source of vitamins and minerals. Fresh and frozen vegetables have more vitamins and less added salt. Rinsing canned vegetables will remove much of the salt.

Unless otherwise noted, the serving size for vegetables (one vegetable exchange) is:

1/2 cup of cooked vegetables or vegetable juice
1 cup of raw vegetables.

Artichoke (1/2 medium)	Cauliflower	Rutabaga
Asparagus	Eggplant	Sauerkraut 🥓
Beans	Greens	Spinach, cooked
(green, wax, Italian)	(collard, mustard, turnip)	Summer squash
Bean sprouts	Kohlrabi	(crookneck)
Beets	Leeks	Tomato (one large)
Broccoli	Mushrooms, cooked	Tomato/vegetable
Brussels sprouts	Okra	juice 🥓
Cabbage, cooked	Onions	Turnips
Carrots	Pea pods	Water chestnuts
	Peppers (green)	Zucchini, cooked

Starchy vegetables such as corn, peas, and potatoes are found on the Starch/Bread List.

For free vegetables, see Free Food List.

🥓 *400 mg or more of sodium per serving.*

List 4 — Fruit Exchanges

Each item on this list contains about 15 grams of carbohydrate and 60 calories. Fresh, frozen, and dry fruits have about 2 grams of fiber per serving. Fruits that have 3 or more grams of fiber per serving have a 🌾 symbol. Fruit juices contain very little dietary fiber.

The carbohydrate and calorie content for a fruit serving is based on the usual serving of the most commonly eaten fruits. Use fresh fruits or fruits frozen or canned without sugar added. Whole fruit is more filling than fruit juice and may be a better choice for those who are trying to lose weight. Unless otherwise noted, the serving size for one fruit serving is:

1/2 cup of fresh fruit or fruit juice
1/4 cup of dried fruit.

Fresh, Frozen, and Unsweetened Canned Fruit

Apple (raw, 2 in. across)	1 apple
Applesauce (unsweetened)	1/2 cup
Apricots (medium, raw)	4 apricots
Apricots (canned)	1/2 cup, or 4 halves
Banana (9 in. long)	1/2 banana
🌾 Blackberries (raw)	3/4 cup
🌾 Blueberries (raw)	3/4 cup
Cantaloupe (5 in. across)	1/3 melon
(cubes)	1 cup
Cherries (large, raw)	12 cherries
Cherries (canned)	1/2 cup
Figs (raw, 2 in. across)	2 figs
Fruit cocktail (canned)	1/2 cup
Grapefruit (medium)	1/2 grapefruit
Grapefruit (segments)	3/4 cup
Grapes (small)	15 grapes
Honeydew melon (medium)	1/8 melon
(cubes)	1 cup
Kiwi (large)	1 kiwi
Mandarin oranges	3/4 cup
Mango (small)	1/2 mango
🌾 Nectarine (1½ in. across)	1 nectarine
Orange (2½ in. across)	1 orange
Papaya	1 cup
Peach (2¾ in. across)	1 peach, or 3/4 cup
Peaches (canned)	1/2 cup, or 2 halves
Pear	1/2 large, or 1 small
Pears (canned)	1/2 cup or 2 halves

Persimmon (medium, native)	2 persimmons
Pineapple (raw)	3/4 cup
Pineapple (canned)	1/3 cup
Plum (raw, 2 in. across)	2 plums
🌾 Pomegranate	1/2 pomegranate
🌾 Raspberries (raw)	1 cup
🌾 Strawberries (raw, whole)	1-1/4 cup
Tangerine (2-1/2 in. across)	2 tangerines
Watermelon (cubes)	1-1/4 cup

Dried Fruit

🌾 Apples	4 rings
🌾 Apricots	7 halves
Dates	2-1/2 medium
🌾 Figs	1-1/2
🌾 Prunes	3 medium
Raisins	2 Tbsp.

Fruit Juice

Apple juice/cider	1/2 cup
Cranberry juice cocktail	1/3 cup
Grapefruit juice	1/2 cup
Grape juice	1/3 cup
Orange juice	1/2 cup
Pineapple juice	1/2 cup
Prune juice	1/3 cup

🌾 *3 grams or more of fiber per serving*

List 5 — Milk Exchanges

Each serving of milk or milk products on this list contains about 12 grams of carbohydrate and 8 grams of protein. The amount of fat in milk is measured in percent (%) of butterfat. The calories vary, depending on what kind of milk you choose. The list is divided into three parts based on the amount of fat and calories: skim/very lowfat milk, lowfat milk, and whole milk. One serving (one milk exchange) of each of these includes:

	Carbohydrate (grams)	Protein (grams)	Fat (grams)	Calories
Skim/Very Lowfat	12	8	trace	90
Lowfat	12	8	5	120
Whole	12	8	8	150

Milk is the body's main source of calcium, the mineral needed for growth and repair of bones. Yogurt is also a good source of calcium. Yogurt and many dry or powdered milk products have different amounts of fat. If you have questions about a particular item, read the label to find out the fat and calorie content.

Milk is good to drink, but it can also be added to cereal, and to other foods. Many tasty dishes such as sugar-free pudding are made with milk (see the Combination Foods list). Add life to plain yogurt by adding one of your fruit servings to it.

Skim and Very Lowfat Milk

skim milk . . . . .1 cup
1/2% milk . . . . .1 cup
1% milk . . . . .1 cup
lowfat buttermilk . . . . .1 cup
evaporated skim milk . . . . .1/2 cup
dry nonfat milk. . . . . .1/3 cup
plain nonfat yogurt . . . . .8 oz.

Lowfat Milk

2% milk . . . . .1 cup fluid
plain lowfat yogurt (with added nonfat milk solids) . . . . .8 oz.

Whole Milk

The whole milk group has much more fat per serving than the skim and lowfat groups. Whole milk has more than 3¼% butterfat. Try to limit your choices from the whole milk group as much as possible.

whole milk . . . . .1 cup
evaporated whole milk . . . . .1/2 cup
whole plain yogurt . . . . .8 oz.

List 6 — Fat Exchanges

Each serving on the fat list contains about 5 grams of fat and 45 calories.

The foods on the fat list contain mostly fat, although some items may also contain a small amount of protein. All fats are high in calories and should be carefully measured. Everyone should modify fat intake by eating unsaturated fats instead of saturated fats. The sodium content of these foods varies widely. Check the label for sodium information.

Unsaturated Fats

Avocado . . . . .1/8 medium
Margarine . . . . .1 tsp.
*Margarine, diet . . . . .1 Tbsp.
Mayonnaise . . . . .1 tsp.
*Mayonnaise,
    reduced calorie . . . . .1 Tbsp.

Nuts and Seeds:
    Almonds, dry roasted . . . . .6 whole
    Cashews, dry roasted . . . . .1 Tbsp.
    Pecans . . . . .2 whole
    Peanuts . . . . .20 small or
                              10 large
    Walnuts . . . . .2 whole
    Other nuts . . . . .1 Tbsp.
    Seeds, pine nuts, sunflower
        (without shells) . . . . .1 Tbsp.
    Pumpkin seeds . . . . 2 tsp.

Oil (corn, cottonseed,
    safflower, soybean, sunflower,
    olive, peanut) . . . . .1 tsp.
*Olives . . . . .10 small or
                              5 large
Salad dressing,
    mayonnaise-type . . . . .2 tsp.
Salad dressing,
    mayonnaise-type, reduced-calorie . . .1 Tbsp.

*Salad dressing
    (all varieties) . . . . .1 Tbsp.
Salad dressing,
    reduced-calorie . . . . .2 Tbsp.

(Two tablespoons of low-calorie salad dressing can be considered a free food.)

Saturated Fats

Butter . . . . .1 tsp.
*Bacon . . . . .1 slice
Chitterlings . . . . .1/2 ounce
Coconut, shredded . . . . .2 Tbsp.
Coffee whitener, liquid . . . . .2 Tbsp.
Coffee whitener, powder . . . . .4 tsp.
Cream (light, coffee, table) . . . . .2 Tbsp.
Cream, sour . . . . .2 Tbsp.
Cream (heavy, whipping) . . . . .1 Tbsp.
Cream cheese . . . . .1 Tbsp.
*Salt pork . . . . .1/4 ounce

---

*If more than one or two servings are eaten, these foods have 400 mg. or more of sodium.

400 mg. or more of sodium per serving.

48

Free Foods

A free food is any food or drink that contains less than 20 calories per serving. You can eat as much as you want of those items that have no serving size specified. You may eat two or three servings per day of those items that have a specific serving size. Be sure to spread them out through the day.

Drinks:
Bouillon 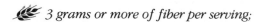 or broth without fat
Bouillon, low-sodium
Carbonated drinks, sugar-free
Carbonated water
Club soda
Cocoa powder, unsweetened (1 Tbsp.)
Coffee/Tea
Drink mixes, sugar-free
Tonic water, sugar-free

Nonstick pan spray

Fruit:
Cranberries, unsweetened (1/2 cup)
Rhubarb, unsweetened (1/2 cup)

Vegetables:
(raw, 1 cup)
Cabbage
Celery
Chinese cabbage
Cucumber
Green onion
Hot peppers
Mushrooms
Radishes
Zucchini

Salad greens:
Endive
Escarole
Lettuce
Romaine
Spinach

Sweet Substitutes:
Candy, hard, sugar-free
Gelatin, sugar-free
Gum, sugar-free
Jam/Jelly, sugar-free (2 tsp.)
Pancake syrup, sugar-free (1-2 Tbsp.)

Sugar substitutes (saccharin, aspartame)
Whipped topping (2 Tbsp.)

Condiments:
Catsup (1 Tbsp.)
Horseradish
Mustard
Pickles, dill, unsweetened
Salad dressing, low-calorie (2 Tbsp.)
Taco sauce (1 Tbsp.)
Vinegar

Seasonings can be very helpful in making food taste better. Be careful of how much sodium you use. Read the label and choose those seasonings that do not contain sodium or salt.

Basil (fresh)
Celery seeds
Cinnamon
Chili powder
Chives
Curry
Dill

Flavoring extracts (vanilla, almond, walnut, peppermint, butter, lemon, etc.)
Garlic
Garlic powder
Herbs
Hot pepper sauce
Lemon

Lemon juice
Lemon pepper
Lime
Lime juice
Mint
Onion powder
Oregano
Paprika
Pepper

Pimento
Spices
Soy sauce
Soy sauce, low sodium ("lite")
Wine, used in cooking (1/4 cup)
Worcestershire sauce

---

3 grams or more of fiber per serving;   *400 mg or more of sodium per serving*

Combination Foods

Much of the food we eat is mixed together in various combinations. These combination foods do not fit into only one exchange list. It can be quite hard to tell what is in a certain casserole dish or baked food item. This is a list of average values for some typical combination foods. This list will help you fit these foods into your meal plan. Ask your dietitian for information about any other foods you'd like to eat. The *American Diabetes Association/American Dietetic Association Family Cookbooks* and the *American Diabetes Association Holiday Cookbook* have many recipes and further information about many foods, including combination foods. Check your library or local bookstore.

Food	Amount	Exchanges
Casseroles, homemade	1 cup (8 oz.)	2 starch, 2 medium-fat meat, 1 fat
Cheese pizza , thin crust	1/4 of 15 oz. or 1/4 of 10″	2 starch, 1 medium-fat meat, 1 fat
Chili with beans , (commercial)	1 cup (8 oz.)	2 starch, 2 medium-fat meat, 2 fat
Chow mein , (without noodles or rice)	2 cups (16 oz.)	1 starch, 2 vegetable, 2 lean meat
Macaroni and cheese	1 cup (8 oz.)	2 starch, 1 medium-fat meat, 2 fat
Soup:		
Bean ,	1 cup (8 oz.)	1 starch, 1 vegetable, 1 lean meat
Chunky, all varieties	10¾ oz. can	1 starch, 1 vegetable, 1 medium-fat meat
Cream (made with water)	1 cup (8 oz.)	1 starch, 1 fat
Vegetable or broth	1 cup (8 oz.)	1 starch
Spaghetti and meatballs (canned)	1 cup (8 oz.)	2 starch, 1 medium-fat meat, 1 fat
Sugar-free pudding (made with skim milk)	1/2 cup	1 starch
If beans are used as a meat substitute:		
Dried beans , peas , lentils	1 cup (cooked)	2 starch, 1 lean meat

3 grams or more of fiber per serving;   *400 mg or more of sodium per serving*

Foods for Occasional Use

Moderate amounts of some foods can be used in your meal plan, in spite of their sugar or fat content, as long as you can maintain blood-glucose control. The following list includes average exchange values for some of these foods. Because they are concentrated sources of carbohydrate, you will notice that the portion sizes are very small. Check with your dietitian for advice on how often and when you can eat them.

Food	Amount	Exchanges
Angel food cake	1/12 cake	2 starch
Cake, no icing	1/12 cake, or a 3″ square	2 starch, 2 fat
Cookies	2 small (1¾″ across)	1 starch, 1 fat
Frozen fruit yogurt	1/3 cup	1 starch
Gingersnaps	3	1 starch
Granola	1/4 cup	1 starch, 1 fat
Granola bars	1 small	1 starch, 1 fat
Ice cream, any flavor	1/2 cup	1 starch, 2 fat
Ice milk, any flavor	1/2 cup	1 starch, 1 fat
Sherbet, any flavor	1/4 cup	1 starch
Snack chips 🧂, all varieties	1 oz.	1 starch, 2 fat
Vanilla wafers	6 small	1 starch, 1 fat

🧂 If more than one serving is eaten, these foods have 400 mg or more of sodium.

The exchange lists are the basis of a meal planning system designed by a committee of the American Diabetes Association and the American Dietetic Association. While designed primarily for people with diabetes and others who must follow special diets, the exchange lists are based on principles of good nutrition that apply to everyone.

©1986 American Diabetes Association, American Dietetic Association.

Exchanges for All Occasions (see Appendix) provides details about exchange lists and additional information on how to use the exchange system.

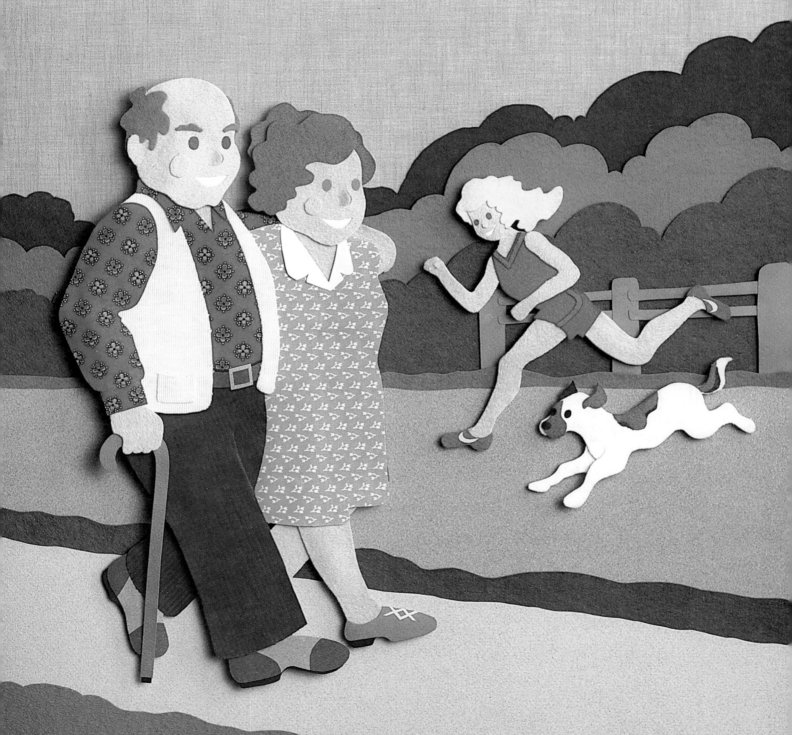

Exercise

Chapter 3
Diabetes and Exercise: Fitting Fitness Into Your Life

Marion Franz, R.D., M.S.

Exercise is important to everyone's health, but it is especially important if you have diabetes! It helps control blood glucose (sugar) levels and weight. The benefits of overall fitness can make many aspects of life easier and more enjoyable.

Although many people agree that exercise is important, many are reluctant to start a regular exercise program. Some argue that their daily work routine provides enough activity. However, in our mechanized society, work and home activities rarely provide enough of the type of activity that is beneficial.

Others feel they do not have the time, money or ability to exercise or are reluctant because they do not know how to begin to exercise or put together an exercise program. You may be worried about precautions related to your diabetes as you begin an exercise program.

This chapter will help you understand those things and will help you get started toward enjoying the benefits of exercise.

What are the benefits of exercise?

The person with diabetes will experience the same benefits and enjoyment everyone else gains from exercise:

1. **Improved fitness.** The World Health Organization defines fitness as the ability to carry out daily tasks with vigor and alertness, without undue fatigue, and with ample reserve energy to enjoy leisure pursuits; and the ability to respond to physical and emotional stress without excessive increase in heart rate and blood pressure.

The basic components of fitness are flexibility, muscle strength and endurance, and cardiorespiratory endurance (your heart and lungs work more efficiently). Flexibility is important because it keeps our bodies mobile and helps to prevent injury to muscles and joints. Muscle strength and endurance help us to perform our daily tasks with less strain and increased capacity for physical work. Muscle strength also helps prevent injuries, and appearance improves as muscles become firmer. Cardiorespiratory endurance is important because it helps reduce the risk of heart disease and helps maintain high energy levels for daily activities.

2. **Psychological benefits.** Exercise helps in coping with stress, building self-confidence and improving self-image. You have more energy to do things, are more relaxed, and feel less tense and more active.

3. **Reduced body fat.** As fitness improves, you increase the amount of muscle and decrease the amount of fat stored on your body. You become leaner, which improves your outward appearance.

4. **Weight control.** Exercise can help you maintain your weight if you are lean, or help you lose weight if you are overweight. Weight loss can occur with exercise if food intake is kept the same or decreased. Exercise helps burn calories, not just during exercise but for many hours afterward. Exercise increases your metabolic rate (how fast your body uses energy) by 25 percent for up to 15 hours after an exercise session. This means you burn more calories than a sedentary person, even when you are not exercising. Appetite is also reduced by a regular exercise program. Weight loss from exercise will be mostly fat loss, as opposed to the losses of body water and lean body tissue that so often occur from dieting alone.

Extra Benefits of Exercise If You Have Diabetes

Diabetes is not a reason to avoid physical activity. On the contrary, it is an additional reason to incorporate exercise into your lifestyle. In addition to the above benefits, the person with diabetes receives many other benefits from exercise, such as:

1. Exercise can lower blood glucose (sugar) levels and improve the body's ability to use glucose.

2. Exercise increases the blood glucose lowering effect of injected insulin, so regular physical activity decreases the amount of insulin you need. Physical training can also help reverse the resistance to insulin that occurs as a result of obesity.

3. Exercise improves risk factors related to heart disease and decreases the risk of developing heart disease, which is a major threat to people with diabetes. This includes the lowering of the amount of fat (cholesterol and triglycerides) in the blood, which is related to the development of heart disease. It increases the amount of high density lipoprotein cholesterol (HDL), the type of cholesterol which is protective against heart disease.

4. Exercise lowers blood pressure. High blood pressure (hypertension) contributes to many of the chronic problems that occur with diabetes.

5. Exercise combined with a reduction in daily caloric intake will often control non-insulin-dependent (Type II) diabetes, without the need for medication.

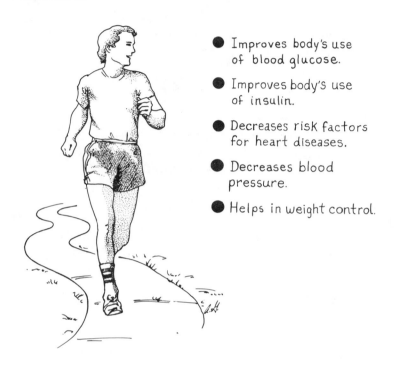

- Improves body's use of blood glucose.
- Improves body's use of insulin.
- Decreases risk factors for heart diseases.
- Decreases blood pressure.
- Helps in weight control.

What precautions need to be taken to exercise safely?

To safely enjoy all the benefits of exercise, certain precautions must be taken. When beginning an exercise program it is important to get an okay from your doctor, especially if you are over 30 or have had diabetes for ten years or more. It is important to build up endurance gradually to avoid heart problems. Because exercise requires the heart to pump faster than normal in order to supply working muscles, a heart attack can occur if heart disease is present.

Problems related to diabetes such as eye, kidney, or nerve damage may be worsened by inappropriate or strenuous exercise. For example, if you have eye problems, exercises that involve straining, such as weight lifting, can cause bleeding in the eyes. And if you have nerve damage or poor blood circulation to your feet, walking and running can cause foot sores that you will not feel, possibly leading to serious damage before you notice the problem.

The next two sections will describe information specific to insulin-dependent (Type I) and non-insulin-dependent (Type II) diabetes.

Insulin-Dependent Diabetes and Exercise

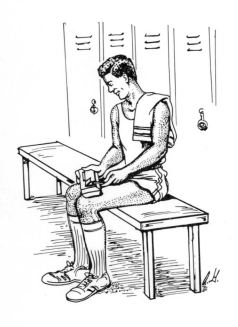

Before starting any exercise program, be sure your diabetes is under good control. It is important to start slowly and gradually build up endurance.

Exercise may initially cause blood glucose levels to change unpredictably. The level of fitness of the person also can affect blood glucose stability — the regular exerciser will have fewer management problems than the occasional exerciser.

The key to ensuring stability of blood glucose levels is to do self blood glucose testing before, during and after exercise. Keep a record of the test results, time of exercise, how long since you last ate, what you ate, and what type of exercise you did and how long you did it. Discuss your records with your health care providers and together develop guidelines for adjusting food intake and insulin injection amounts and times.

Guidelines presented in this chapter are very general, but will give you information that will help you work with your health care provider to get you started on a regular exercise program. To safely enjoy all the benefits of exercise, certain principles must be followed.

For the person with insulin-dependent diabetes, there are five general guidelines that you need to be aware of when planning an exercise program:

1. The effect of exercise in Type I diabetes will depend on the availability of insulin to the muscle cells. When control of diabetes is good or if there is only a mild increase in blood glucose levels without ketosis (ketones), exercise results in a decrease in blood glucose levels and insulin requirements. If blood glucose is not well controlled, exercise will act as a stress on your body and will drive blood glucose levels even higher. When insulin deficiency is severe and diabetes control poor, the production of glucose by the liver and the breakdown of fat to ketones exceeds the ability of the muscles to use them. As a result there is an increase in blood glucose levels and ketones accumulate, thus worsening diabetes control.

When blood glucose is high (generally greater than 300 mg/dl) as a result of insufficient insulin (poor control), glucose use by the muscle doesn't occur. The exercising muscle still needs glucose and will send a message to the liver to produce or release stored carbohydrate. As a result, more glucose is released into the blood, raising rather than lowering the blood glucose level during exercise. It is, therefore, very important to be sure your diabetes is under reasonable control before beginning an exercise session. This is another reason to monitor blood glucose levels.

2. Exercise improves the blood glucose lowering effect of injected insulin. Carefully finding out how exercise affects your blood glucose levels will decrease the risk of having an insulin reaction. Be aware of the peak action times of your insulin, and allow for the greater lowering of blood glucose levels that exercise can cause at these times. An ideal time for exercise is following a meal, when you will have plenty of glucose available. If you do exercise when your insulin is peaking, think ahead and be sure to eat enough carbohydrate to provide the necessary glucose during the entire time you will be exercising. [Blood glucose levels usually remain unchanged or may be slightly elevated during the first 40 minutes of exercise. This is due to glucose released from the liver after the breakdown of glycogen (stored carbohydrate).]

3. Exercise can influence the rate at which insulin is absorbed from the injection site into the blood. Choose your injection site according to the type of exercise you will be doing. For example, if you are planning to play tennis or golf within an hour, do not inject insulin into your arms, because the muscle activity will force the insulin into your bloodstream faster than usual, causing low blood glucose. Avoid your legs as an injection site if you will be walking or running within an hour. The stomach or buttocks is a better choice than the arms or legs when immediate strenuous exercise is planned.

4. You may also need to increase food as a result of exercise. This extra food should be eaten before exercise as well as during activities that last a long time. The extra food you eat to provide glucose during exercise should not be subtracted from your meal plan. If exercise is a regular part of your schedule, food for it should be figured into your meal plan. Well trained people who regularly exercise at about the same time each day will usually need less food than people who exercise only occasionally.

As stated before, the best way to know how much food you need is to test blood glucose levels before, during, and after exercise. The effect of exercise on blood glucose level differs from person to person, because everyone exercises at different intensities and uses insulin and food differently. **The guidelines given in the table "Food Adjustments for Exercise" are only general recommendations.** They can help you plan food for exercise and make food changes based on your own blood glucose level. It is very important that you monitor your blood glucose level and adapt these guidelines to your needs.

5. Blood glucose levels continue to decrease after exercise. It is important to test your blood glucose soon after exercise and again about an hour later if you feel symptoms of an insulin reaction. It can take your body up to 24 hours to replace the glycogen (carbohydrate stored in muscles and the liver and used for energy) that was used during exercise.

Further guidelines and tips are given in Chapter 27 for people taking insulin who participate in sports or more strenuous endurance exercise.

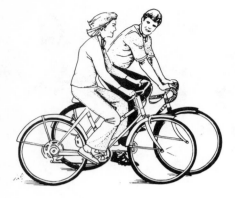

General Guidelines for Making Food Adjustments for Exercise

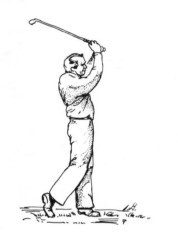

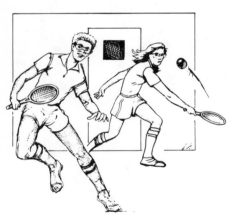

Type of Exercise and Examples	If Blood Glucose Is:	Increase Food Intake By:	Suggestions of Food to Use
Exercise of **short** duration and of low to moderate intensity **Examples:** Walking a half mile or leisurely bicycling for less than 30 min.	less than 100 mg	10 to 15 gms of carbohydrate per hour	1 fruit or 1 starch/bread exchange
	100 mg or above	not necessary to increase food	
Exercise of **moderate** intensity **Examples:** Tennis, swimming, jogging, leisurely bicycling, gardening, golfing or vacuuming **for one hour**	less than 100 mg	25 to 50 gms of carbohydrate before exercise, then 10 to 15 gms per hour of exercise	½ meat sandwich with a milk or fruit exchange
	100 to 180 mg	10 to 15 gms of carbohydrate per hour of exercise	1 fruit or 1 starch/bread exchange
	180 to 300 mg	not necessary to increase food	
	300 mg or greater	Don't begin exercise until blood glucose is under better control.	
Strenuous activity or exercise **Examples:** Football, hockey, racquetball or basketball games; strenuous bicycling or swimming; shoveling heavy snow	less than 100 mg	50 gms of carbohydrate, monitor blood glucose carefully	1 meat sandwich (2 slices of bread) with a milk and fruit exchange
	100 to 180 mg	25 to 50 gms of carbohydrate, depending on intensity and duration	½ meat sandwich with a milk or fruit exchange
	180 to 300 mg	10 to 15 gms of carbohydrate per hour of exercise	1 fruit or 1 starch/bread exchange

Adjusting Insulin for Extended Exercise

When exercising strenuously over an extended period of time, such as all morning, all afternoon or all day, it may be difficult to avoid low blood glucose by just increasing food intake. In such cases one can reduce the dosage of the insulin that will be acting during the time of activity. In effect, the exercise will take the place of the missing insulin, and together with food intake will keep blood glucose in the normal range. You can adjust your insulin by using the following guideline:

Decrease insulin *acting during the exercise time* by 10 percent of the *total* insulin dose. Examples are given below for exercise lasting all morning, all afternoon or all day:

Examples: Insulin dose: 4 Regular, 24 NPH before breakfast
2 Regular, 6 NPH before evening meal
Total dose = 6 + 30 = 36 units

10 percent of total dose = 3.6 units (36 x .10), which can be rounded to 4 units.

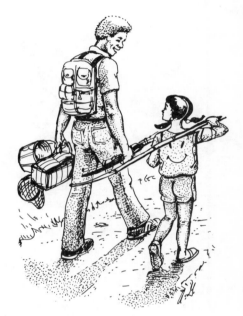

Rapid-acting insulin acts during the morning hours. For cross-country skiing all morning, decrease the morning Regular by 10 percent of the total insulin dose. The morning insulin would then be 0 Regular (4 minus 4) and 24 NPH.

Intermediate-acting insulin taken before breakfast will act during the afternoon hours. For canoeing all afternoon, the morning insulin would be 4 Regular and 20 NPH (24 minus 4).

For an activity lasting the entire day, such as downhill skiing, both the Regular and NPH would be decreased, so the morning insulin would be 0 Regular (4 minus 4) and 20 NPH (24 minus 4).

Again, blood glucose testing before and after physical activity will allow you to make adjustments in these general recommendations. Furthermore, be aware of specific warning signs of an approaching insulin reaction, both during and after activity. If possible, test your blood glucose when you notice such symptoms to make sure they are symptoms of low blood glucose. It is important to always have a source of carbohydrate available during and after exercise, especially exercise that lasts for a long time. Also make sure that others are aware of your diabetes and know what to do if you need help.

Non-Insulin-Dependent Diabetes and Exercise

Exercise can also improve control of blood glucose and reduce fat stores for people with non-insulin-dependent (Type II) diabetes. Regular activity combined with a weight-loss diet will often control Type II diabetes. If you use insulin or a diabetes pill, the dosage can usually be reduced and in some cases eventually eliminated as a result of regular exercise and weight control. *If you use insulin or a diabetes pill to help control blood glucose levels, you must be aware of the precautions listed in the section on "Insulin-Dependent Diabetes and Exercise."* However, since your body is still producing some insulin, your blood glucose levels will not be as unstable with exercise as they may be in an insulin-dependent person.

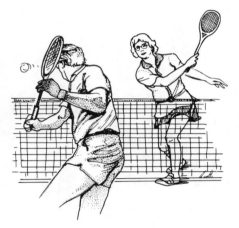

Regular exercise helps the management of Type II diabetes because working muscles use glucose more effectively. Insulin must attach to the surface of individual cells in order to lower blood glucose or promote its other effects in the body. Exercise seems to increase the number of sites on each cell where insulin can attach. This thereby increases the body's sensitivity to insulin. Consequently the insulin or diabetes pill dosage can usually be reduced.

Regular exercise also decreases the amount of cholesterol and triglycerides in the blood, which reduces the risk of heart disease. Exercise increases the amount of HDL cholesterol in the blood, which helps protect against heart disease. Heart disease is a major threat in diabetes, and exercise is one important way of reducing that threat.

Exercise can also be a way to burn up excess calories and to help with weight loss. There are approximately 3,500 calories stored in one pound of body fat, so to lose one pound of fat you must reduce your caloric intake by 3,500 calories or increase your activity level by 3,500 calories or do a combination of both. By decreasing your caloric intake by 500 calories a day and adding 250 calories of activity, you can have a total reduction of 5,250 calories in a week for a loss of 1½ pounds of fat.

The table "Using Up Calories" will give you an idea of how much exercise you need to do to burn 250 calories, as well as the number of calories burned in one hour of various activities. These caloric estimates are general averages; how many calories you actually burn depends on how hard and how skillfully you perform the activity.

A bonus to this caloric reduction is that a regular exercise program also increases your resting metabolic rate, which is the number of calories your body burns when at complete rest. These calorie-using effects last well beyond the actual exercise period.

Using Up Calories

Activity	Time Needed to Use 250 Calories	Calories Used Per Hour of Activity
Rest and Light Activity		
(50-200 calories per hour)		
Lying down or sleeping	3 hrs., 8 min.	80
Sitting	2 hrs., 30 min.	100
Driving an automobile	2 hrs.	120
Fishing	1 hr., 50 min.	130
Standing	1 hr., 45 min.	140
Domestic work	1 hr., 23 min.	180
Moderate Activity		
(200-350 calories per hour)		
Bicycling (5½ mph)	1 hr., 10 min.	210
Walking (2½ mph)*	1 hr., 10 min.	210
Gardening	1 hr., 8 min.	220
Canoeing (2½ mph)	1 hr., 4 min.	230
Golf	1 hr.	250
Lawn mowing (power mower)	1 hr.	250
Bowling	55 min.	270
Lawn mowing (hand mower)	55 min.	270
Rowboating (2½ mph)	50 min.	300
Swimming (¼ mph)	50 min.	300
Walking (3¾ mph)	50 min.	300
Dancing (slow step)	50 min.	300
Softball	45 min.	325
Badminton	40 min.	350
Horseback riding (trotting)	40 min.	350
Square dancing	40 min.	350
Volleyball	40 min.	350
Rollerskating	40 min.	350
Vigorous Activity		
(over 350 calories per hour)		
Mini-trampoline	38 min.	400
Ditch digging (hand shovel)	38 min.	400
Shoveling	38 min.	400
Ice skating (10 mph)	38 min.	400
Wood chopping or sawing	38 min.	400
Tennis, singles	35 min.	420
Waterskiing	32 min.	460
Dancing (fast step)	30 min.	490
Jogging	26 min.	585
Skiing (downhill)	25 min.	600
Squash and handball	25 min.	600
Soccer	25 min.	600
Singles racquetball	20 min.	775
Skiing (cross-country)	15 min.	900
Running (10 mph)	15 min.	900

*Walking or jogging = 100 calories per mile — cover 2.5 miles for 250 calories

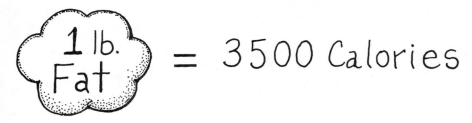

1 lb. Fat = 3500 Calories

Most weight lost during exercise is body water which must be replaced by drinking fluids.

Exercise does not automatically cause weight loss, however. At first there may be an increase in lean body mass (muscle), which may result in a small increase in body weight. In fact, with exercise you may simply lose some of your fat tissue and increase lean body mass, which will make you feel better and may make your clothes fit better. If you do want to lose weight, you will have to reduce caloric intake along with your exercise program.

You may lose several pounds during an exercise session, especially in hot and humid weather. This is NOT fat loss. It is body water lost from sweating and must be replaced by drinking plenty of fluids. If you do not replace the water lost during exercise, you can become dehydrated. If you exercise when dehydrated, you might suffer heatstroke, and possibly even death.

The most efficient way to burn fat when exercising is to: 1) exercise at a level that results in no shortness of breath (low intensity), and 2) exercise continuously for at least 20 to 30 minutes (long duration). Exercise of short duration (under 2 to 3 minutes) and high intensity (shortness of breath) uses stored carbohydrate (glycogen) as the major energy source. Low intensity, long duration exercise uses stored fat as the major energy source. You will use a lot more calories in 20 or more minutes of moderate activity than you would in a few minutes of very intense activity.

Some exercises that are often recommended for weight loss include brisk walking, jogging, swimming, skating, cross-country skiing, bicycling, jumping rope, aerobic dance, and jumping or running in place on a mini-trampoline. All these exercises are forms of "aerobic" (with oxygen) exercise, meaning that you can do them for a long time without running out of breath. And they all involve the use of large muscle groups, which means that you will have many muscles using glucose and burning calories. If you want to use exercise to help you lose weight, you should exercise for at least 20 to 30 minutes five to six days a week.

In summary, exercise is important for people with Type II diabetes because it:
- Increases the body's sensitivity to insulin.
- Improves blood glucose control.
- Reduces risk of heart disease.
- Promotes weight loss.

How to Begin

It is important that you know how to exercise correctly and safely. Doing the right types of exercise correctly will reduce your chances of injury while you are improving your health and blood glucose control.

If you have concerns about starting an exercise program, check with your doctor. Start slowly and build up endurance gradually to avoid heart problems. "An Example of a Gradually Increased Exercise Program" (page 64) is a good guideline for building up slowly.

For general fitness and blood glucose control, choose activities that are aerobic. Aerobic activities require large amounts of oxygen, and usually involve movement of the arms and legs, which contain a large part of the body's total muscle mass. Aerobic exercise uses a lot of energy and if done for long periods of time uses many calories. When performed correctly for long enough periods of time, aerobic exercises strengthen the heart and lungs. This occurs because the heart and lungs are required to work harder for a longer period of time to supply the exercising muscles with blood and oxygen. This makes the heart and lungs more efficient at rest and when performing less strenuous tasks.

Anaerobic activities are the opposite of aerobic exercise. (Anaerobic means without oxygen.) Anaerobic activities are performed at a high intensity for a short period of time, such as sprinting or running up a hill or stairs. These activities exceed the ability of the heart and lungs to deliver and process oxygen, and exhaustion quickly sets in. They do not have the qualities of increasing weight loss, improving endurance, and helping control blood glucose.

What IS an exercise program?

When you design your exercise program, divide it into three periods: warm-up, training (aerobic exercise), and cool-down. All are important. The pattern will look something like this:

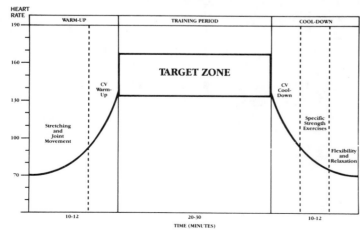

Reprinted with permission from the SHAPE manual.

63

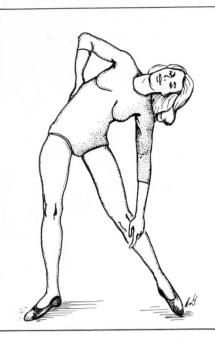

Warming Up

Your warm-up period should last about 10 to 12 minutes and prepare your body for exercise. Begin by stretching and flexing the muscles that are most often the tightest — neck, shoulders, upper and lower back — and so on down to your ankles. Stretching properly can prevent injury and reduce muscle soreness. Stretch slowly, gently but firmly. Hold for 10 to 20 seconds and then relax. Don't bounce when you stretch, because the muscles will resist stretching and can be injured. Don't stretch to the point of pain.

Next do a cardiovascular warm-up, which will probably mean slowly starting into your aerobic exercise and building up to your training level (explained below).

Cardiovascular Conditioning—Aerobic Activity

This will be the main event of your exercise program, and it is where you will build your endurance and overall fitness level. These improvements are known as the "training effect."

Three essential ingredients needed to achieve a training effect are: intensity, duration and frequency.

1. **Intensity** refers to how hard you work during exercise. To get the maximum heart and lung benefits from your exercise program, your heart must reach and maintain a certain number of beats per minute. To measure your heart rate, count your pulse at the wrist by pressing lightly with the first two fingers at the base of the thumb of the opposite hand. Count the pulse beats for ten seconds and multiply by six to find the number of beats per minute. Take your pulse during or immediately after you stop exercising, and count only for ten seconds, because the heart rate will slow down drastically after just 15 seconds.

To improve fitness, the pulse rate must be kept within your individual target zone for at least 20 to 30 minutes of aerobic exercise. This target zone is between 70 and 85 percent of the maximal heart rate, which is the fastest your heart can beat during an all-out effort. Although the maximal heart rate does vary from person to person, it can be roughly estimated by subtracting your age from 220. Because maximal heart rate decreases with age, the training target zone also decreases with age. Exercising at an intensity higher than the target zone will probably shorten your exercise session because you will become fatigued. It will also increase your chances of muscle injury or heart problems.

Target heart rates (beats per ten seconds) have been calculated in the table below:

Target Heart Rates

Heart Beats per ten seconds

Intensity	Age: 15	20	25	30	35	40	45	50	55	60	65	70
60%	20	20	19	19	18	18	17	17	16	16	15	15
75%	25	25	24	23	23	22	22	21	20	20	19	19
85%	29	28	27	27	26	25	25	24	23	22	22	21

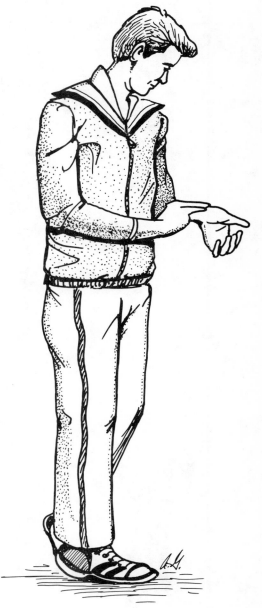

When you first start an exercise program, try to keep your pulse between 60 and 75 percent of your maximum rate. Gradually increase your intensity over several weeks until you are exercising at 75 to 85 percent of your maximum.

As your fitness level increases, you will find that you have to exercise harder to keep your pulse rate in the target zone. This is because your heart and lungs have become more efficient and are better able to handle the intensity of exercise.

A less accurate method of determining exercise intensity that you might want to use after you become more experienced is to observe your depth and rate of breathing while you exercise. You should be breathing deeper and faster than usual to take in the large amounts of oxygen that are needed, yet you should not be huffing and puffing. A good guideline is whether you are able to carry on a conversation during the activity. If you can't, you are exercising at too high an intensity.

2. **Duration** is the length of time you exercise continuously at your target heart rate zone. Heart and lung capacity improves considerably when you exercise regularly for 20 to 30 minutes — preferably 30 minutes. Longer periods of exercise also are beneficial, but the benefits are more related to weight control or preparation for competition than to basic heart and lung fitness.

As you begin your exercise program, limit your workout to 10 to 15 minutes of continuous aerobic exercise at the lower end of the target zone. Gradually increase the duration as you feel capable. Increase the duration of your workouts before you increase the intensity. In other words, exercise longer, not harder.

3. **Frequency** is the number of times you exercise per week. To be effective, an exercise program must be performed at least three to four times per week. Sessions should be spread throughout the week to allow your body to recover. Some additional improvement occurs when exercising five days per week rather than three or four. However, there is no significant change in training gains from exercising six or seven days per week, and you will markedly increase your chance of injury. If you want to exercise every day for weight control, choose different activities that use different muscle groups — jogging and bicycling would be an example.

To summarize the aerobic activity part of your exercise program, you should build up gradually until you can exercise at 70 to 85 percent of your maximal heart rate, for 20 to 30 minutes at a time, from three to five days per week.

Cooling Down

The cooling down period begins with a cardiovascular cool-down. This is a tapering off of your aerobic activity. Gradually decrease your heart rate by slowing down the activity.

Next is the time for specific muscle strengthening exercises. You might want to do some general calisthenic-type exercises or even work with weights. This is the time to do sit-ups for strengthening stomach muscles and for push-ups to strengthen the upper body.

Complete the cool-down with more stretching exercises, similar to the ones done during warm-up. Vigorous exercises tend to shorten muscles, and it is helpful to stretch them out again. It is often helpful and enjoyable to add a relaxation period with deep breathing exercises after stretching. The cool-down period should last approximately 10 to 12 minutes — longer if you add the relaxation time.

An Example of a Gradually Increased Exercise Program

If you find a particular week's pattern of exercise tiring, repeat it before going on to the next pattern. You do not have to progress to 30 minutes of exercise in 12 weeks. Remember to do stretching exercises before the walking warm-up and after the walking cool-down.

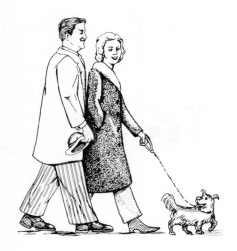

	Warm-up (Slow walking)	Exercise (Brisk walking)	Cool-Down (Slow walking)	Total Time
WEEK 1				
Session A	5 min.	5 min.	5 min.	15 min.
Session B	5 min.	5 min.	5 min.	15 min.
Session C	5 min.	5 min.	5 min.	15 min.
Continue with at least three exercise sessions during each week.				
WEEK 2 (each session)	5 min.	7 min.	5 min.	17 min.
WEEK 3 "	5 min.	9 min.	5 min.	19 min.
WEEK 4 "	5 min.	11 min.	5 min.	21 min.
WEEK 5 "	5 min.	13 min.	5 min.	23 min.
WEEK 6 "	5 min.	15 min.	5 min.	25 min.
WEEK 7 "	5 min.	18 min.	5 min.	28 min.
WEEK 8 "	5 min.	20 min.	5 min.	30 min.
WEEK 9 "	5 min.	23 min.	5 min.	33 min.
WEEK 10 "	5 min.	26 min.	5 min.	36 min.
WEEK 11 "	5 min.	28 min.	5 min.	38 min.
WEEK 12 "	5 min.	30 min.	5 min.	40 min.

Designed by the National Heart, Lung, and Blood Institute. Reprinted from the publication, "Exercise and Your Heart."

YOU Are Ready to Get Started!

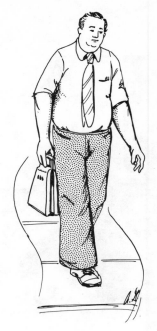

- Get your doctor's approval. This is particularly important if you are over age 30, have had diabetes for more than ten years, or have other physical problems, concerns or questions about exercise.

- Choose an exercise program consisting of activities that you enjoy and that fit your lifestyle. Exercise should be enjoyable, not a chore!

- Invest in a good pair of exercise shoes. This is important for anyone beginning an exercise program, but especially for people with diabetes. Buy shoes that are comfortable and suited to the type of exercise you will be doing. Be careful to avoid blisters or other foot problems during exercise. Treat them immediately if they occur and obtain help from your health care provider if they do not heal promptly.

- Drink plenty of water before, during and after exercise. Dehydration can kill!

- Start slowly. Learn how to measure your heart rate during exercise and **gradually** work up to exercising at 70 to 85 percent of your maximum.

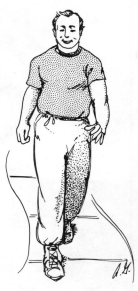

- Make the exercise an enjoyable and necessary part of your life. It should be practical — suited to you and your schedule. Exercise at the time of day that feels good to you. People with Type I diabetes usually find that it helps their blood glucose control if they exercise at about the same time each day.

- Test your blood glucose frequently to find out how exercise affects you. Obtain help from your health care provider if you need to adjust your food intake or medication.

- Warm up and cool down adequately in every exercise session. Hold stretches for ten seconds and do not bounce or strain. Gradual warm-ups and cool-downs and proper stretching are keys to injury prevention.

- If you want to lose weight, use a combination of a diet designed with your dietitian and exercise of long duration and moderate or even low intensity. Choose more than one type of aerobic exercise and do them on alternate days so that you can exercise almost every day.

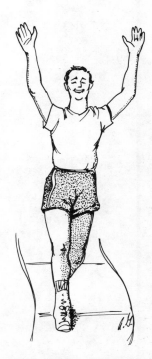

- Try to increase your activity in daily living, changing sedentary routines into mini-exercise sessions. Take the stairs instead of the elevator, walk to the store instead of driving, park a little ways from your destination and walk the rest. Together, these behaviors can add up to significant caloric consumption.

- Make a commitment to exercise and stick with it. An exercise partner can help you stay with it and add to the enjoyment. Just telling others about your exercise program can provide motivation to keep you going.

- You will lose the benefits of exercise very quickly — in a matter of days — when you stop doing it. If you have a layoff period, gradually work back to your previous level of fitness.

- Most importantly, remember to have fun and feel good about yourself. You need to hear "cheering from within." This will be what keeps you going!

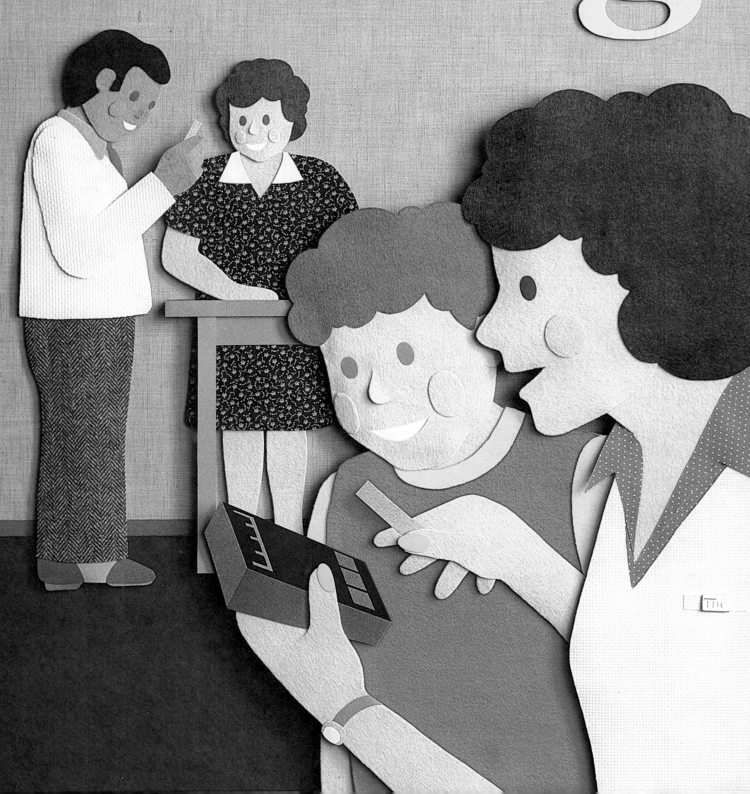

Testing

Chapter 4
Controlling Diabetes: The Importance of Testing

Judy Ostrom Joynes, R.N., M.A.

Diabetes researchers and health care providers are becoming more and more convinced that testing the level of glucose (sugar) in your blood is one of the most important things you can do to control your diabetes. This is because you and your health care providers can use the results of glucose testing to make important decisions about medication, meal planning, and exercise.

The purpose of "monitoring" blood glucose (keeping track of test results) is so you and your health care provider can take action to keep your blood glucose levels as close to normal as possible. Studies show that keeping blood glucose levels close to normal seems to be the best way to prevent complications of diabetes. Children seem to follow normal growth and development patterns, the short-term problems of low blood glucose and high blood glucose occur less often, and the long-term problems affecting the small and large blood vessels are minimized.

You will need to decide whether you want to do blood glucose testing rather than rely on the older and less useful method of testing urine glucose. In this chapter we will explain both types of testing and will discuss the pros and cons of each. We will also explain why it is important to test the urine for ketones if the blood glucose level is high.

How is it possible to test the amount of glucose in the blood?

The oldest method of finding out if there is too much glucose in the blood is by testing the urine. In Chapter 1 we mentioned the ancient technique of placing urine near an ant hill to see if the ants would be attracted by the sugar crystals. Another old and crude method was to actually taste the urine to see if it was sweet. Fortunately there are now much better methods that use strips of chemically treated paper to test the urine. And most recently, methods have been developed that allow a person with diabetes to directly test his or her blood using a chemically treated paper strip that can be visually compared to a color chart or read by a machine that shows a very accurate level of glucose.

But before we discuss how to test your blood or urine, let's review the way glucose gets into the blood and urine. In Chapters 1 and 2 we described how the body digests food, turning much of it into glucose. Glucose then passes through the walls of the intestines into the circulating blood. The glucose travels throughout the body in the bloodstream. When enough insulin is available, the glucose can be taken in by the cells of the body and used for energy. But if no insulin is made by the pancreas (Type I diabetes) or if the insulin is not effective in moving glucose into the cells (Type II diabetes), then glucose builds up in the blood.

The kidneys, which are at the lower back near the spine, remove waste products from the blood by filtering it. This creates urine to carry the waste products out of the body. When blood glucose is in a normal range, almost no glucose is filtered from the blood and removed from the body in the urine. But if the level of glucose in the blood gets too high, the kidneys try to reduce the amount of blood glucose by washing larger amounts into the urine. This is why a "positive" urine test for glucose can be taken as a sign of high blood glucose.

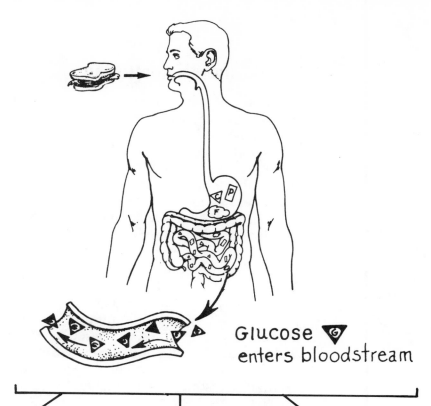

Glucose ▽G
enters bloodstream

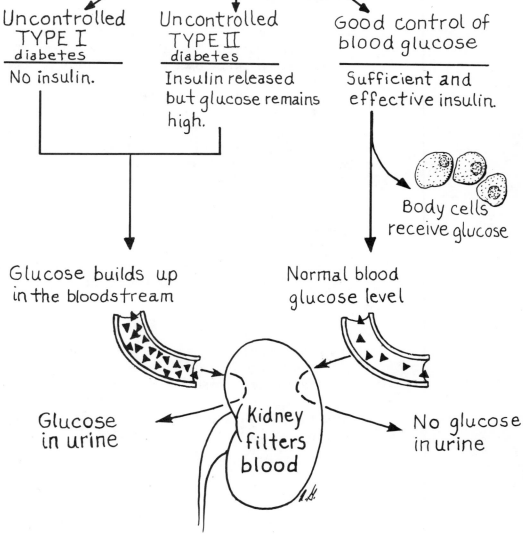

Uncontrolled
TYPE I
diabetes

No insulin.

Uncontrolled
TYPE II
diabetes

Insulin released
but glucose remains
high.

Good control of
blood glucose

Sufficient and
effective insulin.

Body cells
receive glucose

Glucose builds up
in the bloodstream

Normal blood
glucose level

Glucose
in urine

Kidney
filters
blood

No glucose
in urine

Blood Glucose Monitoring

Blood Glucose Monitoring is the best way to check daily blood glucose levels.

Before the 1960's, the only way to directly test the level of glucose in a person's blood was to do an expensive test in a laboratory. But in the late 1960s, methods began to be developed by which a person could test blood glucose levels at home. In the late 1970s, these methods became reasonably easy to perform and their cost was reduced enough so that they became practical for everyday use. Small calculator-like machines called "blood glucose monitors" were developed that could use a ray of light to "read" blood glucose test strips. Devices were also developed to help people remove a small drop of blood for each test.

Blood glucose monitoring has now been improved to the point that it is the best method of testing for almost all people with diabetes. It is especially valuable for pregnant women with diabetes (Chapter 17), people who use an insulin pump (Chapter 8), people who have an altered renal threshold (explained later in this chapter), and people with insulin-dependent diabetes. We at the International Diabetes Center believe that blood glucose monitoring is the most reliable method of testing for anyone who wants to achieve the best possible control of his or her diabetes.

There are now a variety of products on the market that can be used in blood glucose monitoring. There are lancets (finger prickers) and holders which can be used to obtain almost painlessly a small drop of blood for testing. There are different types of test strips (stix) that can be read by visually comparing the changing color to a color chart after blood has been applied to the test strip. There are different types of instruments called blood glucose monitors that can read these test strips and show the exact blood glucose level. A blood glucose monitor is even available that can be used by the blind—it has an electronic voice that reports the glucose level.

While not all these instruments and products are needed by everyone who wants to do blood glucose monitoring, even the basic supplies make it a more expensive method than urine testing. This procedure is slightly more difficult to learn than urine testing, but even young children can test their blood with proper instruction. The accuracy of blood glucose monitoring is so superior, however, that we rarely suggest patients use urine testing.

If you decide to use blood glucose monitoring, first receive proper instruction from your health care provider. Your main choice will be whether to use the visual blood tests, the monitor-read blood tests, or a combination of the two methods. Some people like to leave their monitor at home and just carry the bottle of strips to obtain visual readings while at school or work.

The visually read blood testing method does not give a specific number reading for milligrams of glucose per deciliter of blood (mg/dl). The color chart contains ranges, such as 80-120 mg/dl, 120-180 mg/dl, etc. By comparing the color of your test with the color of the color chart square it is closest to, you can estimate about where in the range your blood glucose level falls.

Some people prefer to have a specific number reading that tells them their blood glucose level in mg/dl. The same strips that can be visually read can also be placed in a blood glucose monitor to obtain an accurate mg/dl reading. The procedure is different for different types of monitors, but the general procedure is described in Chapter 5.

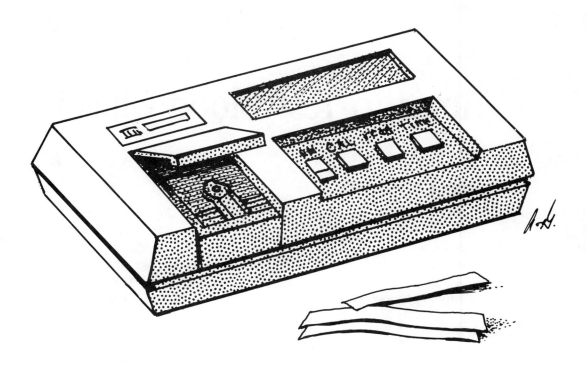

Many people with diabetes now use blood glucose monitoring to obtain blood glucose level readings as many as six times a day. It is helpful to test before meals and at bedtime, before and after exercise, whenever you feel symptoms of low or high blood glucose, or just whenever you need to be reassured that you are in control of your diabetes. The times of day at which testing is done vary from person to person. Your health care providers will make recommendations based on whether you are taking insulin and how often, and how stable your blood glucose level is. General guidelines for testing times are as follows:

- If you are taking insulin to help control Type I or Type II diabetes, it is most helpful to test your blood before breakfast, lunch, dinner, and your evening snack.
- If you have Type II diabetes, are not taking insulin, and your blood glucose level stays close to or within the normal range, it may only be necessary to test two days per week. On these days, test once before breakfast, once before a main meal, and once two hours after a main meal.

Times to Test Blood Glucose

If Taking Insulin

Before meals.
Before bedtime.
Before and after exercise.
When feeling symptoms of an insulin reaction.
When feeling like blood glucose is high.
When feeling ill.
Test more often when ill.
Test urine ketones if blood glucose is 240 mg/dl or higher.

If Not Taking Insulin

Test two days per week. On testing days, test before breakfast, before a main meal, and two hours after a main meal.
More often if control is not good.
Test often when ill; you may need insulin for a short time to help control blood glucose.

Urine Testing

Urine tests are a reflection of what the blood glucose level has been during the time the urine has been accumulating in the bladder (a sac-like organ that stores urine produced by the kidneys). The advantages of urine testing are that it is easy to learn how to test the urine and the tests are not very expensive. The basic disadvantage of urine testing is that the results do not give a very good reading of what the actual blood glucose level is at the time you are doing the urine test. This limits the usefulness of urine testing in making decisions about medication, food intake and exercise—all things that will affect your blood glucose control.

One reason for the lack of accuracy with urine testing is that the urine test method assumes that the kidneys will begin removing extra glucose as soon as the blood glucose level exceeds normal range. The trouble is that not everyone's kidneys work that way. Some people can have a positive test when their blood glucose is within the normal range and others can have a negative test when their blood glucose is elevated.

The blood glucose level at which the kidneys begin removing extra glucose from the blood is called the "renal threshold" (renal means kidney and threshold means a limit above or below which something will happen). An average renal threshold is about 180 mg/dl; this means that a urine test would not be positive until blood glucose went higher than 180 mg/dl. (Remember, the normal blood glucose range is 60 mg/dl to 160 mg/dl.) However, one study showed that when 65 people with diabetes were given urine tests and blood glucose tests, 50 percent had positive urine tests when their blood glucose level was actually quite normal—135 mg/dl or less. Another study found that 38 percent of a group of children with diabetes had negative urine tests even though the average of their blood glucose levels was quite high—233 mg/dl. These variations in renal threshold make urine test results misleading for many people.

Urine testing results are misleading for many people with diabetes.

Another problem with urine testing is that it does not give you any information about low blood glucose. When a urine test is negative, you only know that your blood glucose is probably not high. You do not know if it is at the high end of the normal range or at the low end. This lack of information makes it hard to make decisions about your blood glucose. If it is at the high end of normal, you would eat less than usual before exercising and eat your usual snacks and meals. But if it is low, you would not want to exercise or go to bed without first having an extra snack to prevent a reaction. Because they do not have this information about low blood glucose, some people with diabetes purposely run positive urine tests to avoid reactions. This practice is very dangerous in the long run, because it increases the risk of long-term complications of diabetes.

As you can see, there are several problems with using urine testing as part of a program to control blood glucose levels. It is not a completely useless method, however. Some people with Type II diabetes that can be controlled by diet and exercise and a few people with very stable Type I diabetes can use urine testing to estimate blood glucose. You and your health care provider will consider two main things when deciding whether to use urine testing:

1. Can you really achieve **good** blood glucose control using urine testing?
2. Are you capable of performing the blood glucose testing procedure?

Why Is It Better to Test Blood Glucose Rather than Urine Glucose?

Blood

Very accurate if performed correctly.

Results show current level of glucose in blood.

Results show whether symptoms are due to low blood glucose and tell if extra food should be eaten.

Records of tests are very helpful in working to improve blood glucose control.

Can be performed quickly without need for privacy.

Can be used to plan food intake before, during, and after exercise.

Urine

Inaccurate; results depend on person's renal threshold.

Results do not show current level of blood glucose, but rather an average result since previous urination.

No help in avoiding reactions or deciding if reaction is occurring.

Records are helpful, but even if they are negative the person may have dangerously high or low blood glucose levels.

Person must find bathroom and be able to urinate in order to test.

Not useful for planning exercise or adjusting food intake.

Testing Urine for Ketones

Whether or not you decide to use urine testing or blood glucose monitoring, there is another test that you must know how to perform. This test involves checking the urine for ketones, which are formed in large quantities when the body uses too much fat for energy. When the body uses glucose as its main energy source, the glucose is completely burned up by the cells. But when there is not enough insulin or the insulin is not effective in moving glucose into the cells, the body switches over to burning an excessive amount of fat.

The ketones that are left behind when the body burns fat can make the body very sick if they accumulate in the blood. The kidneys try to remove the ketones just as they remove extra glucose from the blood. But if the body must burn large amounts of fat for energy, the kidneys cannot remove enough ketones from the blood. The body cells are then bathed in blood that has too high of an acid level because of the ketones. The sickness that is caused by having too many ketones in the blood is called ketoacidosis ("keto" for ketones, and "acid-osis" meaning an abnormal acid condition). Ketoacidosis can be a very serious sickness, causing stomach pain, nausea, vomiting, dehydration, unconsciousness, and even death if it is not treated promptly and correctly. It is explained more completely in Chapter 8.

A positive ketone test means you need to take action to prevent trouble.

It is important that you test your blood or urine glucose often, because either of these tests will tell you if you should check for ketones in your urine. If your urine glucose test shows ½% or higher, you should do a urine test for ketones. And if your blood glucose test is 240 mg/dl or higher, you should check a urine sample for ketones. The procedure for testing urine for ketones is as follows:
1. Pass ketone testing strip through the stream of urine.
2. Time test according to the directions on the package.
3. Compare test strip to package color chart.
4. Record the results.

The urine ketone test will tell you whether you have zero ketones present, a trace of ketones, or a small, moderate, or large amount of ketones. Discuss with your health care provider the steps you are to take if your blood glucose level is high and your ketone test is positive. In general, a positive ketone test is like a flashing red light—a sign that you need to take action to prevent trouble. This may mean phoning your health care provider for advice.

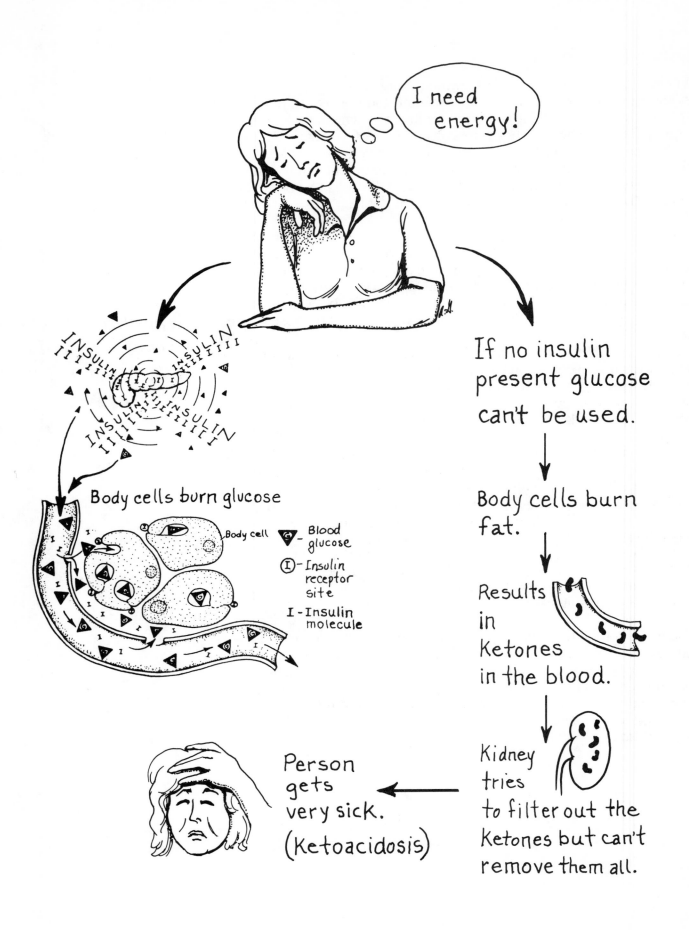

So far we have discussed routine tests that you can do to make sure your diabetes is in good control. There is another very valuable test that your health care provider can do to gain a more complete picture of your diabetes control. This is called a **glycosylated hemoglobin** or **hemoglobin A1C** test. It can be used with your daily testing records to make decisions about possible changes in your diabetes management.

Glycosylated Hemoglobin, or Hemoglobin A1C Test

"Glycosylated hemoglobin" is a phrase that means "glucose attached to the protein hemoglobin which is contained in the red blood cells." "Hemoglobin A1C" is the specific type of protein that is often measured to find out how much glucose has become attached over a period of six to eight weeks. By doing a very sophisticated laboratory analysis of a sample of your blood, your health care provider can obtain a value that will indicate how well your diabetes has been controlled over the past couple of months. See Chapter 8 for more information on how results of this test can be used to improve diabetes control.

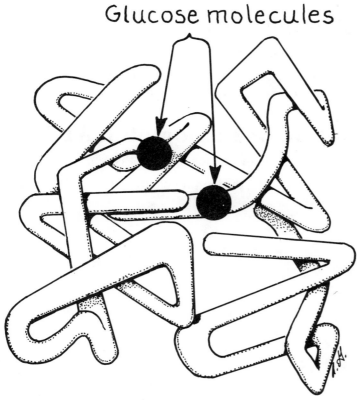

Glucose molecules

Glycosylated Hemoglobin

Summary of Tests

Blood Glucose Monitoring

Tests level of glucose (sugar) present in blood at time of test.

Single drop of blood is placed or smeared on test strip, then color change is read by visually comparing to a color chart or by placing strip in a meter.

Normal blood glucose range is 60-160 mg/dl.

Goals for people with diabetes:

Before meals — 80-120 mg/dl.
One hour after meals — under 200 mg/dl.

Urine Testing for Glucose

Tests amount of glucose filtered into urine by kidneys — indirect estimate of whether blood glucose has been high during time urine was being formed.

Very few people can achieve good diabetes control using urine testing.

Urine Testing for Ketones

Very important test to detect the development of ketoacidosis.

Should be performed when blood glucose is 240 mg/dl or higher or urine glucose is 1/2% or higher. Also test for ketones whenever feeling ill.

Glycosylated Hemoglobin, or Hemoglobin A1C

Laboratory test of average blood glucose level over previous two months.

Should be done every three months, or more often during pregnancy or if blood glucose control has been poor.

Summary

The information presented in this chapter covers the various types of tests that can be done to monitor diabetes control. These tests range from the routine blood glucose and urine ketone tests that show current control to the glycosylated hemoglobin test to evaluate control over one to two months.

It is important that you learn about these tests so that you can work with your health care provider to make decisions that will allow you to control your diabetes. This will not only help you stay healthy from day to day, it can make a big difference in whether or not you have a healthy future.

NOTES

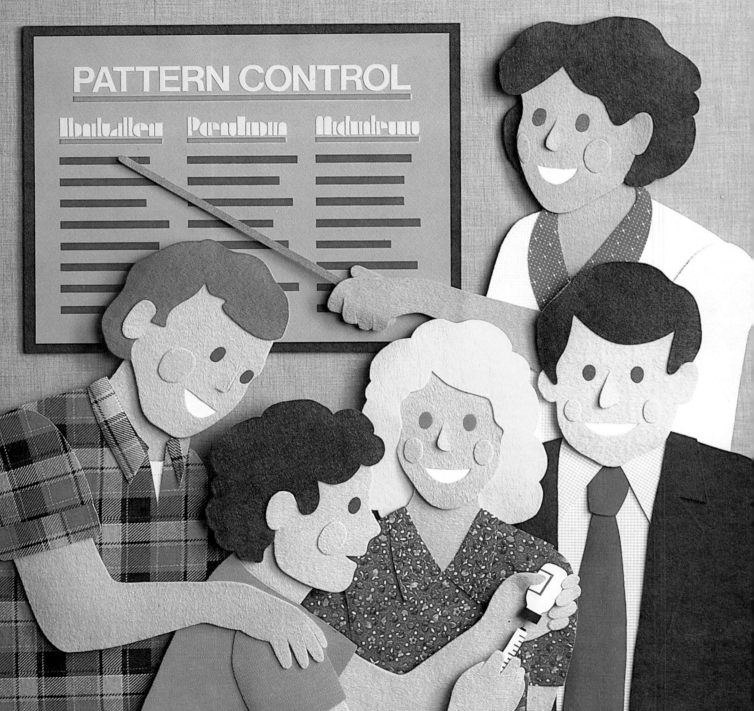

Chapter Five
Diabetes Skills: Learning and Sharpening Your Management Abilities

Lucy Mullen, R.N., B.S.

You are the key to the success of the daily management of your diabetes. Your ability to learn and sharpen skills needed in diabetes management will allow you to improve your diabetes control.

Diabetes skills include: knowledge of your medication, ability to prepare and inject insulin, blood glucose monitoring, urine testing for ketones, and pattern blood glucose control.

Knowledge of Your Medication

Basically what you need to know about your medication is what you are taking, the dosage, and when to take it. If you have non-insulin-dependent (Type II) diabetes and are taking a diabetes pill, you will need a prescription from your doctor to get your medication from the pharmacist. You still must know the name of your medication, your dosage, when to take it, and what the time action of the pill is. Write this information down in several places and keep a copy in your billfold.

If you have insulin-dependent (Type I) diabetes or if your doctor has prescribed insulin to help control your Type II diabetes, there are more facts to know about your medication. You do not need a prescription to purchase insulin (in most states), so you need to know what to ask for. Know the manufacturer of your insulin (Lilly, Squibb-Novo, etc.), the type (Regular, NPH, etc.), and the concentration (U-100 or U-40). Look at the bottle of insulin; the manufacturer is written on the top, the concentration is in the upper left hand corner, the type is written across the middle of the label, and the expiration date is along the side (see illustration). If you can't remember all this, bring your old bottle to your pharmacist, or write the information on a card and keep it in your billfold.

Along with knowing which insulin is prescribed for you, you need to know which syringe to purchase. You need the proper syringe to match your insulin concentration. If you are taking U-100 insulin, you must use U-100 syringes.

Once you know what to buy, you must know how to take care of your supplies. Extra insulin should be stored in the refrigerator. Insulin that is opened and that you are using daily should be kept at room temperature. Keep it out of direct sunlight and away from heat and cold.

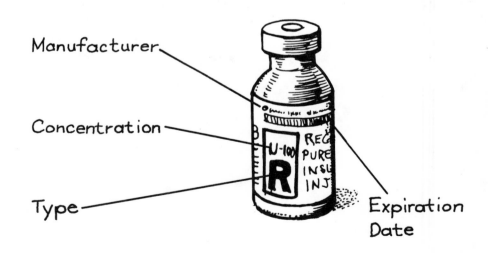

When you have the right insulin and syringe you can get ready to draw up your insulin. Pick up the syringe and practice working it. It consists of a needle, a measuring gauge, and a plunger. The plunger moves back and forth to allow you to measure the correct amount of insulin. You are ready!

If your doctor has prescribed a single type of insulin:

1. Wash your hands.

2. Roll the bottle of insulin between your hands to mix the contents. Do not shake. This will cause air bubbles, which will cause incorrect measurement but are not dangerous if injected.

3. Remove the protective covering from the needle.

4. Pull down on the plunger and measure an amount of air in the syringe equal to your insulin dose.

5. With the bottle in the upright position, inject the needle into the rubber stopper. Push down on the plunger and air will flow into the bottle. This air makes it possible to draw insulin out of the bottle.

6. Now turn the bottle upside down on top of the needle. Make sure the tip of the needle is covered with insulin.

2.

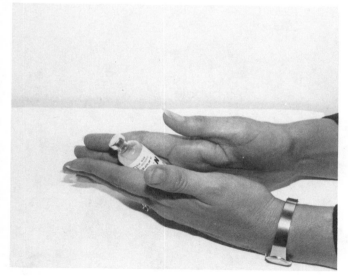

6.

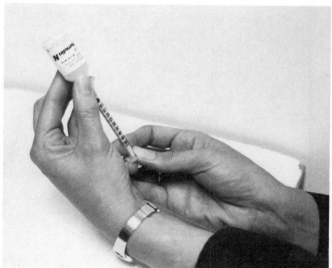

7. Pull down on the plunger, allowing the insulin to enter the syringe.

8. Push the plunger back up. The insulin will return to the bottle.

9. Repeat steps 7 and 8. You are removing air bubbles from the insulin in the syringe to make sure you inject the correct amount.

10. Pull the plunger down to the required amount of insulin. Look to see that there are no air bubbles in the syringe.

11. Remove the syringe from the bottle.

12. Place the syringe on a flat surface without letting the needle touch anything. The needle is sterile and you want to keep it that way.

13. Go to page 89 for instructions on how to inject insulin.

10.

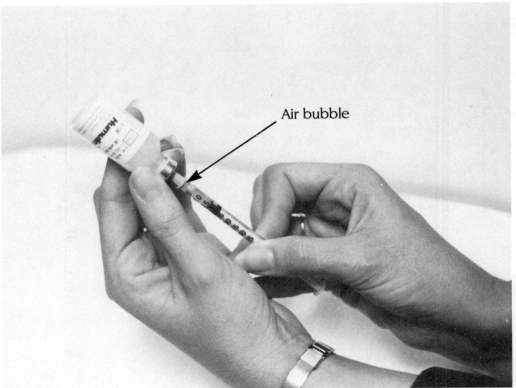

Air bubble

Mixing two types of insulin:

You can mix two types of insulin in one syringe so that you only have to inject once. Make sure you have the correct insulins and know your prescribed dosage for each one. To prevent errors, mark the short-acting insulin by winding a rubberband around it.

1. Wash your hands.

2. Roll the intermediate- or long-acting insulin between the palms of your hands to mix the contents. Do not shake. This will cause air bubbles, which will cause incorrect measurement.

3. Remove the protective covering from the needle.

4. You need to inject air into both bottles of insulin in order to be able to remove the insulin. With the bottle of intermediate- or long-acting insulin in the upright position, draw up the amount of air equal to your dosage of that insulin and inject into the bottle. Remove the syringe.

5. Draw up the amount of air equal to your dosage of short-acting insulin and inject into the upright bottle.

2.

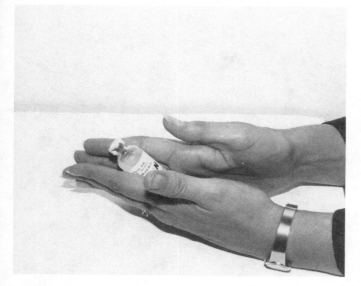

4.

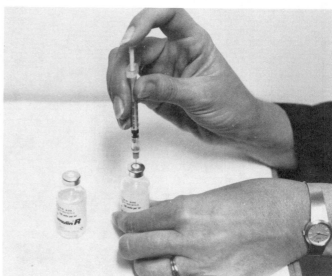

89

6. Turn the bottle of insulin upside down on top of the needle.

7. Pull the plunger halfway down the syringe, allowing insulin to flow into the syringe.

8. Push the plunger upwards and the insulin will flow back into the bottle.

9. Repeat steps 7 and 8 to make sure there are no air bubbles in the insulin in the syringe.

10. Pull the plunger down to the required dose of short-acting insulin. Check to see that there are no air bubbles, then remove the syringe, which now contains your dose of short-acting insulin.

11. Insert the needle of the syringe into the upside down bottle of intermediate- or long-acting insulin. (Remember, air has already been placed inside this bottle.)

12. Pull the plunger down to the required amount of intermediate- or long-acting insulin. Remember to add the units of short-acting insulin to the units of intermediate- or long-acting insulin to arrive at the total number of units for this step.

13. Remove the needle from the bottle and place it on a flat surface where it will not touch anything.

You are now ready to inject the mixed doses of insulin.

10.

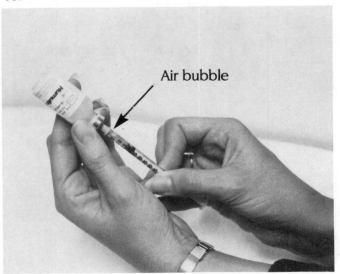

Air bubble

12.

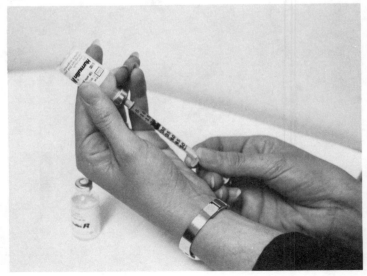

Choosing and Preparing the Injection Site

There are many different areas on the body (sites) that can be used for injecting your insulin (see illustrations below). Any place where there is fatty tissue can be used. You will be injecting the needle into the fatty tissue, which is called subcutaneous tissue or "Sub-Q." There are many sites that can be used, which include the back of the arms, the top and outside area of the thighs, the abdomen except for a 1-inch area around the belly button, and the buttocks. All sites should be used in a planned rotation among sites.

Some individuals develop skin problems if the same small area is used repeatedly for injections. Two problems may develop—the skin at the site may begin to break down (atrophy), causing an unsightly depression in the skin; or the skin at the site may become scarred or swollen (hypertrophy). To avoid these problems, develop a system for keeping track of the sites you use for injecting and rotate them in a planned manner.

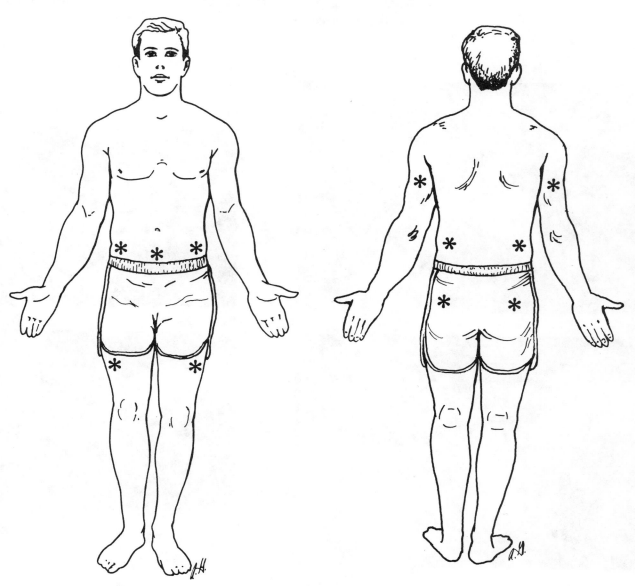

Injecting Insulin

1. The site you have selected should be clean.

2. With one hand, pinch the skin together to keep the tissue from moving.

3. With your other hand, pick up the syringe, holding it like a dart.

4. With a dart-like motion insert the needle into the pinched skin at a 45 to 90 degree angle (see photos). Remember, you want to inject into the subcutaneous fatty tissue. If you have a normal amount of fatty tissue, use a 90 degree angle. For very small children or extremely thin adults a 45 degree angle may be necessary.

5. Once the needle is inserted, push down the plunger to inject the insulin.

6. Withdraw the needle from the skin, covering the injection site with your finger to prevent insulin from leaking out of the tissue.

7. Place the cover back on the needle and discard the syringe.

8. Write down in your record book the amount of insulin injected, the time, and the site used.

2.

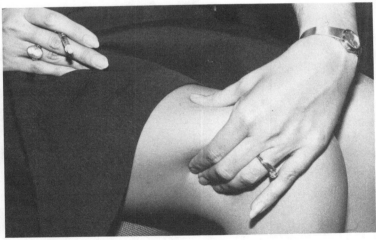

4a.   90 degree angle

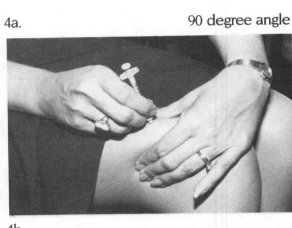

6.

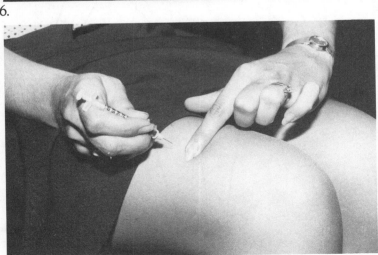

4b.

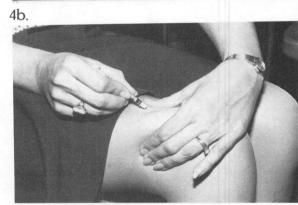

45 degree angle

Monitoring Blood Glucose

There are two ways to test blood glucose levels: by visually comparing a test strip to a color chart, or by inserting a test strip into a blood glucose testing meter. See Chapter 4 for a discussion of how each works and why each is used. When testing visually a drop of blood is placed on a small chemically treated pad on a paper strip. The pad turns color when exposed to glucose. The color pad is then compared to a color chart of blood glucose levels which is on the test strip bottle.

The instrument for measuring blood glucose is called a "reflectance meter." It uses light to "read" the color change on the same test strips which can be read visually. The darker the color of the test pad the less light is reflected, allowing the meter to display a number which is your blood glucose level.

For both methods of testing you will need a blood-letting device. There are many on the market. The devices consist of a lancet and a holder. Puncturing the skin with one of these devices is almost painless if they are set properly. Ask your health care provider to demonstrate several so you can choose the best for your needs.

Blood-letting device

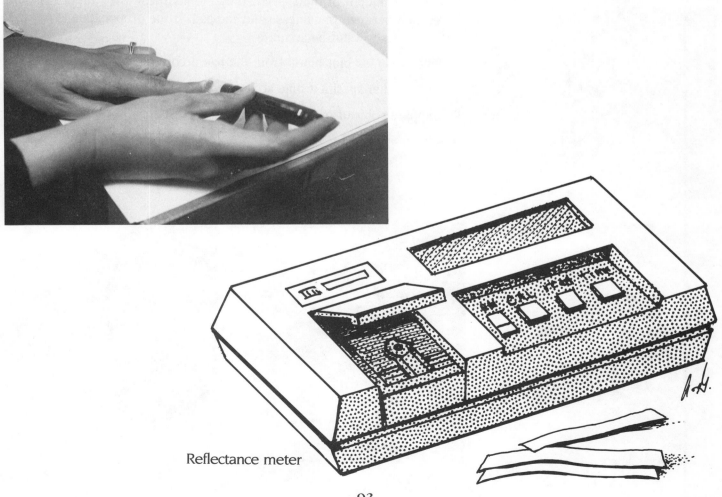

Reflectance meter

93

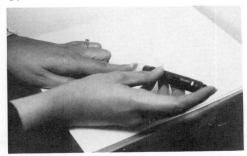

3.

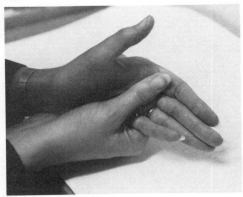

4a.

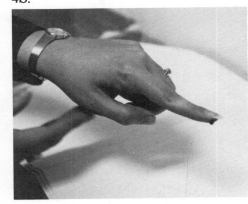

4b.

Visual Testing Method

1. The ear lobes, sides of the fingertips, or toes may be used to obtain a drop of blood. Rotate these sites. (Do not use your toes if your doctor has told you that you have poor circulation or loss of sensitivity in your feet.)

2. Prepare the site by washing with soap and warm water. The warm water will increase the blood flow to the area. Dry the area thoroughly. Any moisture or sugar from food left on the site may make the blood glucose reading inaccurate. It is best not to use alcohol to clean the skin. If not completely dry the alcohol can change the blood glucose reading and cause discomfort.

3. Puncture the skin with the blood-letting device.

4. Gently massage the hand or other area to bring a large drop of blood to the puncture site. When a large drop accumulates allow it to hang from the site.

5. Place the large hanging drop of blood on the test pad. Be sure to cover the entire pad with blood. Follow the product's instructions. With some products the blood must be dropped on the pad and with others it can be smeared.

6. Wait the amount of time specified by the instructions to allow a chemical reaction between the glucose and the pad. If the proper time is not used, the results will not be accurate.

7. Wipe, wash, or blot blood from the pad according to product instructions.

8. Wait another specified time according to instructions.

9. Compare color of pad with color scale on test strip bottle.

10. Write your blood glucose level in your record book.

5.

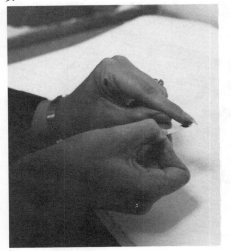

7.

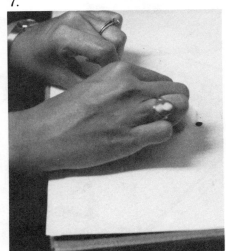

9.

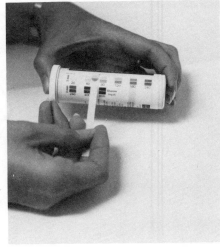

Meter method

1. Choose site.

2. Wash site with warm water and soap, and dry thoroughly.

3. Puncture site.

4. Place drop of blood on pad so that the entire surface is covered.

5. Time chemical reaction according to product directions.

6. Wipe, wash, or blot blood according to directions.

7. Place strip in meter.

8. Wait for number readout to appear on display unit.

9. Record results.

3.

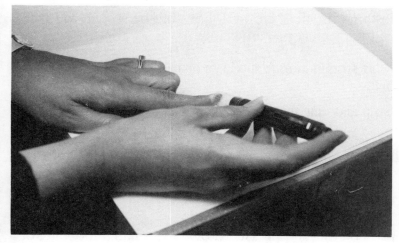

4.

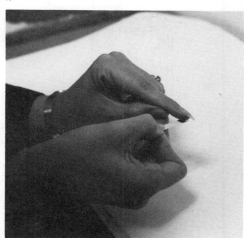

6.

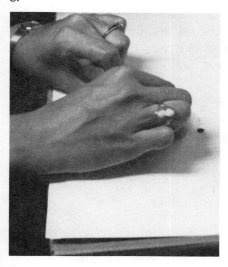

8.

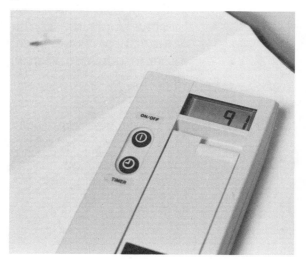

Urine testing

As was discussed in Chapter 4, urine testing is not an accurate method of monitoring blood glucose levels. However, even though blood testing is more accurate, you and your health care provider may decide it is more appropriate for you to test urine. In the past this was a common method, but now with the availability of the much more useful method of blood glucose monitoring, urine glucose testing is seldom recommended.

Urine Ketone Testing

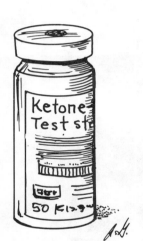

As was explained in Chapter 4, it is important to test for ketones when you are ill or when your blood glucose level is 240 mg/dl or above. The presence of ketones in the urine is an early warning of the possible development of ketoacidosis (see Chapter 8). Ketone test strips come in individual foil wrappers or in bottles. Once a bottle of test strips has been opened, it will expire in four months. General intructions for testing urine for ketones follow, but be sure to follow the directions on the product you are using:

1. Dip a ketone test strip in a urine specimen or pass the strip through a stream of urine.

2. Remove the strip and time the reaction according to the directions on the product.

3. The pad will change colors if ketones are present. Compare the test strip to the color chart on the package.

4. Record the result.

If ketones are present, they are measured by trace, small, moderate, or large. Discuss with your health care provider the steps you are to follow if your blood glucose level is elevated and your ketone test is positive. A positive ketone test is like a flashing red light signaling that your diabetes is getting out of control. You may need to give yourself more insulin, or you may need to call your health care provider for advice.

Pattern Diabetes Control

It is important to record and use your blood glucose testing results to make sure you are in control of your diabetes. At first you will just want to use your test results and notes of any changes in food intake or exercise to discuss your diabetes control with your health care provider. But as you learn more about how to manage your diabetes you will probably want to be able to make minor changes without having to visit or call your health care provider.

Pattern control is a successful method used by many people to make changes to maintain the best possible blood glucose control. This skill takes time and practice to learn and requires working closely with your health care provider. It involves using blood glucose testing results over several days to decide if adjustments are needed in food or insulin. Pattern control is not something that can be learned just by reading about it. This skill must be practiced and your decisions checked with your health care provider at first.

You should be familiar with the time actions of the insulin or insulins you are taking. You can use this information together with your blood glucose testing results and food and exercise records to decide which insulin dose could be increased or decreased slightly to control blood glucose at a specific time of day. Your routine may change during vacations or on holidays or weekends, so it is important to be aware of any changes before you change your insulin dosage.·

Pattern control must be practiced and your decisions checked with your health care provider at first.

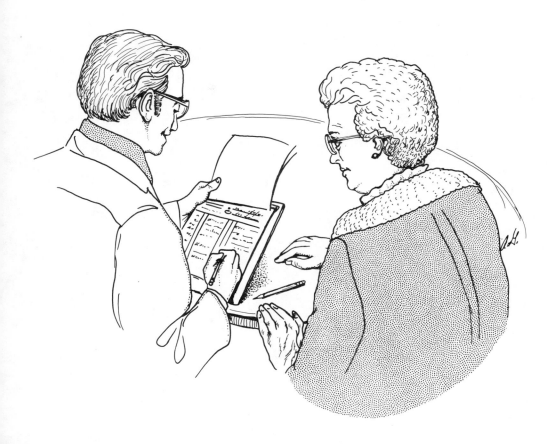

Summary

Knowing what to do to manage your diabetes is very important. But it is equally important to perform tasks correctly. Work with your health care team to build your skills and review them regularly. Not only will they become easier to perform, but your diabetes control will be improved as your skills improve.

NOTES

EMOTIONAL Adjustment

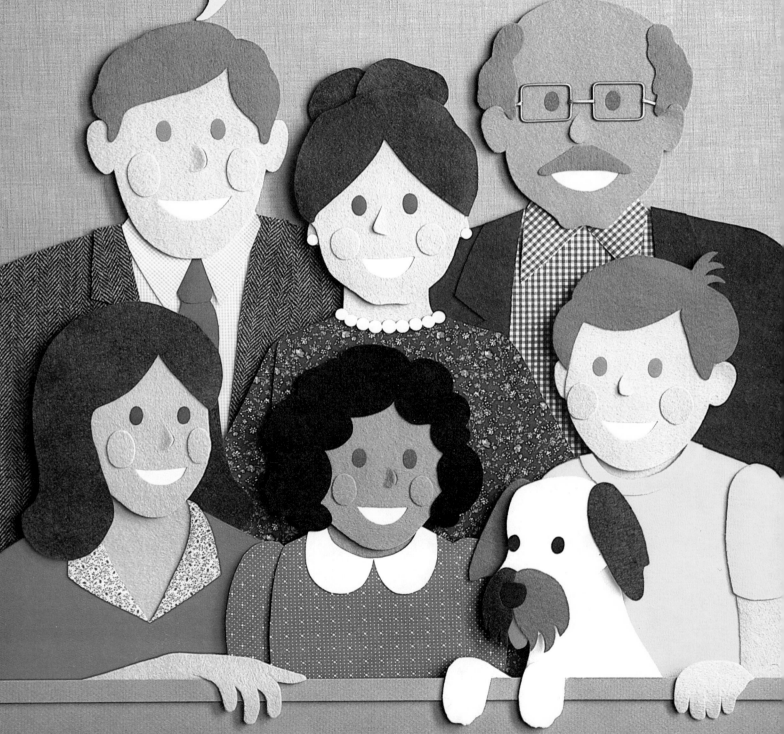

Chapter 6
Emotional Adjustment to Diabetes

Randi Birk, M.A., Licensed Psychologist

When the doctor says that you or your child, spouse, parent, or close friend has diabetes, your world is suddenly changed to include new and very special concerns, considerations, and challenges. It's difficult to make lifestyle changes but it is often harder to adjust emotionally to those changes. Sometimes emotions can get out of control just as diabetes can get out of control—and often the two go together. This chapter will discuss some common feelings about diabetes and suggest ways of making these feelings part of a healthy process of adjustment to living with diabetes. The result will be a happy and productive lifestyle for your whole family.

If you have only recently learned that you or someone close to you has diabetes, you may be feeling somewhat overwhelmed and frightened—perhaps numb! You may have hoped this was a bad dream from which you would awaken. As the reality sinks in, you will probably experience a variety of emotions that range from anger, "Why me?" or "Why my child?" to relief, "Thank goodness diabetes is controllable!".

As you and your family struggle to cope with diabetes, you enter the adjustment process. Many emotions will surface, often repeatedly. Identifying and then accepting these emotions helps adjustment to occur. This chapter will explore some of the feelings you may experience throughout the adjustment process.

What does it mean to 'adjust emotionally?'

When we think of adjustment many words come to mind. Webster's dictionary uses words such as settle, resolve, and adapt. Others have suggested change, acceptance, and coping in describing adjustment. There is no one correct definition. However, in looking at "adjustment to diabetes," the ultimate goal is to "live well with diabetes."

Ideally, a balance is achieved between living fully and managing diabetes.

We can identify two aspects of living well with diabetes—"living well" and "diabetes." Both parts are extremely important and clearly affect one another. Ideally a balance is achieved between living an active, full, productive life and managing one's diabetes. However, at times that balance may be tipped to one side or the other. For example, a person might resist making the necessary changes in his or her previous lifestyle that would allow for good diabetes management. While he or she may temporarily be living fully, diabetes management suffers. Or on the other hand, one may be so concerned about diabetes that unnecessary limits are placed on active living. In neither of these situations is the person really living well with diabetes. Eventually this will affect both diabetes management and the rest of the person's life.

How you adjust emotionally will help determine how well you balance diabetes management and living fully. In some ways adjustment, like insulin, can be viewed as a "key." For just as insulin is the key that allows the cells in our bodies to use food for energy, emotional adjustment is the key that helps you use medical technology and information about diabetes to live fully while managing diabetes. Because adjustment is so important, we will discuss the process of adjusting to diabetes and the feelings that may be involved. And remember, the whole family and other loved ones will experience this process of adjustment and the emotions described—not just the person with diabetes.

Denial (Disbelief)

"This isn't really happening."
"I don't have to change, diabetes isn't forever."
"It's not that serious."
"I don't have to feel anything about my diabetes."

One of the first feelings many people experience is disbelief. "This can't be happening to me!" When you suddenly learn that you have diabetes, you may have frightening and confusing thoughts and feelings. Particularly at first, there are many unknowns about diabetes and the future. Until you experienced it personally, you probably had very little accurate information about diabetes. This lack of knowledge can affect your feelings about the disease.

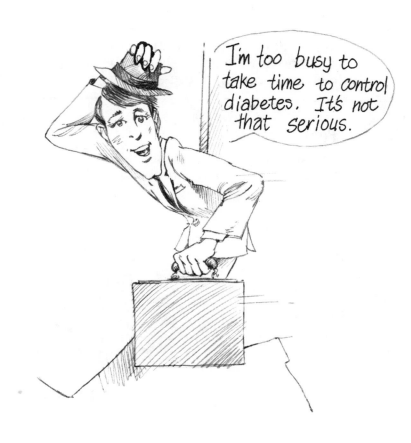

It is natural to avoid or deny the unpleasant and scary feelings and to deny the reality of having diabetes. This denial or disbelief can be healthy and protective at first. It insulates you from all the scary, confusing feelings that would be overwhelming if you let them in all at once. It "buys time" for you to get used to your situation and the required changes, as you are ready and able to deal with them.

We all use denial in everyday living. It is the belief that the accidents, natural disasters, assaults, etc., that we read or hear about daily won't happen to us that allows us to go about the business of living fully without constant worry. This is healthy and useful. However, sometimes denial becomes unhealthy and affects how we take care of ourselves. For example, when we smoke or drink too much, or overeat, or don't wear seatbelts and feel that *we* won't get lung cancer, liver disease, heart problems, or have an accident, we take extra risks based on a belief that we are somehow specially protected. Similarly, if you persist in denying your diabetes, or feel that changes are not necessary for good diabetes management, then you won't care for yourself properly. You then suffer the consequences of feeling ill, lacking energy, and risking future health.

Sometimes the loved ones of a person with diabetes deny the diabetes or feelings about it because they too have fears that can be overwhelming. If this continues, the person with diabetes can get the message that his or her diabetes is not real or serious and that proper management is not necessary.

Fear

"What will this mean for my life?"
"What's going to happen?"

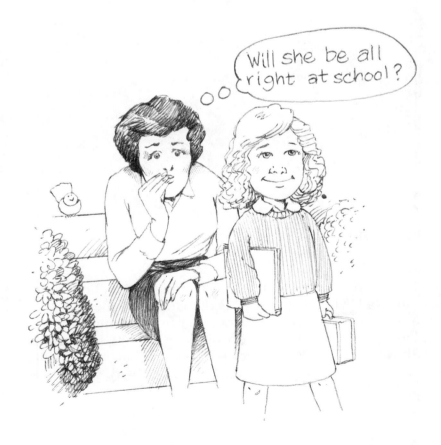

As denial grows weaker, the reality of a situation becomes increasingly clear. You or your loved one has diabetes, and you are going to need to make some changes. But what does it all mean? Will you/they still be able to live a full life? Although you probably now have a few more facts about diabetes than before it was diagnosed, it's all still quite new. It is difficult to put aside the false and negative stories you may have heard or read, or perhaps even past experiences with a family member whose diabetes was poorly controlled.

Diabetes is serious. It does require change, and that's scary. It is common to feel a loss of control over your body during the time right after diagnosis. Your body, which you trusted without question, has betrayed you by failing to function as it should. Being in the hospital at this time can add to the fear. And you don't yet have the information you need to regain control of your body and your life. You might feel anything from mild nervousness to downright terror, and the intensity of your fear may change from time to time.

But just as denial was useful at first, fear also has a purpose. It is fear, along with the discomfort of being out of control, which can motivate you to seek the answers you need to live well with diabetes. Limited and appropriate fear, which is really just respect for consequences or danger, motivates us to proceed carefully in life. However, too much fear over a long period of time can also lead to a feeling of hopelessness. And when you have no hope, you have no reason to care for yourself, feeling "it doesn't matter anyway."

When family members or others feel overly fearful about their loved one's diabetes, they sometimes react by becoming overly protective. They may unnecessarily restrict activities or situations in which he or she could safely be involved. They may also become overly demanding that the person be very strict about following his or her diabetes management plan. Over time, this can cause the person to actually accept less responsibility for his or her management. It can also lead to rebellion against those rigid demands and the loved one who is making them.

Anger

"Why me?"/"Why my child?"
"Why do I have to do all this stuff?"
"It isn't fair!"

Everyone who has diabetes or loves someone who has diabetes feels anger at one time or another. It is natural to feel angry when changes happen in our lives that are unwanted, unexpected, undeserved and beyond our control. Diabetes is all those things. It demands that you make changes in your life and requires extra attention and energy for day to day management.

It is healthy and normal to feel angry once in a while. In daily living our anger often gives us the energy we need to deal with or remove ourselves from an unpleasant situation. Since you can't remove yourself from the condition of having diabetes, your anger will affect how you deal with it. It can help you gain energy to meet the challenge of your diabetes management. It is very important to recognize your anger and accept that it is all right to be angry for a while.

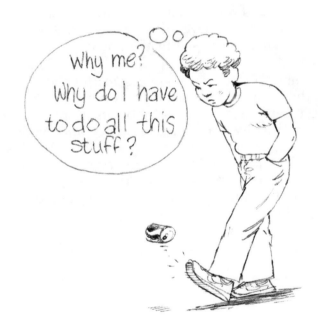

How much anger is felt, how long it is felt, and how anger is directed varies from person to person and within a person from time to time. As with the other emotions we have discussed, anger can become unhealthy if it is felt too strongly, for too long a period, or is directed in a harmful manner. For example, sometimes anger at diabetes is misdirected at family members, causing them to be treated unkindly. Sometimes a person's anger with diabetes continues for so long or is so strong that it interferes with daily management, causing personal harm.

Loved ones also feel anger as a normal part of their adjustment process. But again, when it is felt too strongly, or for too long, or directed at the person with diabetes instead of at the diabetes, it can hurt that person's ability to live well with diabetes.

Guilt

"What did I do to deserve this?"
"If I just hadn't eaten so much sugar..."
"The diabetes must have come from my side of the family."

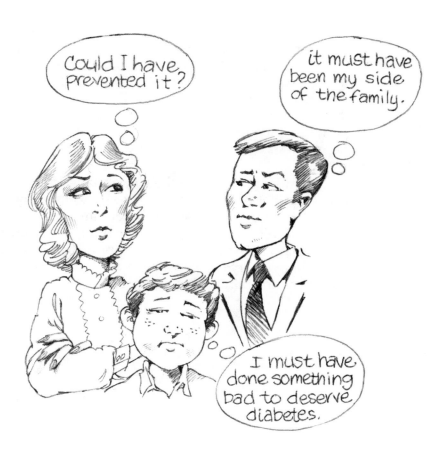

Guilt is an emotion we feel when we think we are responsible for something bad happening. You may have this feeling because of a misunderstanding of diabetes. For example, if someone mistakenly thinks that diabetes is caused by eating too much sugar or is inherited from just one parent, that person might feel guilty if he or she had always had a sweet tooth and then developed diabetes, or if his or her parent had diabetes and now his or her child does. If you believe that people "get what they deserve," you might wonder what wrong you have done to deserve diabetes.

Some guilt is healthy and useful. We all need to have a conscience in order to live responsibly in society. Feelings of guilt can serve as a sign that we have slipped in the goals we set for ourselves, such as to follow a meal plan, to quit smoking, or to test blood glucose (sugar) regularly. The intensity of our guilt and how we respond to it is important. If you feel somewhat guilty about "cheating" on your diet, and you accept that you're human and made a mistake and will try to do better, your guilt has proved to be healthy and appropriate. However, if you feel too guilty, you may give yourself messages that you are "bad" or "a failure." These messages are likely to make you miserable and depressed, with little concern for correcting the mistake and improving your diet or working toward other goals.

Parents feel responsible for their children's wellbeing and may therefore feel guilty that they couldn't prevent the child's diabetes or that they can't get him or her to maintain better control. Guilt such as in the examples above is based on ideas that are untrue or unclear, and therefore the guilt is not realistic or helpful. Since the reasons for these feelings of guilt may be beyond our control or are in the distant past, the guilt accomplishes nothing but frustration, self-criticism, and depression.

When family members feel guilty about a loved one's diabetes, they may treat that person differently to try to make up for his or her diabetes. Parents, spouses, or other family members sometimes feel guilty and react by becoming overindulgent. They may set few limits, lower expectations for positive, appropriate, responsible behavior, and otherwise try to make up for the loved one's misfortune. This can have very unhealthy consequences.

Depression

"I feel so sad."
"I just don't feel like doing anything."
"I feel so alone, no one understands."

After you have tried a number of ways to cope with diabetes—you've tried avoiding or denying it, you've been afraid and have sought information, you've been angry—and you realize diabetes will not go away, you may feel depressed, sad, defeated, or resigned.

Depression is a normal response to being unable to change a situation we don't like. Diabetes and the changes that it requires are forever, and you can't make them go away. It is understandable and healthy for you to feel depressed for a while. In fact, recognizing and accepting your sad feelings are important to your adjustment to diabetes. During the time you are sad, you often make the necessary change in your self-image to include diabetes. This is a very important part of adjustment. It helps you focus on your new limits and the changes you must make. You learn to accept your new life, like many others before you.

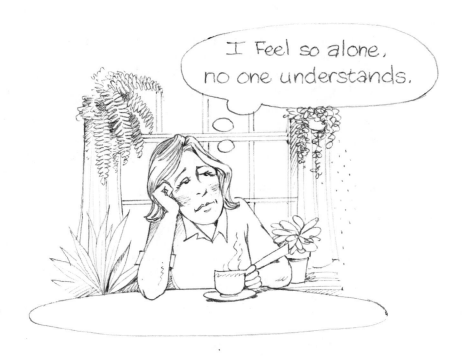

Everyone has had to accept some limitations in life and at times has felt sad or depressed because of them. For example, a person may have wanted to be athletic, artistic, tall, beautiful, or rich. If it doesn't turn out that way, that person may at times feel sad. However, by accepting his or her limits, that person is able to move on and make realistic choices about life, making the most of his or her strengths.

Of course, depression can become unhealthy if it lasts for a long time or is very severe. People who are severely depressed often lack energy, have little appetite, and experience changes in their sleeping patterns. They may feel isolated, and this may cause them to further avoid others, which adds to their feeling of isolation. In addition, people who are very depressed usually feel hopeless. Therefore, they may not take care of themselves, since it does not appear to them to matter what they do.

When family members feel depressed about their loved one's diabetes for a long period of time, they can convey a message of hopelessness, which can affect how the person cares for himself or herself.

Here are some clues to help you identify what you may be feeling:

- Do you feel that you can avoid your diabetes treatment plan without consequences?
- Do you hope that if you ignore your diabetes it will somehow go away?
- Do you feel that you are no different now than you were before you developed diabetes, and that *you don't need to change?*
   If so, you may be feeling disbelief, denying that you truly have diabetes, that it is permanent, that it is serious, or that it's going to take time to adjust to.

- Are you absolutely rigid about your meal plan and injection times?
- Do you feel that diabetes has so many possible complications that your situation is hopeless?
- Do you resist allowing your child with diabetes to sleep overnight at a friend's house or go to camp?
   If so, you may be feeling fear.

- Do you feel life is terribly unfair?
- Do you find yourself irritable with family members, friends, or health care team members for no apparent reason?
- Do you refuse to follow the recommendations of your medical team?
   Perhaps you are angry.

- Do you want to do things for your child to somehow make up for his or her diabetes?
- Do you expect less of your family member with diabetes because he or she already has enough to deal with?
- Do you feel like a failure when even one blood glucose test is high?
   Then you may be experiencing guilt.

110

- Do you feel sad and tired all the time?
- Do you avoid other people because no one seems to understand you anymore?
- Have you stopped enjoying activities you used to think were fun?
    If so, you may be depressed.

Dealing with Emotions and Feelings

Denial, fear, anger, guilt, depression—these are just some of the feelings you may have about diabetes. They are not unique to individuals or families with diabetes. Everyone feels these emotions from time to time. These emotions are in themselves neither good nor bad, healthy nor harmful. Each one can be helpful and useful to you as you strive to live well with diabetes, but each also can become unhealthy and interfere with your life. Understanding how that might happen can help you avoid or recognize problems if they develop.

What determines if an emotion is healthy or unhealthy?

An emotion becomes unhealthy when it upsets the balance you are striving for—that is, living well with diabetes. For example, people who for a long time deny they have diabetes, or that it is serious, or that it is forever, will manage their diabetes poorly. An equally unhealthy imbalance will result if a person is extremely fearful and unnecessarily restricts his or her activities.

Two factors largely determine whether an emotion will interfere in your life: its intensity, or how strongly you feel it; and its duration, or how long you feel it. Feeling is not an all or nothing process. For example, you do not feel guilty either about everything or about nothing, but rather experience guilt within a range between those extremes. And you will likely feel different amounts of an emotion at different times. You might feel very depressed at one point, mildly sad at another, and not at all depressed on a third occasion. When you do experience an emotion to an extreme degree, for example intense fear, your ability to maintain the balance of living fully and managing diabetes is reduced.

How long you experience an emotion is also important. It is very normal and healthy for people to be angry when they learn that they or a loved one has diabetes. However, if they continue to feel anger about the disease several years later, this is clearly unhealthy because it will interfere with the long-term management of diabetes.

Is there a time limit on how long an individual can feel an emotion before it becomes unhealthy, or an amount beyond which an emotion is too strong? No. Just as there isn't one right insulin dosage or caloric intake for everyone, there isn't one right length of time or intensity to feel emotions. Each person will respond differently, and it is important to recognize and accept those differences. However, as with food and insulin, extremes may be a problem.

How can you recognize when your emotions have become a problem?

If you are aware of the balance you want to maintain, then you can be aware when that balance is tipped. If your diabetes is out of control or if there is a problem area within the rest of your life—conflict within your family, difficulties in school or at work, problems with friends, or limitations in your activities—it is time to ask yourself some questions.

If you are aware of the balance you wish to maintain in life, you will be aware when that balance is tipped.

Why are you experiencing this difficulty? If your diabetes is out of control, have you experienced a change in medication, food or activities that is temporarily affecting your blood glucose, or is this a long-term problem? Problems in the rest of your life will not always be related to your diabetes. For example, you may simply be having difficulty with a school subject or dislike your new boss. However, there are also times when your feelings about diabetes will affect how you interact with family members, friends, and employers, and which activities you choose to participate in or limit.

What can you do once you determine that some of your feelings have become an obstacle to living well with diabetes? Identifying that there is a problem is a healthy, positive first step. Next you must try to identify what you are feeling.

Often when you know **what** you are feeling, you can change **how** you express this feeling. For example, once you realize you are really angry at your diabetes and not at your spouse, you can work toward expressing anger in a way that won't hurt you or others. You might release this anger through sports or exercise, or talk it out with family members, friends, or clergy. If you recognize that it is fear that stops you from letting your child become independent, or guilt that keeps you from setting limits for him or her, you might be able to take a deep breath and let go—a little at a time—or feel better about setting some realistic expectations.

These changes may not be easy and they won't happen overnight. You **can** change what you feel and how you express your emotions. Sometimes you might need help. It is often more difficult to struggle with feelings alone. Support from others can be critical. You need to accept and actively seek emotional support from family, friends, and your health care team. Some people find it very rewarding to join a support group made up of others experiencing similar feelings or challenges. Contact your local diabetes chapter or the International Diabetes Center for information about support groups in your area.

Support from others can be critical in coping with emotions.

If you have identified a problem related to your feelings about diabetes and have struggled with this problem alone or talked with family and friends and have realized that it is something with which you need help, it is time to seek professional help. Counselors, social workers, and psychologists are skilled professionals who can help you identify your feelings and work toward a more healthy expression of those feelings. This could be a key to successfully coping with diabetes in oneself or one's family. The earlier this action is taken, the easier it will likely be to work out a solution.

Acceptance

"I don't always like watching how much food I eat, but I understand how important that is to me."

"I have diabetes, so I guess I am going to have to make some changes."

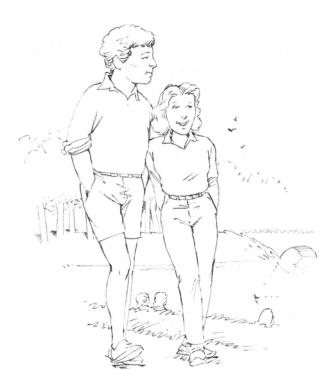

Hopefully—sometimes sooner, sometimes later—you will come to the point that you "accept" your diabetes. That doesn't mean you like having diabetes, want it, or feel happy that you or a family member has it. It only means that you fully admit to yourself and others that you or a loved one has diabetes. You admit that it is part of you or them. At that point, you are able to choose to make the necessary changes that good diabetes management requires. But at the same time you avoid setting unnecessary limits or restrictions. You have achieved that balance described earlier and are "living well with diabetes." It is desirable for everyone to be able to accept the limitations or challenges he or she is given in life. With this acceptance, you can then focus not on your limitations but rather on your strengths.

Does everyone experience the same process of adjustment in order to reach acceptance?

While most people experience many of the feelings we have described, each person is unique, and his or her emotional responses will also be unique. The adjustment process is not a neat, orderly, predictable process that everyone moves through in the same way. We do not proceed from one feeling to another and then magically arrive at acceptance and live happily ever after.

Is acceptance forever?

Not exactly. Just as a smooth pond will occasionally and temporarily experience rippling, there will be occasional "ripples" in your acceptance. There will be times, perhaps, when the long-term "forever" aspect of diabetes temporarily becomes too much. Or when an important decision or life event causes you to be faced again with some of the old fears or anger or sadness about your diabetes. It is not unusual to every once in a while return to some of the feelings you experienced during your initial adjustment. Sometimes you might repeat the whole process, again returning to acceptance.

Other feelings often come with acceptance. Feelings such as pride. You can feel proud of yourself—proud that you are coping well, taking excellent care of yourself, and meeting your challenges. You feel in control of your diabetes and your life. You are the driver rather than the helpless bystander. You can feel hope, not necessarily that a cure for diabetes will be found tomorrow, but that the growing knowledge and understanding of the disease will help you live fully and well with diabetes.

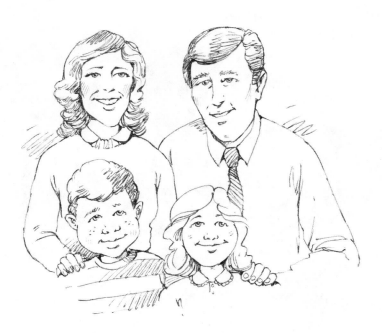

Motivation

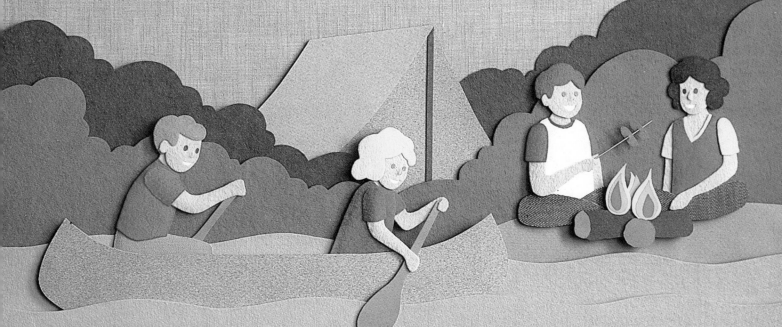

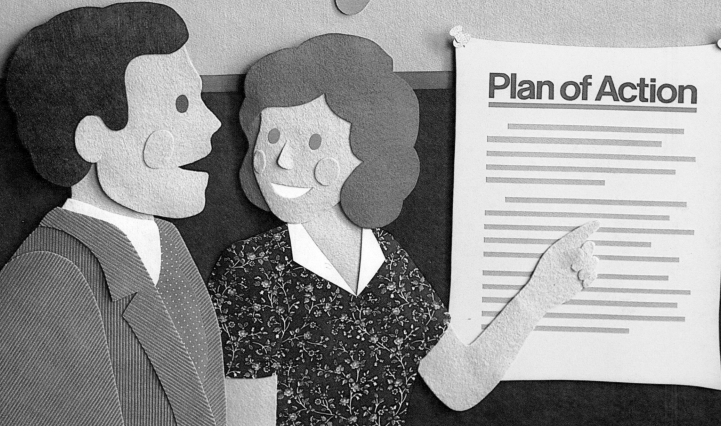

Plan of Action

Chapter 7
Motivating Yourself to Control Diabetes

Catherine Feste*

Knowing what to do and doing it are two very different issues. Some people know they shouldn't smoke—yet they do smoke. Some people with diabetes know how to eat and exercise to have good control of their blood glucose—yet they don't follow their meal or exercise plan. Why? One way to describe this failure to act is the lack of **motivation**.

Motivation is the action component of education. Knowledge alone is simply stored information. Knowledge plus action equal an educated person—a motivated person.

That seems like an easy equation. We all know, however, that taking action is not easy. The path of least resistance is always easier. We all differ in how easy or difficult we find it to take action. Experience has told us that some people get diabetes, learn what they need to know, then simply make the appropriate lifestyle changes and carry on with their lives. Other people never seem to accept diabetes. Although they learn what behaviors they should follow, they resist making lifestyle changes. How would you describe your ability to take action to control diabetes?

Along with a good general understanding of what diabetes is and how it should be managed, you need specific individualized recommendations from a knowledgeable medical team. This manual and your medical team can only make recommendations. You make the final choices. Will you be a storehouse of information or will you choose to be an educated, motivated person?

If you choose to use your information to take action, you will need support to keep your efforts going. This chapter is designed to show you sources of support to help you be a motivated, healthy person. We will start by discussing the concepts of choice, goal setting, rewards, stress management, and belief.

$$\frac{\text{Knowledge} + \text{Action}}{\text{Motivation}}$$

*Ms. Feste is a motivation specialist. She has had diabetes since she was ten years old.

Choice

You are the most important decision-maker in your diabetes management. You listen to and read important information and then decide what you will do. Instead of viewing your decision making as a burden, view it as an indication that you are in control. When some people rebel against having diabetes they seem to be saying, "I don't want to be controlled by anyone or anything outside of me. I don't want to be told what to do." This is precisely why people with diabetes need to take charge of the decision-making so that they are in control. We believe in this advice: You control your diabetes. Don't be controlled by it. Here is an illustration:

Sue is 18 years old and has diabetes. She was invited by a friend to go boating. They planned to be gone all day. Although Sue and her friend packed a lunch, Sue did not pack extra food for snacks or in case her blood glucose got low. Sue thought, "I want to be normal. I'm not going to 'give in' to diabetes by bringing along a lot of extra food and juice!"

By 3 p.m. the increased activity was causing Sue to be hypoglycemic. Since she had no carbohydrate along to bring her blood glucose up to normal, she had to ask her friend to take her to a store on the other end of the lake. At the store Sue bought some juice to help her. However, because she had neglected to bring food with her, she had suffered an uncomfortable insulin reaction. She had also caused her friends to interrupt their fun to hurry and get help for her. Sue felt embarrassed and angry. She felt, as she often does, that diabetes controls her life.

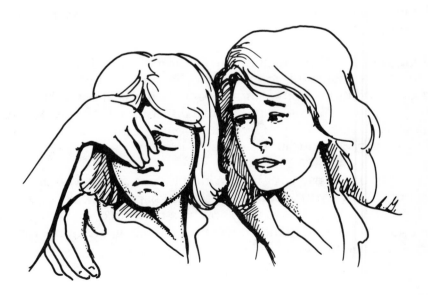

Debbie feels differently. Debbie is 12 years old and has diabetes. One day she and another friend planned to go shopping all day. As Debbie got ready to leave her home she thought, "Since we'll be in shopping centers, food will always be available. I won't really need to bring food with me because I can buy my lunch and snacks." As Debbie thought further she reasoned, "It's better to be safe than sorry. I'll just stick some raisins in my purse."

About mid-afternoon, Debbie and her friend decided to take the bus to another shopping center. As she rode on the bus, Debbie began to feel lightheaded and sweaty. She was starting to have an insulin reaction! Confidently, she reached into her purse and pulled out her raisins. Within minutes she felt fine again. When the bus arrived at the shopping center Debbie and her friend stopped for a snack. Then they continued to enjoy a fun day of shopping and chatting. Debbie does not allow diabetes to control her life because she controls her diabetes.

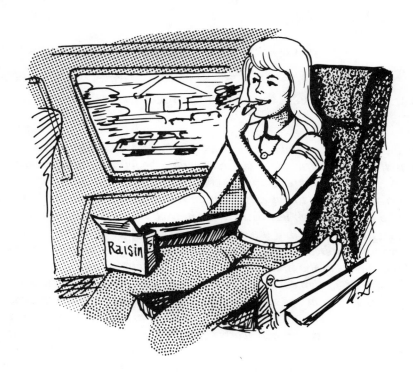

Percentage of Time YOU are in Control of Diabetes

If you decide that you want to be in control, then begin by taking responsibility for the choices you make. The line below indicates the degree to which one's diabetes is managed, from poor management to excellent management. Where do you want your diabetes management to be?

_0%_   _?_   _100%_

To decide this, consider the following:
1. Build in leeway for those times when you may choose less than excellent management (occasional over-eating, not enough exercise, or sleeping an extra hour on Saturdays, etc.).
2. Consider consequences of your actions. If you say you are satisfied with having your diabetes well managed 50 percent of the time, what are the possible consequences of such management (or lack of management)?
3. Set goals to help you achieve diabetes management at the level you have chosen.

To illustrate how you take this decision process to action, consider the following example:

Bill has decided that he would like to have his diabetes under good control. To help himself make specific goals, he first decides the level of management he wants. His business breakfasts and lunches sometimes result in less than perfect meals. Also, Bill chooses to eat extra food in restaurants from time to time. He feels that he wants enough leeway to allow himself freedom at these times. However, he also believes that the consequences of poorly controlled diabetes lead to serious complications, so he chooses to have well managed diabetes about three-fourths of the time, or a level of 75 percent.

Next he applies 75 percent to all the behaviors which his health team have recommended. His team has recommended that he test his blood four times per day. Seventy-five percent of four is three, so he sets his testing goal at three times every day and occasionally working in the fourth test. As Bill looks at his calendar, he figures that 75 percent of a 30-day month is 22 days. This means that on 22 days he will follow his meal plan precisely, but eight days per month he will allow a business breakfast or social dinner to interrupt his meal plan. Bill does the same for his exercise prescription and for taking his insulin. In setting a goal for taking insulin it is not an issue of whether or not to take the insulin. The goal-setting issue centers around consistency in timing. Bill takes his insulin 100 percent of the time but with his 75 percent goal he allows himself to sleep in an extra hour every Saturday and sometimes on Sunday.

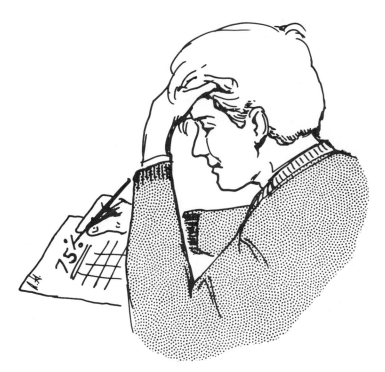

Next Bill must evaluate. *His evaluation covers two basic areas: diabetes management and quality of life. With the help of daily blood testing records and periodic laboratory tests, Bill and his medical advisers can evaluate whether his plan is achieving the desired result of good diabetes management.*

The other issue is quality of life. Bill must answer this for himself. Is the 75 percent level too rigid? Is it disturbing the quality of his life? Bill concludes that for him 75 percent is a good level. He realizes that before he set specific goals he used to say to himself: "I'll just go off my routine once in a while." He discovered that "once in a while" was getting to be every other day! Bill made another important discovery: Good habits are as easy to follow as bad habits. After awhile he found his new behaviors easy to follow because they'd become habits.

Now you decide your level of diabetes management. Take a hard and realistic look at your lifestyle and your commitment to well-managed diabetes. After choosing your level (from 0 to 100 percent) apply it as Bill did in the example. Make a copy of the blank **Plan of Action** on the next page and fill in one or more goals you want to achieve. Fill in the rest as you read this chapter. Once you have completed the plan you will have practiced an important motivational skill: **Goal Setting**.

The remaining skills in motivation are aimed at helping you achieve your goals and maintain your new behaviors.

Plan of Action

My GOALS are: _____

_____

_____

Obstacles which prevent my attaining these goals include: _____

_____

_____

I can overcome my obstacles by modifying my behavior and/or my environment in the following way(s):

_____

_____

_____

_____

To keep me going I can get a real BOOST from the following people, activities, experiences, reading, "things:"

_____   _____

_____   _____

_____   _____

_____   _____

When I successfully resist temptation or modify my behavior or break an old, bad habit, or reach my goal I will reward myself with:

_____

_____

Diabetes danger signals are those signs which indicate that I am sliding off my routine and need to get back on. These signals include weight gain, high sugars, not testing, etc. My signals are: _____

_____

©Copyright 1981. Catherine Feste

Done Well? Reward Yourself!

Rewards are a good tool to include in your motivation tool box. Behavior which is rewarded is likely to be repeated. Remember to **reward behavior, not results**. Results such as weight loss are sometimes slow to occur. People need encouragement along the way. So reward your good behaviors, and the results will come.

Another pitfall in rewarding results occurs when people only reward good test results. Since blood glucose can rise or fall because of factors beyond your control (stress, illness, menstruation) it is unfair to base rewards on blood glucose testing results. People should not be made to feel that their worth as a person is related to test results. This sometimes leads to the falsification of test results, both by children and adults.

Reward behaviors, not results.

Children want and need approval from parents, teachers, and other authority figures in their lives. When they see that normal blood glucose results are rewarded with praise and approval and that high blood glucose results bring disapproval, they quite understandably are tempted to give false results. Adults also want to appear as if they are "following doctor's orders" and may be embarrased to reveal less than ideal test results. Rewards, then, should be given for the testing behavior, which provides results (low, normal, or high; not bad or good) that can be used to monitor and improve diabetes control.

If eating, exercising, and medication behaviors are being well rewarded, then positive test results ought to be a natural outcome.

What kinds of rewards do you give?

Each individual should choose his or her own rewards. Children will no doubt need to negotiate this with their parents. Some people put stars on their calendar each day that they achieve their goal. When they have reached a predetermined number of stars (5, 10, 15) they give themselves a reward (money, time to oneself, tickets to a favorite event, a special outing, etc.).

This system of rewards need not continue forever. It is especially helpful when one is attempting to make a significant change in one's behavior (changing from testing once a week to several times a day, or changing from loosely following a meal plan to following it closely.) Usually, after two to three months of following a desired behavior the person is well on the way to establishing a new habit. Rewards can help you get there.

Stress Management

Are you managing your stress? Or is it managing you? Stress is one of the major obstacles to motivation. The most common methods of coping with stress are eating, drinking, and smoking. These coping methods are harmful to anyone, but they are especially harmful for people with diabetes because they can cause blood glucose levels to rise, thus disturbing diabetes management. Stress alone can cause blood glucose to rise, so it is important for people with diabetes to get stress under control and not to use any coping methods which further threaten diabetes control or overall health.

What are your methods of controlling stress? There are many positive methods, including exercise, laughter, relaxation techniques, meditation, music, writing, or talking about your stress. The methods vary from person to person. One important similarity in successful coping methods is a firm belief by the person that "I can cope. I will make it. I am in control." A famous psychologist, Dr. George Vaillant, said, "Stress does not kill us so much as ingenious adaptation to stress facilitates our survival." Stated plainly: We survive by inventing healthy ways of coping with stress.

What are your "ingenious adaptations," or healthy coping methods?

Let's apply the concept of ingenious adaptation to some advice given by many stress management experts: Stress is not in events, it is in our perception of events. The following illustrations show how the same event can be perceived differently.

Wow! Was that roller coaster ride ever fun! Let's go again!
Versus
That was the scariest experience I've ever had! I'll never do that again!

What a day! I must have been interrupted 20 times by that darned telephone!
Versus
The phone rang off the hook today. Business is really good!

Now that I have diabetes I can no longer enjoy the good things in life.
Versus
Now that I have diabetes I have a special reason to live a really healthy lifestyle and take good care of myself!

I wish insulin had never been discovered! It's really a "bummer" that I have to take shots every day of my life!
Versus
Without insulin I would die. By taking a couple of shots each day I can lead a full and happy life. I'm really thankful insulin was discovered.

The examples could go on and on. The same event can be perceived quite differently. Now, to apply "ingenious adaptation," we must realize that perceptions can change or be adapted. Think of examples in your life when this has been true. Quite commonly perceptions change with age. As an example, let's say that there was a cave in your home town. As a small child you may have viewed it as a scary place and you stayed away from it. As a teenager you may have viewed it as a fascinating place and you spent hours exploring it. And if you are a parent you may again view it as a scary place and you forbid your children to go near it! These changes in perception happen naturally with the maturation process. Now let us explore how we can make changes (adaptation) occur in perceptions.

Parents influence their children's perceptions. One of the most striking examples can be seen in how two 10-year-old children were told that they have diabetes.

A boy was told by his mother and doctor that he had diabetes, which meant that he couldn't be in sports or play with his friends like he used to because he was sick.

A girl (me) was told she had diabetes. Then her mother explained that diabetes would teach her all about good nutrition. Diabetes would cause her to be very healthy and a very strong person. In fact, she told her daughter, diabetes would make the whole family healthier and closer.

The boy grew up feeling that diabetes was a terrible burden. I grew up thinking of diabetes as the major influence on my positive lifestyle. The "ingenious adaptation" for me is a positive attitude.

Parents influence their children's perceptions of diabetes.

Parents influence their children's attitudes. Adults influence their own attitudes. To ingeniously adapt your attitude (perception), practice the following technique. It is practical, easy, and it works!

Positive Self-Talk

(Psychologists call it "cognitive restructuring.")

Give yourself positive messages. Very simply: Coach yourself. Feed yourself positive, "I can do it" sorts of messages. And, if you hear negative, "I'll never make it" sort of messages, adapt them to make them positive. Below are illustrations:

Negative

I'll never be able to learn enough to stay healthy.

Positive

I can live very well with diabetes. Knowledgeable medical professionals, sophisticated new equipment and my own education all will work together toward a positive, healthy future.

Negative

Now that I have diabetes our annual ski vacation is ruined.

Positive

I'm lucky I've received a good education in diabetes. I can figure out how to balance my food, insulin, and exercise so our skiing trip won't be affected by my diabetes.

Believe in Yourself!

The stress management/motivation technique of positive self-talk leads us to one of the most important concepts of our discussion: **Belief**. The mind does affect the body. Another way of saying this is: "Expectations become self-fulfilling prophecy." When we believe that something will happen, we consciously and subconsciously help to make it happen.

At the International Diabetes Center we have observed that the people who are the healthiest are the ones who believe in health and, consequently, pursue healthy behaviors. Belief serves as the basis for action. Consider the following example:

Expectations become self-fulfilling prophecy.

When I was a teacher I took a group of high school students on a three-day canoe trip. Because I have a positive belief in health it never occurred to me that diabetes would be an obstacle to keep me from the canoe trip. I put my syringes and insulin in an airtight container so they would float if the canoe tipped over. I also packed dried fruit and other nonperishable food items to supplement the trail food. I was ready!

The morning came for us to board the bus which would take us to the beginning point of our canoe trip. Imagine my surprise when a 15-year-old student brought a note from home which read: "Please excuse Jim from the canoe trip. He cannot go because he has diabetes." Imagine Jim's amazement when he learned that I, the teacher, had diabetes!

This true story illustrates the difference between positive and negative belief. Jim's negative belief of "I can't do a lot of things because I have diabetes" (an idea he may have gotten from his parents or medical team) prevented him from exploring ways to go on the canoe trip. And my positive belief of "I can" helped me to figure out how.

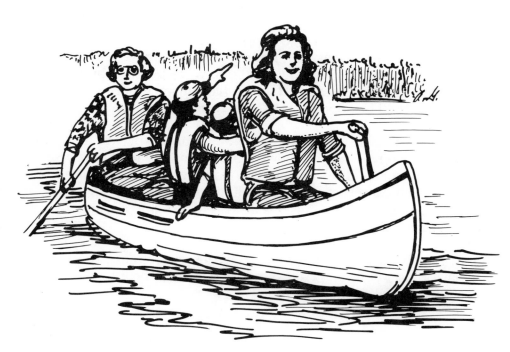

So far we have examined briefly the following concepts and techniques of motivation:

Choice, Goal Setting, Reward, Stress Management, and Belief

The final area is the one which will serve as a continual resource to help you maintain your goals, manage your stress, and sustain your belief. It is the development and use of your **Support System**.

A support system is a collection of people, activities, and events which support you and reinforce your efforts. Several common examples include: parents finding support for their child-rearing efforts by talking with other parents, a person with newly diagnosed diabetes finding support by talking with someone who's lived well with diabetes for many years, and a person moving from one house to another finding support when a group of friends show up to help move furniture.

Sociologists tell us that support is an important factor in healthy human development. People who sense that they are well supported in life can cope more effectively with life's stresses. Stress management expert Dr. Hans Selye suggests an interesting use of support in stress management. He recommends that people give support to others and that in helping others we help ourselves. Give support and also make sure that you get support.

To help you maintain your goals, find specific support for each specific goal. For instance, a goal of regular exercise can be supported by taking a class in exercise or arranging with a friend to exercise regularly. A goal of following one's meal plan can be supported by visiting your dietitian, buying a good cookbook with exchanges figured out, arranging with a friend to swap recipes and menu ideas, planning menus for a whole week, and finding friends (with or without diabetes) who are similarly interested in weight control and good nutrition. Just the realization that you have many friends interested in eating well will be supportive of your healthy lifestyle.

Again, find support. It's there, so look for it and expect to find it for each goal you have set for yourself. Also, continue to give yourself positive messages. They will support your behaviors and sustain your belief. When exercising give yourself messages like: "It feels good to exercise! Exercise burns calories, lowers blood glucose, and increases my energy and vitality!"

Now think of your own messages. Have a positive message for every behavior. As an overall positive message for your healthy lifestyle consider the following:

Look to this day
for it is the very life of Life.
In its brief course lie all
the verities and realities
of your existence.
For yesterday is but a dream
And tomorrow is only a vision
But today well-lived makes
every yesterday a dream of
Happiness
and every tomorrow a vision of
Hope
Look well, therefore, to this day
It is the life of Life!

Sanskrit

NOTES

Section II

Information to Help You Live *Well* With Insulin-Dependent (Type I) Diabetes

Your Health Care Plan
Insulin
Nutrition
Possible Complications

(Information in this section will also be helpful for individuals with non-insulin-dependent diabetes who are taking insulin or diabetes pills to help in controlling blood glucose levels.)

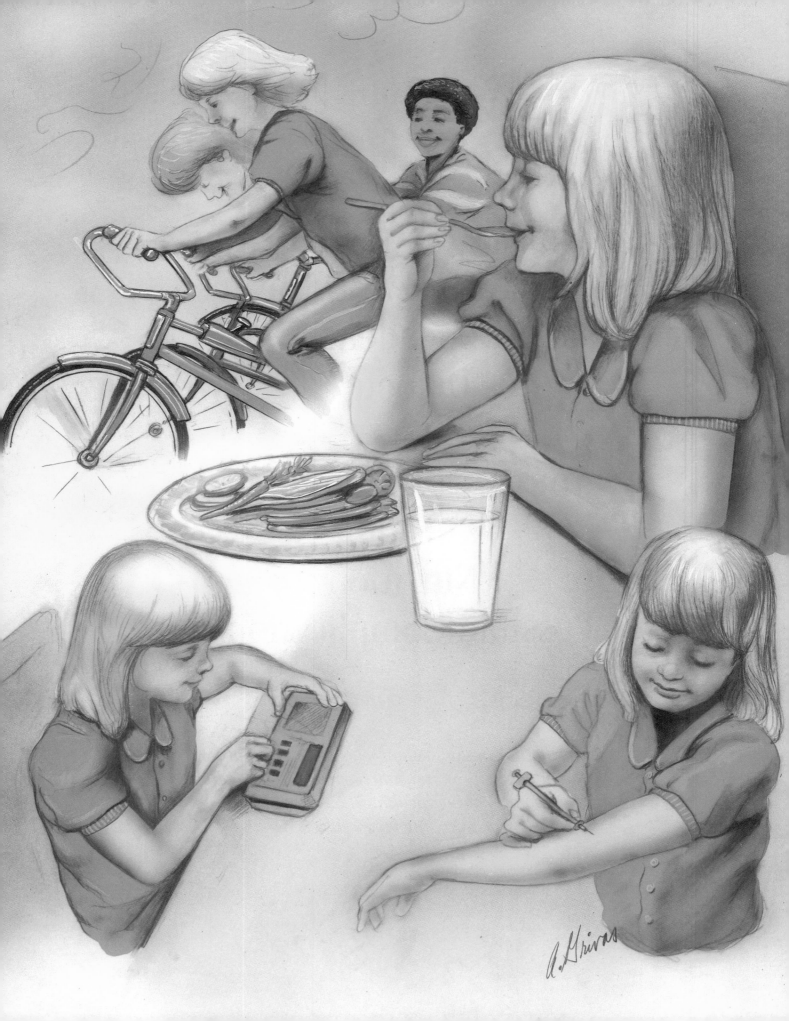

A. Grivas

Chapter 8
Your Health Care Plan for Insulin-Dependent (Type I) Diabetes

Martha Spencer, M.D.

Insulin-dependent (Type I) diabetes is now a disease that can be controlled. The exciting challenge is for individuals to work with their health care providers to find out just how healthy they really can be!

Type I diabetes used to be and still is sometimes called "juvenile" or "brittle" diabetes. Both of these terms are inaccurate. Juvenile diabetes is a misleading term because Type I diabetes can occur at any age, although it is most likely to occur in young individuals. Brittle diabetes refers to wide and uncontrollable swings in blood glucose (sugar), which used to be fairly common but is now less frequent because of improved insulins, availability of self blood glucose monitoring, and more attention to nutritional goals. Another major improvement is that people with diabetes are better informed and can work as a part of the health care team to improve their diabetes control.

Type I diabetes usually occurs in children and in adults less than 40 years old. There is little or no insulin produced by the pancreas, so insulin must be given by injection for survival. Type I diabetes occurs in only about 10 to 15 percent of all persons with diabetes. It occurs in about one out of every 600 children in the United States.

Type I diabetes has an enormous effect on a person's and family's daily life. Each person reacts differently to the physical and emotional stresses of diabetes and must be treated on an individual basis. This chapter will explain how you can work as part of your health care team to plan your diabetes management. It will also explain the importance of regular updates of that plan and frequent checking for early signs of long-term complications.

Diagnosis

The onset of Type I diabetes is usually sudden, with symptoms of thirst, frequent urination, tiredness, and weight loss despite eating large amounts of food. Children may start bedwetting. Often a urinary infection is suspected. The total time between the onset of symptoms and the diagnosis may be only a few days or weeks. Occasionally, onset will be more gradual, with small amounts of glucose in the urine and poor weight gain.

Some children, especially the very young, may have stomach pain and vomiting as a result of the onset of diabetes. These children need immediate treatment and may require hospitalization. Their blood glucose is usually very high, and large amounts of ketones are present in the urine. These findings confirm the fact that there is not enough insulin for the body to use glucose effectively for energy. The body must rely on fat for energy, which results in too many ketone acids in the blood, and may result in ketoacidosis. This is a medical emergency and if not treated immediately can lead to death.

Treatment

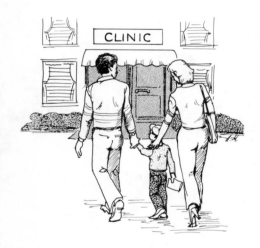

Once Type I diabetes is detected, it is important to begin treatment as soon as possible. In the past, everyone was hospitalized when Type I diabetes was diagnosed. Now, specialized health care teams in diabetes clinics can start insulin therapy and teach people how to manage diabetes during a series of clinic (outpatient) visits. When outpatient health care is available, and the diabetes has been detected before the person becomes seriously ill, hospitalization is not necessary.

The key points of these first visits (or days in the hospital) are to learn what diabetes is and how to inject insulin, test blood glucose and urine ketones, plan meals, and recognize and treat symptoms of low and high blood glucose. The treatment of diabetes is a complex process and the management plan must be individualized for each person. When diabetes is detected, each person should receive a complete physical examination, nutritional history, and assessment of activity level. It is also necessary to identify sources of stress which could affect blood glucose, as well as sources of emotional support for the person and family. With the information gathered, a meal plan and insulin schedule can be designed according to the person's activity level and time schedule. Together, the meal plan, activity plan, and insulin schedule are called the **Health Care Plan**.

The diabetes health care plan must be compatible with each person's lifestyle. Ideally, each person with diabetes should work with an experienced diabetes health care team, which may consist of a nurse educator, dietitian, social worker or counselor, and the physician. In smaller communities, some of these team members may not be available. Where services are limited, your doctor may wish to work in cooperation with a diabetes center near your area. What is most important is that all aspects of a person's life are considered in determining the health care plan.

Goals of the Health Care Plan

Keeping in mind the seriousness of diabetes, the major goal of the health care plan is to keep body metabolism as close to normal as possible. In people who do not have diabetes, the blood glucose level before meals will be between 60-120 mg/dl and after meals below 160. Goals for people with diabetes are to keep fasting blood glucoses between 80-120 mg/dl, and one hour after meal blood glucoses under 200 mg/dl. Other important considerations are maintaining normal blood fat levels, normal weight and growth in children, a healthy weight in adults, no episodes of ketoacidosis, and no serious insulin reactions.

Achieving and maintaining these goals is a challenge. It may require lifestyle changes for many families. As a person with diabetes, it is important that you and your family learn all you can about diabetes, assume major responsibility in daily diabetes management, and work with your health care team.

You must learn when, how, and whom to contact when you have questions or problems. Part of sharing responsibility with your health care team is to be seen on a regular basis for routine health care and re-evaluation of your health care plan. Your health care team is not there just to treat you when you are sick, their focus is on helping you stay well and live fully.

Insulin

In Type I diabetes, the body cannot make its own insulin. Since insulin is necessary to sustain life, it must be replaced. Insulin taken by mouth is destroyed by the stomach, so it must be given by injection under the skin. See Chapter 5 for instructions on preparing and injecting insulin.

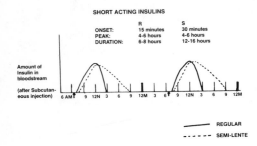

SHORT ACTING INSULINS

	R	S
ONSET:	15 minutes	30 minutes
PEAK:	4-6 hours	4-6 hours
DURATION:	6-8 hours	12-16 hours

Amount of
Insulin in
bloodstream

(after Subcutan-
eous injection)

——— REGULAR
- - - - - SEMI-LENTE

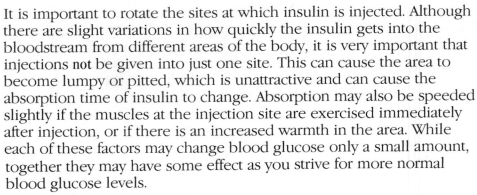

INTERMEDIATE ACTING INSULINS

	LENTE (L)	NPH
ONSET:	3 hours	3 hours
PEAK:	9-12 hours	7-12 hours
DURATION:	18-28 hours	18-24 hours

Amount of
Insulin in
bloodstream

NPH & LENTE

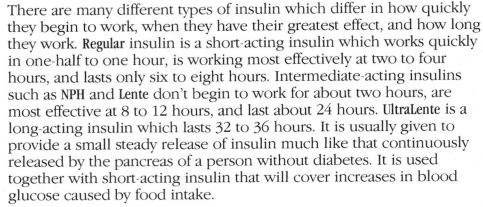
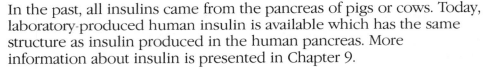

LONG ACTING INSULINS

	ULTRALENTE (U)	PZI
ONSET:	3-4 hours	3-4 hours
PEAK:	16-18 hours	14-20 hours
DURATION:	30-36 hours	24-36 hours

Amount of
Insulin in
bloodstream

ULTRALENTE & PZI

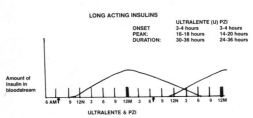

It is important to rotate the sites at which insulin is injected. Although there are slight variations in how quickly the insulin gets into the bloodstream from different areas of the body, it is very important that injections **not** be given into just one site. This can cause the area to become lumpy or pitted, which is unattractive and can cause the absorption time of insulin to change. Absorption may also be speeded slightly if the muscles at the injection site are exercised immediately after injection, or if there is an increased warmth in the area. While each of these factors may change blood glucose only a small amount, together they may have some effect as you strive for more normal blood glucose levels.

There are many different types of insulin which differ in how quickly they begin to work, when they have their greatest effect, and how long they work. **Regular** insulin is a short-acting insulin which works quickly in one-half to one hour, is working most effectively at two to four hours, and lasts only six to eight hours. Intermediate-acting insulins such as **NPH** and **Lente** don't begin to work for about two hours, are most effective at 8 to 12 hours, and last about 24 hours. **UltraLente** is a long-acting insulin which lasts 32 to 36 hours. It is usually given to provide a small steady release of insulin much like that continuously released by the pancreas of a person without diabetes. It is used together with short-acting insulin that will cover increases in blood glucose caused by food intake.

In the past, all insulins came from the pancreas of pigs or cows. Today, laboratory-produced human insulin is available which has the same structure as insulin produced in the human pancreas. More information about insulin is presented in Chapter 9.

Initial insulin doses will vary a great deal depending on age, weight, and blood glucose level. The initial insulin doses will be modified according to each person's individual response to insulin, activity pattern, meal plan, and level of stress.

The successful use of any insulin schedule requires that you understand a great deal about how exercise, food, and stress affect your blood glucose. A combination of short-acting and intermediate-acting insulins are usually given twice daily, the first injection 30 minutes before breakfast and the second 30 minutes before supper. Usually about two-thirds of the total daily insulin is given in the morning and one-third in the afternoon or before supper. Intermediate-acting and long-acting insulins should be given at about the same time each day. Short-acting insulin is most effective when injected at least one-half hour before meals, so it can act in time to prevent too much of an increase in blood glucose and to allow better use of the food by the body.

If your doctor has asked you to mix two different types of insulin for injection, it is especially important that you receive instruction in how to prepare and measure the doses to receive the correct amount of each insulin (see Chapter 5).

The natural course of Type I diabetes is that at first the pancreas is making very little insulin. Often, this function may temporarily recover, causing a rapid decrease in the need for injected insulin. This may occur two weeks to six months after the onset of diabetes and is called the "honeymoon period." It may last weeks or even months. During this time a single injection of intermediate-acting insulin may meet the person's needs, and sometimes no insulin is needed. In children, 1 to 2 units of insulin may be given daily to reduce the disappointment when the full insulin schedule must be resumed.

In addition to the insulin schedules already mentioned, there are many others which may be used to obtain the blood glucose goals that you and your doctor have identified. Your doctor will usually prescribe the simplest insulin schedule and progress to a more complex insulin schedule if and when the need arises. There is no **one** right insulin dosage or schedule. Each must be individualized and adjusted when necessary. Insulin requirements do change, particularly in children because of growth, illness, and seasonal changes in activity.

Intensive Insulin Therapy: Multiple Insulin Doses and the Insulin Pump

Some individuals may require three or more daily injections of Regular insulin as well as an intermediate (NPH, Lente) or long-acting insulin (UltraLente) given at various times throughout the day to control blood glucose. This is one way doctors have been successful in controlling so-called "brittle" diabetes.

The use of an insulin pump to deliver insulin is another method that has been used to improve diabetes control. An insulin pump is a battery-powered microcomputer a little larger than a deck of cards. The pump is worn on the outside of the body, and instructions to deliver different amounts of insulin at different times of the day can be entered through a keyboard on the pump. Pumps were first used in the 1970s. Even though they have been available for a number of years, pumps are not commonly used; however, some people find them helpful.

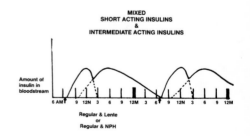

Only short-acting (Regular) insulin is used in a pump. The insulin is contained in a syringe or reservoir inside the pump which is filled every two to three days. The insulin is delivered to the body through a small plastic tubing, which is attached to a needle inserted into the skin and taped in place. The needle and tubing are replaced when the pump is refilled with insulin.

The theory of using multiple insulin doses or an insulin pump is that a small amount of insulin (called the basal insulin) can be delivered continuously during the day and night to allow normal basal (resting) metabolism. With the pump the basal insulin is Regular insulin. With multiple doses the basal insulin is the intermediate or long-acting insulin. Then before meals, a larger dose of Regular insulin (called a bolus) is given to allow the body to properly use the food and prevent too large a rise in blood glucose level. This combination of a basal insulin rate and boluses of insulin mimics the way a healthy pancreas responds to a rise in blood glucose.

An insulin pump is usually used when maximum control of diabetes is desired, such as during pregnancy. Some individuals like them because they provide a more flexible lifestyle, although the best control is achieved when meals and activity are kept fairly consistent. In general, meal times should not vary by more than an hour and meal sizes should remain consistent so that it will be easier to judge insulin requirements. Snacks may not be needed during the day, but an evening snack is important to prevent low blood glucose during the early morning hours.

Wearing an insulin pump does not allow the wearer to forget about diabetes. In fact, the pump is a constant reminder of diabetes. A person wanting to use an insulin pump must be highly motivated and knowledgeable about nutrition, exercise, insulin action and adjustments, physical and emotional stress, and how all affect blood glucose levels. The person must test blood glucose at least four times a day to make sure the pump is functioning properly and normal blood glucose levels are being achieved. The wearer must also follow the necessary pattern of changing the pump's batteries, filling the syringe or reservoir, programming the pump, and changing the tubing and needle.

As you can see, external insulin pumps are not yet more convenient than injecting insulin several times a day. In the future, insulin pumps may be developed which can monitor blood glucose levels and deliver insulin appropriately. They may also be implanted in the body, much like heart pacemakers. These advances are discussed in the chapter on research, Chapter 25.

Your Meal Plan and Exercise

Your meal plan is one of the most important parts of diabetes control. The health care plan will be based on a relatively consistent food intake. For children, the meal plan is designed for normal growth. For adults, it is designed for maintenance of the individual's desirable weight.

Reduction of saturated fats, cholesterol, and simple sugars in your food intake is encouraged. The meal plan usually consists of three meals and two or three snacks per day. The number of snacks and the timing of meals are designed to take into account your lifestyle. Once a meal plan has been designed, it is important that meals and snacks be eaten at approximately the same time each day. See Chapter 10 for additional information on meal planning.

Activity is the third part of the health care plan. In children it is hard to predict when activity will take place. Unpredictable activity, inability to recognize symptoms of low blood glucose, and variability in appetite all contribute to children having wider swings in blood glucose than are seen in most adults. Individuals with Type I diabetes are encouraged to make exercise part of their lifestyle. Chapters 3 and 27 include guidelines and information to help you design a safe and effective exercise program. Most people who exercise feel better, take better care of themselves, and take an active interest in living a healthy life.

Monitoring

The best way to determine how successfully you are balancing food, insulin, and activity is to measure your blood glucose (see Chapters 4 and 5). The most valuable information is obtained if blood tests are done before each meal and at bedtime. Other times to test are when blood glucose is low (especially when you suspect low blood glucoses at night), when you are ill, or when there is a change in your schedule. However, testing in itself does not improve blood glucose control. Test results must be **recorded and used** with your health care providers' help to learn about and balance the inter-relationships among activity, food, insulin, and stress.

Blood glucose testing results must be recorded and used to maintain good blood glucose control.

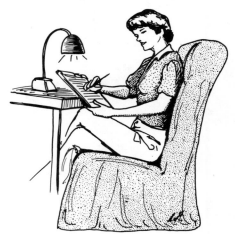

Besides blood glucose testing, it is important to know how to test for ketones in the urine. This must be done whenever your blood glucose is 240 mg/dl or higher, or if you are feeling ill. The presence of ketones in the urine along with high blood glucose means there is not enough insulin to allow the body to continue to use glucose for energy. The body has switched over to using too much fat for energy. This can be due to too little insulin, too much food, or an unusual amount of stress. A blood glucose test of 240 mg/dl or higher and a positive ketone test are a warning that some changes need to be made to prevent ketoacidosis, which will be discussed later in this chapter.

Common Problems with Diabetes

It is difficult for a person with diabetes to duplicate the fine blood glucose adjustments made by a healthy pancreas. It is a challenge to balance food, insulin, and activity. And even when these factors are balanced, unusual emotional or physical stress can result in wider than normal swings of blood glucose. In this section we will discuss how to prevent, recognize, and treat low blood glucose (hypoglycemia) and high blood glucose (hyperglycemia).

The overall goal in managing your diabetes is to maintain blood glucose levels no lower than 80 mg/dl and no higher than 200 mg/dl one to two hours after a meal. It is thought that this is the best way to avoid complications of diabetes. There are three classifications of complications according to how long it takes problems to develop: sudden complications, intermediate complications, and long-term complications.

In this chapter we will discuss sudden complications which can develop in minutes, hours, or days. These are **insulin reactions** and **ketoacidosis**. Intermediate complications which can develop in months or a few years are failure of normal growth (Chapter 10) and problems during pregnancy (Chapter 17). Long-term problems which take years to decades to develop include small blood vessel disease which causes eye and kidney disease, and large blood vessel disease which causes heart disease and stroke. Another long-term complication is damage to nerves, which can lead to a loss of sensitivity and function in some parts of the body. Long-term complications are discussed in Chapter 11.

Low Blood Glucose or Insulin Reactions

The results of low blood glucose are known by several different names: insulin reaction, reaction, insulin shock, or hypoglycemia. All of these terms refer to the body's response to blood glucose that is below 60-80 mg/dl. Hypoglycemia can be caused by one or a combination of three things: too much insulin, too little food, or an increase in activity. Reactions can occur suddenly in a matter of minutes, usually just before meal times, during or after exercise, and at times when your insulin is having its greatest effect.

When your blood glucose gets too low, the body tries to protect itself by releasing a hormone called adrenalin or epinephrine, which is the same hormone released during stressful situations. You may feel shaky, sweaty, dizzy, or suddenly hungry. You or even others who do not have diabetes may have these feelings during a stressful situation. It is important to test your blood glucose if possible to find out if you are having an insulin reaction or just responding normally to stress. If the test reads below 80 mg/dl, treat the reaction by following the instructions in the next paragraphs.

If blood glucose continues to be low, the brain sends out warning signals. You may develop a headache, blurred vision, or numbness or tingling of the lips. People around you may notice that you have become pale, clumsy, confused, or are acting differently than usual. If you have any of these signs, check your blood glucose. If the test reads below 80, treat the reaction by eating 10 grams of a fast-acting glucose food. If you are unable to test your blood glucose, go ahead and treat the reaction. Suitable foods and amounts are listed below:

1 small box (2 Tbsp.) raisins
½ cup regular pop (not diet)
4 or 5 dried fruit pieces
2 large sugar cubes
1 Fruit Roll-Up
5 small sugar cubes
½ cup of any fruit juice
6 or 7 LifeSavers
1/3 bottle Glutose or other forms of glucose
    available at your pharmacy

Hypoglycemia can be caused by:
  1) too much insulin,
  2) too little food,
  3) increased activity,
  4) a combination of the above.

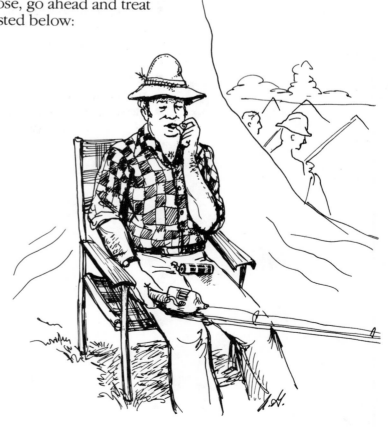

141

Always carry some form of fast-acting glucose.

Remember that it takes a while for the glucose you've eaten to get into your bloodstream and begin to be used by the body. If you don't feel better in 15 to 20 minutes, again eat the same amount of food. If you continue to feel as if you're having a reaction, check your blood glucose. If it is still below 80, repeat the treatment a third time. If there is no response in 15 to 20 minutes, call your health care provider. An untreated reaction can lead to unconsciousness and seizures. Severe hypoglycemia lasting several hours can result in brain damage and death.

Food used for treating reactions is an addition to your regular meal plan. Do not subtract this food from your next snack or meal. Always carry some form of fast-acting glucose with you, especially when you are driving. Eat 10 grams (the amount of carbohydrate in one fruit exchange) of the food at the first sign of an insulin reaction.

The best way to prevent insulin reactions is to make sure your health care plan is achieving a good balance of food, insulin, and exercise. The following points are keys to preventing reactions:

- Test routinely and use the results to make changes to avoid low or high blood glucose levels.
- Eat your prescribed meal plan.
- Do not delay meals or snacks by more than one-half hour. (This includes breakfast on weekends and holidays.)
- Monitor blood glucose and if necessary eat extra food before and during unscheduled or unusually prolonged exercise.
- Be alert to changes in your daily routines that may affect blood glucose level.
- Measure your insulin carefully.
- Take other medications exactly as prescribed.
- Remember, alcohol can lower the blood glucose. Discuss its effects with your health care provider. See Chapter 2 for more information.
- Be aware of early warning signs and always carry some form of glucose so you can treat reactions promptly.

Rebounding

Frequent blood glucose testing provides information that can be used to avoid wide swings in blood glucose levels. These wide swings can occur because of stress hormones that the body releases when the blood glucose level gets too low. These hormones can prevent severe hypoglycemia, but they sometimes keep on raising the blood glucose until the level is above the normal range. When high blood glucose levels are a result of hormone reaction to hypoglycemia, the effect is called rebounding. This was first described by Dr. Michael Somogyi, and is therefore sometimes called the Somogyi effect.

If the person and doctor are not aware that high blood glucose levels are a result of rebounding, the decision may be made to increase the insulin dosage. This can result in too much insulin (over-insulinization), which will only make the problem worse. Sometimes this is the cause of a person's "brittle diabetes." The error can be discovered by testing blood glucose every two hours or so during the day and night to try to find out whether the insulin dosage is actually causing hypoglycemia. Another clue that rebounding is occurring is that the result of increasing the insulin dosage has been to cause higher, rather than lower, blood glucose levels. The dosage may have to be lowered or spread over several injections throughout the day to avoid the rebounding effect.

Another mistake that can result in rebounding is when a reaction is overtreated and then the person takes extra short-acting insulin because of the resulting high blood glucose. Never increase insulin on the basis of one or two high blood glucose tests unless urine ketones are present. Always wait to see if a pattern develops over several days and then if you are not sure how to adjust insulin, or if blood glucose is not controlled by your adjustments, discuss the situation with your health care provider. See Chapter 5 for a discussion of pattern control.

The over-insulinization discussed above may be the cause of frequent insulin reactions that cannot be explained by a skipped or delayed meal or snack or by unusual exercise. The insulin dosage may be too high or need to be given in several injections spread over the day. If a person is having frequent symptoms of low blood glucose, especially hunger, headaches, or irritability, or is gaining weight, again the insulin dosage may be too high. Too much insulin will cause low blood glucose, which will cause the appetite to increase and the person to eat more. Having too much insulin in the blood causes the excess food to be stored as fat, so the person gains weight.

Rebounding can be caused by:
1) *stress hormone response to low blood glucose,*
2) *too high a dosage of insulin, or*
3) *eating too much to treat a reaction and then taking extra insulin because of the resulting high blood glucose.*

Sometimes people with diabetes are extra sensitive to decreasing blood glucose levels. They may have symptoms of a reaction when their blood glucose has fallen from a very high level but is in the normal range or still high. If extra food is eaten to treat these false symptoms, blood glucose will of course rise even higher. If extra insulin is then taken, a rebounding situation will likely develop. This is why it is important to test blood glucose whenever possible to make sure the symptoms are actually a sign that blood glucose is below 80 mg/dl.

Another way that rebounding can cause problems is if the low blood glucose occurs while the person is sleeping, or if the person doesn't feel any symptoms. Stress hormones may then cause a very large increase in blood glucose that may last for several days. Since the person is unaware that the low blood glucose episode was responsible, the insulin dosage may be increased, worsening the rebounding problem. Only rarely does rebounding result in the development of ketoacidosis. Ketones may appear in the urine, but they are a sign that not enough glucose was available during the period of low blood glucose, not a sign that not enough insulin was available to use glucose. Again, it is important to discuss the situation with your health care provider before changing your insulin dosage. Good communication with your health care team and frequent blood glucose testing can prevent repeated rebounding.

Pattern of Rebounding Blood Glucose Levels

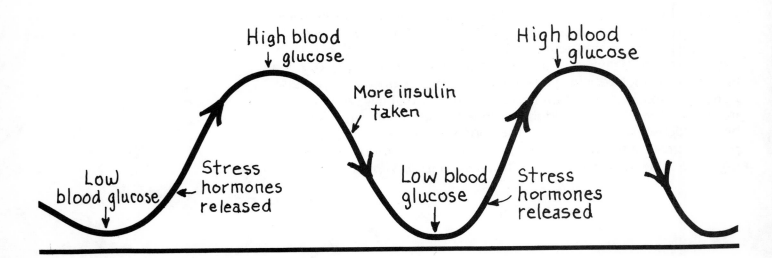

Severe Insulin Reactions

If low blood glucose is not treated with some form of glucose, and if stress hormones are not able to raise the blood glucose level, a severe insulin reaction may develop. The person may become confused, act strangely, and can have convulsions and lose consciousness. The person may refuse food or be unable to eat if these symptoms develop, and the reaction must be treated by someone who knows how to inject a substance called glucagon.

Glucagon is a hormone produced by a group of cells (alpha cells) in the pancreas. It has the opposite effect of insulin—it increases blood glucose. Glucagon can be used to treat an insulin reaction when the person with diabetes is semiconscious or unconscious or for some other reason is unable or refuses to take food or drink by mouth. Glucagon, like insulin, is a hormone that must be given by injection. When injected, glucagon causes glucose stored in the liver to enter the blood, increasing the blood glucose level. Glucagon is a safe medication, and should be kept in the home and wherever a person with diabetes spends large amounts of time.

Glucagon is a prescription medication. Contact your health care provider for a prescription and renewals as needed. Store glucagon in the refrigerator. When properly stored, glucagon is effective for several years. Be sure to periodically check the expiration date on the box so you can replace it before it actually expires.

Periodically review the instructions for injecting glucagon with those who live and work with you. The glucagon kit comes with a syringe already filled with diluting fluid and a small bottle containing the powdered form of glucagon. The diluting fluid must be mixed with the powder before it can be injected. The instructions for mixing and giving glucagon are included in the glucagon kit. It should be injected the same way and in the same parts of the body that you inject insulin. If glucagon is mixed but not used, it will be effective for 30 days if kept refrigerated.

Periodically review the instructions for injecting glucagon with those who live and work with you.

The following instructions are important after a person has been treated with glucagon:

- The person with diabetes usually responds within 15 to 30 minutes. If no response occurs within this period call for emergency assistance.
- An upset stomach, nausea, or vomiting may develop.
- When alert enough to swallow, start offering small amounts of regular pop, soda crackers, or dry toast.
- If the person is able to keep these foods down, offer additional food such as milk and a sandwich.
- If the nausea and vomiting continue, follow the sick-day meal plan described in Chapter 10 and contact the health care provider.
- When the treatment has stabilized blood glucose levels in the normal range, continue to test blood glucose four times a day for the next two days to avoid further episodes. The insulin dose may need to be adjusted if blood glucose tests continue to run low.

Review with your health care provider the events that led up to the severe reaction. Was there something unusual in your lifestyle, food intake, activity pattern, etc.? Consult your health care team for help in making insulin adjustments if necessary.

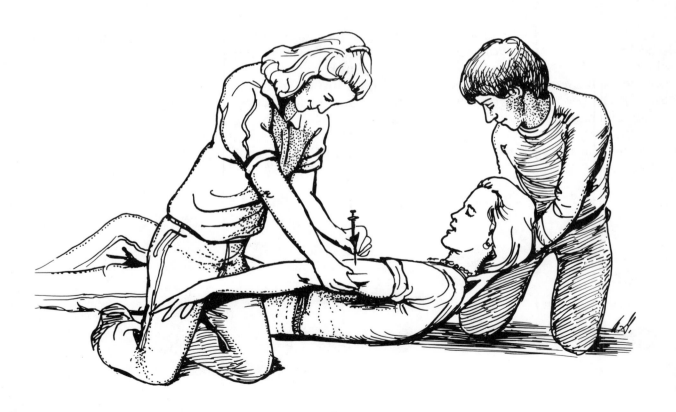

High Blood Glucose and Ketoacidosis

High blood glucose can lead to ketoacidosis. Ketoacidosis develops when there is not enough insulin in the blood to allow glucose to be used for energy. The body then must rely on fat for energy. When the body must use too much fat for energy, the fat can't be broken down completely by the liver, and ketones are formed. At the same time, the high blood glucose leads to high urine glucose and loss of large amounts of body fluid and minerals (potassium and sodium).

Large amounts of ketones make you feel nauseated, so you may not be able to eat your regular meal plan. The high blood glucose causes you to lose large amounts of body fluids through excessive urination, and it is hard to drink enough fluids to completely replace the amount lost. This leads to a drying out of body tissues (dehydration), which is very dangerous. If you are vomiting or have diarrhea, you can become dehydrated very quickly. This is especially true for small children. Signs of dehydration are dry mouth and sunken eyes.

You need immediate medical attention if high blood glucose and urine ketones lead to drowsiness, rapid breathing, or unconsciousness.

When blood glucose is over 240 mg/dl for several days you may experience symptoms of thirst, dry mouth, frequent urination, weight loss, and tiredness. If the high blood glucose persists and the urine becomes positive for ketones, then you may have abdominal pain, nausea, and vomiting. Your face may become flushed and you may have blurred vision. You need immediate medical attention if you go on to become drowsy, start breathing rapidly, or lose consciousness. You may have to be hospitalized.

Ketoacidosis can become very dangerous and cause unconsciousness (diabetic coma) and death if not treated immediately. It can be detected early if you are testing blood glucose regularly. If a blood test is 240 mg/dl or higher, test urine for ketones (see Chapter 4). Call your health care provider if any of the following signs are present:

- Moderate to large ketones in the urine along with high blood glucose levels.
- Severe nausea.
- Vomiting.
- Abdominal pain.
- Rapid breathing.

Ketoacidosis usually develops when there is not enough insulin to handle unusual amounts of stress from illness, infection, or extreme and prolonged emotions. If an illness such as the flu or a bad cold prevents you from eating your prescribed meal plan, it is important to follow the sick-day meal plan described in Chapter 10.

Preventing Ketoacidosis During Brief Illness

- Take your insulin or diabetes pill. Extra insulin may be needed.
- Test blood glucose and urine ketones more frequently, at least four times a day.
- Eat carbohydrates, replacing 50 grams every three to four hours with frequent small feedings, especially if blood glucose is under 240 mg/dl (see page 166 for examples).
- Drink at least one large glass of liquid every hour, taking small sips of water, tea, broth, or other clear liquids.
- If you can't keep any fluid or carbohydrate down, or if symptoms continue for more than one day, contact your health care provider.
- If you begin to breathe rapidly, become drowsy, or lose consciousness, your doctor must be contacted immediately.

What should be done in routine health care visits?

Through routine visits to your health care team every three to four months you can work together to evaluate your blood glucose control and make changes as needed. If your diabetes is not in good control more frequent visits may be necessary. In Chapter 4 we described how you can use your blood glucose testing records to work with your health care providers to maintain good blood glucose control.

We also described the **glycosylated hemoglobin** test, which your doctor can have done in the laboratory. This test provides very valuable information, because it shows what your average blood glucose level has been over the previous six to eight weeks. The glycosylated hemoglobin level for people without diabetes who have been tested in our laboratory is 3.5 to 5.3%. Each laboratory has its own normal level. Your result must be interpreted according to your laboratory's normal value. Your doctor will do this and discuss the result with you. The test results, along with your daily blood glucose records, will allow you and your health care team to evaluate how your health care plan is working. If the levels are higher than expected, your insulin, meal plan, or exercise pattern may need to be adjusted.

Glycosylated hemoglobin measurements do have some limitations. As with any laboratory test, they must be done very carefully to provide accurate results. The test does not reveal if you have had problems with low blood glucose, and is not helpful in pinpointing what you need to change to improve your average blood glucose level. This is why it is important to record accurate daily blood glucose readings and work with your health care team to make changes if necessary.

Blood glucose control is not the only factor that will be checked in routine visits. Your blood pressure will be checked, often two or three times to obtain a reliable result. Your doctor will check your eyes, feet, heart sounds and the condition of your other organs, condition of the tissue at your injection sites, and strength of pulses in different areas of your body. Ask questions about what is being checked and discuss with your doctor how signs of long-term complications can be detected.

If you are an adult your doctor will have additional laboratory tests done approximately once a year to check your cholesterol and triglyceride levels (under 180-200 milligrams is desirable for cholesterol and under 150 milligrams for triglycerides). Blood and urine tests will be done annually to check for signs of kidney damage. It is very important that all these things are checked and prompt action taken if needed. Good blood glucose control and early detection of long-term complications can best be achieved by visiting a diabetes specialist at least once or twice a year.

Education

One of the most important tools you can have to allow you to work with your health care team is diabetes education. The learning process is most successful when approached in three basic stages: "survival skills," in-depth education, and ongoing education.

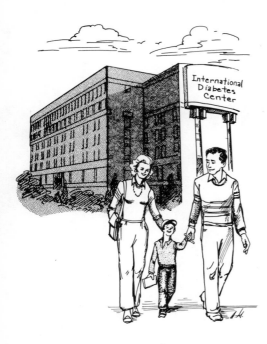

When you are first diagnosed, you need to learn "survival skills." This means learning which insulin to give, how much and how to inject; which foods you need to eat and when; and how to test and record your blood glucose and urine ketones. You also need to learn about the problems of low and high blood glucose, how to recognize, prevent and treat them. You need to learn where to buy your diabetes supplies, how you'll pay for them, and how to store them. This is a lot of information to learn when you're still in shock over hearing you have a disease that will be with you for the rest of your life. Any attempts at learning more about diabetes at this time usually fail.

After a few weeks or a couple months, when you've had a chance to adjust emotionally to your diabetes and are familiar with the routine of managing your diabetes, it will help to learn all about diabetes and how you can live well with it. At this time you will be able to apply what you learn to your own experiences, which will help you remember the information. This is a good time to attend an intensive educational program such as the week-long program offered by the International Diabetes Center (see Appendix for more information). A good program will help you and your family work as a part of the health care team to re-evaluate your health care plan and make any adjustments necessary to improve your diabetes control and/or quality of life.

You will always need to keep updating your knowledge of diabetes. Scientists and doctors are discovering new and better treatment methods every year, so it is important to remain informed about this progress. Your local affiliate of the American Diabetes Association can inform you of programs in your area.

The more you learn about diabetes, the more you will be in control of it, rather than it controlling you.

Your diabetes also will be constantly changing, so you need to learn how to modify your health care plan to allow for these changes. Seasonal activity, work schedules, health problems, life changes, and many other things can affect your diabetes and require changes in your health care plan. Your health care team can help you make changes in your insulin schedule, meal plan, or activity to allow you to control your diabetes without needlessly restricting your lifestyle. The more you learn about diabetes, the more you will be in control of it, rather than it controlling you.

Summary

Studies have shown that the success of the diabetes health care plan is affected by how serious the person is about controlling their diabetes, how well the health care plan is understood and followed by the person, how well the health care plan is adapted to all parts of the person's lifestyle, and how the person adjusts emotionally to diabetes and receives support from others.

The child or adult who has diabetes must not think of himself or herself or be thought of by family members and friends as a "diabetic" who must live a restricted life. He or she is a person who happens to have diabetes, which fortunately can be made a part of a very healthy, productive, and full life.

NOTES

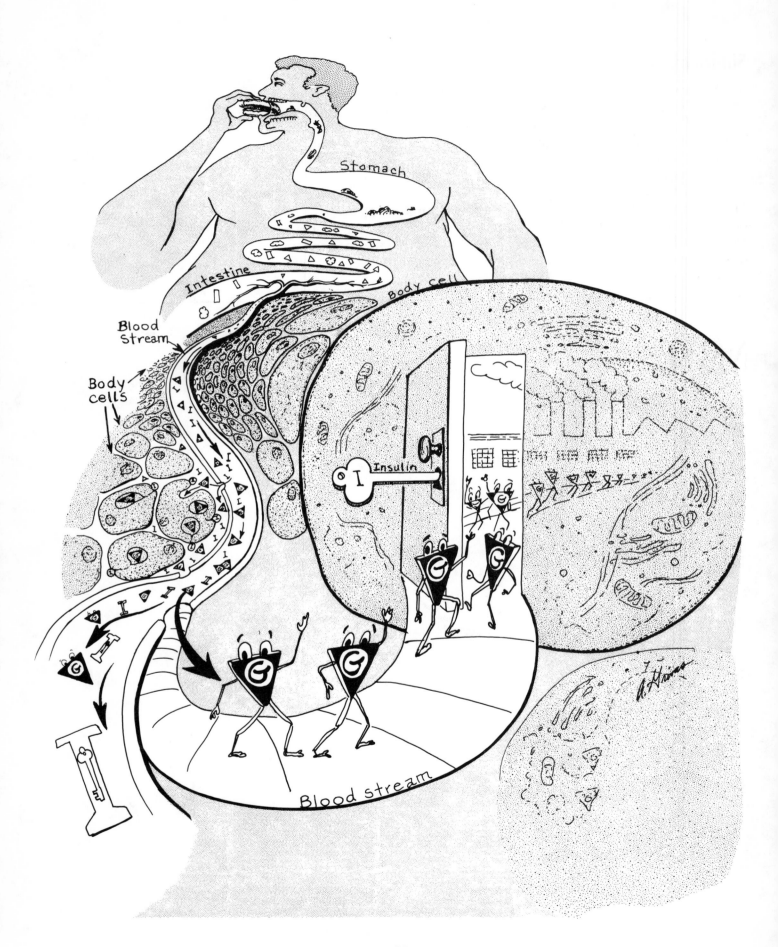

Stomach

Intestine

Body cells

Blood Stream

Body cells

Insulin

Blood stream

Chapter 9
Insulin: The Key to Type I Diabetes Management

Ron Kitzman, R.Ph.

Perhaps you would like to know some more details about insulin and why it is a life-saving medication for people with Type I diabetes. This chapter will first explain what insulin is and how it works. We will then discuss the differences among types of insulins used for injection, and what types of things your doctor will consider when choosing an insulin to be the "key" to your diabetes management program. This information will help you understand why your doctor wants you to use a specific kind of insulin and how that insulin will act in your body. (For instructions on how to inject insulin, see Chapter 5.)

What is insulin?

Insulin is one of many hormones in the body that help cells do their work. Hormones are chemicals made in the body to control specific body processes. Insulin is a protein made up of 51 building blocks called amino acids. These are divided into two connected chains, an A chain and a B chain (see illustration). Insulin is produced in the beta cells of the islets of Langerhans in the pancreas. In addition to insulin, the pancreas makes, stores, and releases many other hormones, digestive fluids, and enzymes.

The production of insulin in the pancreas starts with the formation of a larger hormone called **proinsulin**. Proinsulin contains the A and B chains of insulin connected to an additional set of amino acids called the connecting peptide, or C-peptide. When proinsulin is broken down in the pancreas, it releases one molecule of insulin and the C-peptide separately into the bloodstream.

The action of insulin was explained in Chapter 1, but briefly, insulin acts by assisting in the transfer of glucose from the blood into the body cells, where energy is needed for the cells—and therefore the body— to function. Insulin also aids in the storage of glucose in the form of glycogen in the liver and muscles, which prevents the body from relying on body protein and too much fat for energy. Insulin also helps the body store fat and repair tissue. In these ways, insulin prevents muscle breakdown and excessive weight loss, as well as preventing the buildup of ketones in the blood.

Proinsulin

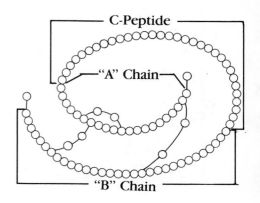

Insulin

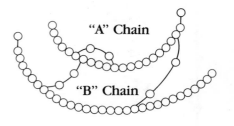

How is injected insulin different from the insulin the body makes?

There are four main ways in which injected insulin differs from insulin made in the human body:

1. Source, or where the insulin came from.
2. Action time, or when and how long it is effective.
3. Concentration, or how much insulin is in a given amount of liquid.
4. Purity, or how many noninsulin hormone parts it contains.

Source

At the present time there are several sources of insulin: beef, pork, and two types of human insulin made in laboratories. When insulin was discovered in 1921, it became possible to inject insulin into people who would otherwise die of Type I diabetes. This insulin was obtained from the pancreases of cows and pigs. Insulin must be injected if it is to work. If it is taken by mouth, the digestive system will destroy the insulin before it can get into the blood. Pork insulin is more similar in structure to the insulin made by the human pancreas than is beef insulin. A mixture of beef and pork insulins is also manufactured. In general, insulin that is most like that made in the human pancreas is less likely to cause problems.

It seems logical that the ideal form of insulin for injection would be identical to the insulin made by the human body. Obviously the human pancreas is not an available source of insulin for someone with diabetes. Recent advances in chemistry and biology, however, have provided two methods of producing human insulin artificially. One way is to instruct bacteria to make human insulin using a "blueprint," called DNA, for human insulin. DNA is a chemical chain which carries genetic information from one generation to the next. The bacteria follow this blueprint to make insulin identical to human insulin. This insulin is retrieved from the bacteria and purified through a complex chemical process and is then available for use by patients with diabetes. Another way of making insulin identical to human insulin is to change a molecule of pork insulin into a molecule of human insulin. Remember, insulin is a made up of a chain of 51 building blocks called amino acids. The pork insulin chain and the human insulin chain differ by only one amino acid. Through a chemical process, the different amino acid can be cut out of the pork insulin chain and replaced by the amino acid which will make the pork chain identical to human insulin.

Source

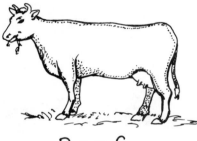

Beef

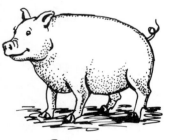

Pork

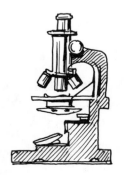

Human

Action Time

Insulin that is released by the pancreas into the bloodstream is immediately active, or available for use by the cells. This is not so when insulin is injected into the fatty tissue under the skin. There are three time actions of injected insulin: rapid-acting, intermediate-acting, and long-acting. The different action times of insulin are a result of the use of zinc or protein in the insulin mixture, which causes the insulin to be absorbed more slowly from the injection site into the blood. Each insulin action time has a general pattern of when the insulin will become active (onset), when it will be working hardest (peak), and how long it will continue to be active (duration). The graphs below show the general action patterns of the different types of insulins.

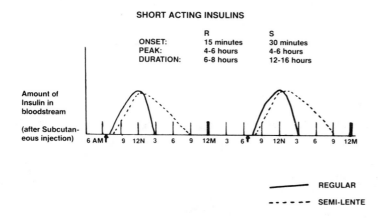

SHORT ACTING INSULINS

	R	S
ONSET:	15 minutes	30 minutes
PEAK:	4-6 hours	4-6 hours
DURATION:	6-8 hours	12-16 hours

Amount of Insulin in bloodstream

(after Subcutaneous injection)

——————— REGULAR

- - - - - - SEMI-LENTE

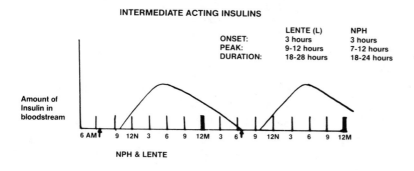

INTERMEDIATE ACTING INSULINS

	LENTE (L)	NPH
ONSET:	3 hours	3 hours
PEAK:	9-12 hours	7-12 hours
DURATION:	18-28 hours	18-24 hours

Amount of Insulin in bloodstream

NPH & LENTE

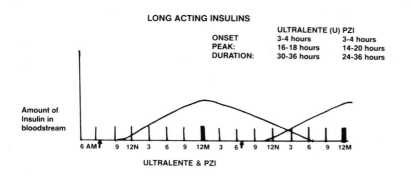

LONG ACTING INSULINS

	ULTRALENTE (U)	PZI
ONSET	3-4 hours	3-4 hours
PEAK:	16-18 hours	14-20 hours
DURATION:	30-36 hours	24-36 hours

Amount of Insulin in bloodstream

ULTRALENTE & PZI

155

Concentration

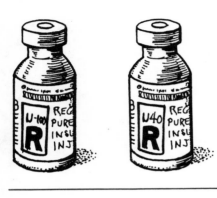

Concentration

The third way injected insulin can differ from the insulin made by the human pancreas is the concentration of the insulin product. There are two basic concentrations of insulins used for daily injections: U-100 and U-40. U-100 means there are 100 units of insulin in each cubic centimeter (cc). Therefore, a 10-cc bottle of U-100 insulin contains 1,000 units of insulin. U-40 is a less concentrated form of insulin. It has 40 units of insulin in each cubic centimeter of liquid. A 10-cc bottle of U-40 insulin contains 400 units of insulin. U-100 is the concentration that is most commonly used in the United States, but U-40 is more common in many other countries.

Since there are different concentrations of insulin, it is important to buy U-100 syringes for U-100 insulin, and U-40 syringes for U-40 insulin. Syringes are clearly marked either U-40 or U-100.

Purity

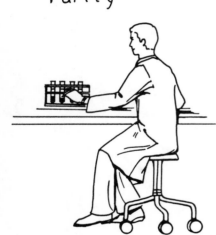

Insulin products have been made increasingly pure (free of proinsulin and other hormone parts) over the years through the use of electrical and chemical laboratory techniques. All insulins sold today are greatly improved in purity, but some are very highly purified and are sometimes helpful if problems result from the use of other insulins.

There are several non-insulin ingredients in a bottle of insulin. They include the diluting solution, a preservative to prevent bacteria from growing, some protein or zinc to increase action time, and ingredients that are used to adjust the acidity of the insulin solution.

Despite the very high quality of today's insulin products, insulins may cause an allergic reaction in some individuals. This can result in a rash, redness, lump (hypertrophy), or sunken area (lipoatrophy) at the injection site. Your doctor will watch for these problems, and if necessary will change your insulin.

If you think you might benefit from switching insulins, ask your health care provider for advice. Never switch to a different insulin type or brand without first discussing it with your doctor. Any change from your current prescription could threaten your diabetes control.

Buying Insulin

It will be easier to buy the right insulin if you become very familiar with your type and brand of insulin and the information on the product label. Do not accept any product that is not the same as the insulin your doctor has prescribed. Bring the prescription or a recently used bottle to the pharmacy, and check the type, brand name and maker, source, concentration, and expiration date before you pay.

Cost can vary from one pharmacy to another, so shop around to get the best buy on your type of insulin. Always buy enough insulin so that you are not in danger of running out if a bottle breaks or is lost. Do not count on being able to buy your brand or strength of insulin if you are traveling, especially outside of the United States. Take enough insulin with you, but do not check it with your baggage, as it could become lost.

Store insulin bottles that you are not using in the refrigerator, and keep opened bottles at room temperature. If insulin is cold when injected, it may sting. Don't allow the insulin to freeze, because this will cause it to become ineffective. Also, don't allow it to be in direct sunlight or temperatures higher than 90 degrees Fahrenheit for long periods of time. Throw away any bottles that have been exposed to temperature extremes.

Insulins of the Future

The many types of insulins available today may seem confusing, but remember, you only need to know about the insulin or insulins your doctor has prescribed. Many experts think human insulins are the insulins of the future, and many physicians routinely start individuals with newly diagnosed diabetes on human insulin.

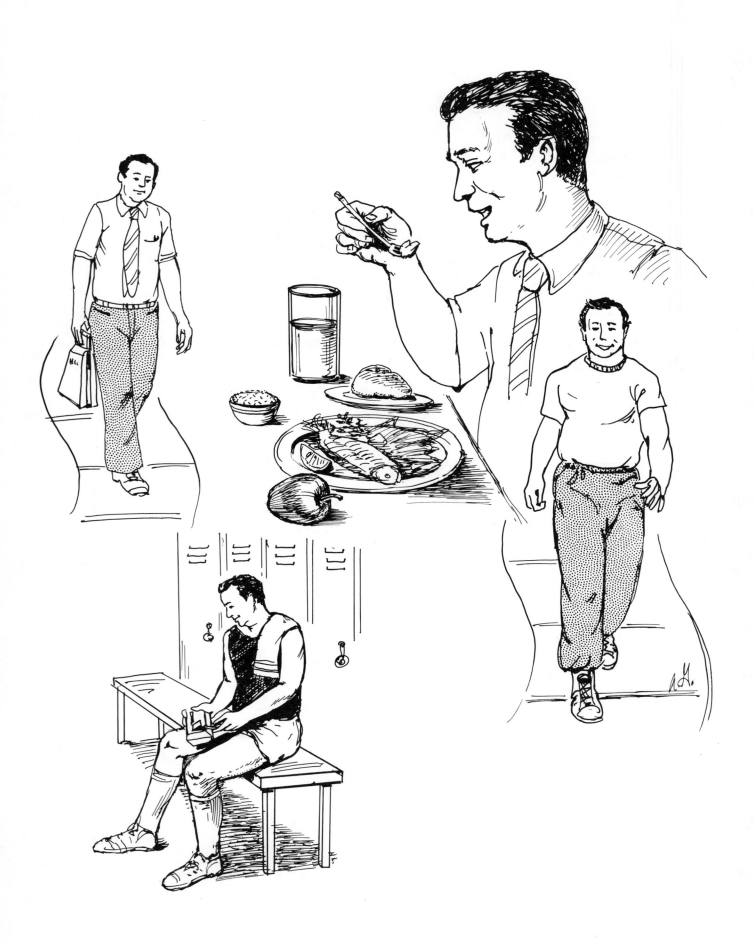

Chapter 10
Consistency: The Nutrition Key in Type I Diabetes

Marion Franz, R.D., M.S.

Meal planning is an essential part of the management plan to control blood glucose and blood fat levels in Type I diabetes. However, it is a mistake to think that you are just eating to control your diabetes. A well-designed meal plan will provide all the nutrients necessary for a healthy lifestyle, with enough variety to be enjoyable and enough flexibility to allow for your personal likes and dislikes. Your meal plan is not a "diabetic diet," it is a way of eating that is recommended for everyone, so your whole family will benefit from eating in a similar manner.

Your meal plan is based on nutritional recommendations made by the American Diabetes Association for persons with diabetes, which include three main changes from the way the average American now eats.
1. Less fat, especially saturated fats and cholesterol.
2. More "naturally-occurring" sugars and starches, with an emphasis on fiber.
3. Less salt (sodium).

The nutrition recommendations also emphasize the need to maintain a reasonable body weight.

Why is an individualized meal plan necessary?

The above recommendations will help everyone eat better as part of a lifestyle of "wellness," but they do not provide specific guidelines for individuals. If you have diabetes, it is essential that your meal plan is individualized, which means it is designed specifically to meet your nutrient and caloric needs as well as your lifestyle. Such a plan can best be developed by working with a registered dietitian (a health professional with the letters R.D. after her or his name). A registered dietitian can help you work the necessary nutritional changes into your lifestyle, so you can manage diabetes and eat well. An R.D. will explain what is important in meal planning and will teach you how to do it. By learning more about nutrition and your meal plan you can add variety to your meal and flexibility to your lifestyle. You will also be better able to solve the problems and situations that you encounter in your daily eating habits.

A registered dietitian can help you work nutritional changes into your lifestyle.

After working with a dietitian to design an individualized meal plan and receive nutrition education, it is important to continue to seek more information and continuing help from your dietitian. As your needs change as a result of growth, weight, activity, or lifestyle changes, it is important to have them reflected in your meal plan. Your meal plan should be reviewed with you at least two to four times a year. Children's meal plans should be reviewed at least twice a year (before and after the school year), but preferably every three months. This will ensure that it is meeting your needs and that you feel comfortable with it. Changes can be made in your meal plan to reflect a healthier lifestyle, or simply to make it more convenient for you.

Consistent food intake and exercise must be balanced with the correct dosages of insulin.

Why is consistency so important?

Your meal plan will reflect your caloric and nutrient needs based on your age, height and weight, activity level, lifestyle, and food preferences. Once your meal plan has been established and you feel you can follow it on a regular basis, your insulin dosage can be adjusted to balance your food intake and regular activity. This is why it is so important to be consistent in following your meal plan. By eating the same number of exchanges at the same times each day and by doing regular blood glucose testing before meals and at bedtime, you or your health care provider can make adjustments in your insulin therapy. This is the best way to keep blood glucose levels as close as possible to the normal range.

Keep in mind that in someone who does not have diabetes, the body matches the amount of insulin it produces to the amount of food eaten. This is what you and your health care provider are trying to duplicate by balancing your food intake, activity, and insulin. If a person without diabetes eats more food one day than the next, the body makes more insulin as needed. Since a person with diabetes can't do this, blood glucose has to be kept in line by a consistent balance of food, activity and insulin.

Since different types of insulin work hardest at different times and act over different periods of time, these things must be considered when your meal plan is designed. It then becomes important for you to be consistent in the times you inject your insulin, since your insulin has been planned to match the amount and time you eat. Food needs to be eaten when the blood-glucose-lowering action of the insulin is the strongest.

Your meal plan will include the number of exchanges you should eat and at what times you should eat them, based on the timing of your injections and type of insulin given. This means you will probably need three meals and at least two to three snacks. Snacks are very important for matching the time action of insulin. An injection of a short-acting and intermediate-acting insulin before breakfast often makes a morning snack necessary, especially for children. The time action of the intermediate-acting insulin will make an afternoon snack necessary; sometimes children do better with two afternoon snacks. An evening snack is important to balance the insulins acting throughout the night.

Planned snacks are very important for matching the time action of insulin.

The insulin schedule can be designed to allow some flexibility in meal times for those whose work or lifestyle interferes with regular food intake. For example, a daily injection of a long-acting insulin with a short-acting insulin injected before meals will allow more flexibility in the timing of meals. Flexibility can also be increased by using an insulin pump (see Chapter 8). A pump allows the wearer to continuously receive a small amount of insulin and a larger amount at meal and snack times; amounts and times can be programmed into the pump by the wearer. However, even when these methods are used, individuals usually do better when their meal times and food intake are as consistent as possible.

Meal planning should also take into account how fast the foods you eat are changed into glucose and absorbed into the bloodstream (see Chapter 2). To help keep your blood glucose normal, try to select foods that will be absorbed slowly. Blood glucose monitoring can help you find out how different foods affect your blood glucose so that you can make appropriate decisions about how to use them in your meal plan.

As you learn more about your meal plan and gain practice in adjusting food, insulin, and activity based on blood glucose tests, you will find yourself gaining more flexibility in meal planning.

Besides your lifestyle, nutritional goals, and food preferences, your meal plan will emphasize the following important considerations:

Regularity of meals. The times of day and number of meals and snacks you eat every day will be based on your needs and desires. Regularity of food intake will help in blood glucose control.

Consistency of food intake. Day-to-day consistency in the number of calories eaten and the way they are spread throughout the day is another major goal. Your meal plan should be adapted to your usual food intake, with emphasis on a healthy and nutritionally adequate result.

Consistent daily exercise improves blood glucose control and overall health.

Activity. Exercise and normal activity levels will affect how your meal plan is designed. Your dietitian will want to know about the types and times of your normal activity (work, school, home) as well as exercise, sports practices and competition. It is helpful if your activity pattern can also be consistent. Not only will it be easier to work your needs into the meal plan, but your body also adapts to a regular training pattern and this can aid in blood glucose control as well. With regular exercise the body becomes more sensitive to the actions of insulin.

You may need to increase your food intake before and perhaps after activity or exercise that you don't do on a regular basis. The best way to decide how much food you need is to monitor blood glucose levels before and after exercise. The effect of exercise on blood glucose levels differs among individuals because everyone's body reacts differently to exercise. For guidelines on how to adjust food based on blood glucose levels, see Chapter 3. With experience you can become a better judge of your needs than your dietitian or physician. It is important to continue to monitor blood glucose even after exercise because blood glucose can continue to drop. The blood glucose lowering effect of exercise may last for several hours, even up to 24 hours. After very strenuous exercise done for a long time, the body must replace the muscle and liver carbohydrate (glycogen) that was used during exercise.

Insulin. As we explained earlier, insulin therapy will be adjusted to your food intake, making consistency important in both food intake and insulin injections. Blood glucose monitoring can be used to make daily adjustments in this balance, but don't react to one high blood glucose by skipping snacks or cutting back on meals. Wait for patterns to develop and then make appropriate changes in food or insulin (see Chapter 5 for information on "pattern control").

Total Daily Calories. It is important that your meal plan has the right number of daily calories to help you reach or maintain desirable weight. Children need enough calories to allow for normal growth as well. And pregnant women need extra calories to meet the needs of the growing baby as well as their own needs.

Dietitians use general guidelines to estimate what a person's caloric needs will be. These are used to design a trial meal plan, which the person follows for a time to see if it does meet his or her needs and tastes. The weight of adults and growth patterns of children are monitored during this time to see if changes in the number of calories are needed.

Children's Growth Needs

For children and young adults, caloric needs will be based on age, height, and activity level. It is important to record height and weight on a growth chart at least every three to six months. If height or weight fails to increase in a child who should be growing, the cause must be investigated. Some possible causes are not enough calories and/or poor control of diabetes.

An example of a height and weight chart is shown below. You can see that the boy being charted was growing in the 75th percentile before developing diabetes. This means that if 100 boys his age were lined up according to height, 75 would be shorter and 25 would be taller than he is. But after this boy developed diabetes, his growth slowed to about the 25th percentile, meaning that out of 100 boys his age, 75 are now taller than he is. This change in growth rate should not happen. The growth chart allows a health professional to detect slowed growth early, when meal plan changes and/or diabetes control can still restore normal growth.

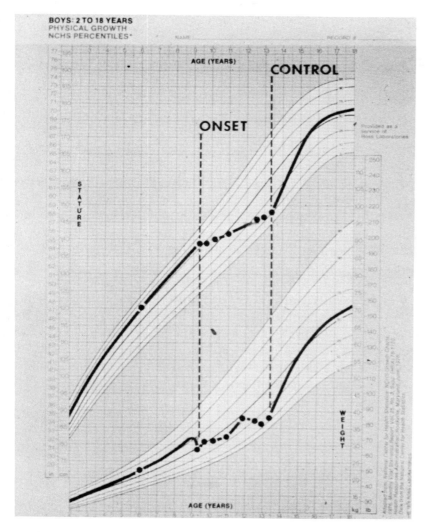

In general, children and young adults need the following number of calories each day. If they are very active or tall for their age they may need more.

Children under 12 years of age: 1,000 calories plus 100 calories per year of age. For example, a 10-year-old would need about 2,000 calories a day.

Boys age 12 to 15: 1,000 calories plus 100 calories per year of age through 11 and then 200 calories per year from age 12 to 15. For example, a 13-year-old boy needs about 2,500 calories a day (1,000 + 1,100 + 400 = 2,500).

Girls age 12 to 15: This will vary depending on the girl's activity level. Caloric needs often drop during the late teen years, so it is important to adjust the meal plan at this time to avoid excess weight.

Young men age 15 to 20: A young man who is moderately active will need about 18 calories per pound of weight per day. Heavy activity will increase his needs to about 20 to 25 calories per pound and if he is relatively inactive his needs will drop to about 15 calories per pound.

Young women age 15 to 20: A moderate activity level requires about 14 to 16 calories per pound of weight per day.

Adult Caloric Needs

To determine how many daily calories an adult needs, it is first necessary to find the person's desirable body weight. The following general guidelines can be used:

For women: 100 pounds for the first 5 feet and then add 5 pounds for each additional inch.

For men: 106 pounds for the first 5 feet and then add 6 pounds for each additional inch.

Frame size: It is important to allow for a person's frame size, which is the general size of the bones, when figuring desirable body weight. Wrist or elbow measurements are often used to find whether a person has a large, medium, or small frame. If the person has a small frame, 10% is subtracted from the above weight, and 10% is added for a large frame.

An estimate of an adult's daily caloric needs can be made once desirable weight is calculated. This is an approximate number, which may change based on the person's activity level and lifestyle. The best way to determine an accurate and acceptable daily caloric level is to monitor the person's weight for several months. If progress is not made toward reaching desirable weight, or if the person who is at desirable weight starts to lose or gain weight, changes can be made in the number of daily calories.

Caloric Estimates:

- **For moderately active adults:** 15 calories per pound of desirable body weight. Higher activity levels will demand additional calories and body weight should be monitored closely to make sure needs are being met.
- **For mostly inactive adults or after age 55:** 13 calories per pound of desirable body weight.
- **For obese or very inactive adults:** 10 calories per pound of desirable body weight.

Losing Weight

If an individual needs to lose weight, the meal plan must include fewer calories than the person burns each day. About 3,500 calories are stored in each pound of body fat. So to lose one pound of fat, the person must either reduce caloric intake, increase energy expenditure, or do a combination of both to equal a 3,500-calorie loss over several days. To lose one pound a week, you would need to consume 500 fewer calories per day than you need to maintain current weight, giving you a 3,500-calorie deficit after seven days. To lose two pounds per week, a 1,000-calorie-a-day deficit is needed. (To gain weight you would reverse the procedure, but continue exercising so that most of the added weight will be lean weight rather than fat.)

Generally we do not recommend daily caloric levels below 1,200 for women and 1,500 for men. At lower levels it is difficult to meet nutrient requirements, and it becomes such a limited diet that it is difficult to follow.

The best way to lose weight is to combine extra energy expenditure with a cutback in caloric intake. The extra energy you burn could come from a regular exercise program or from changes in routine activities to make them more active, such as taking the stairs instead of the elevator, walking or biking to the store instead of driving, etc. See Chapter 3 for information about exercise and Chapter 13 for information about percent body fat and weight loss.

The best way to lose body fat is to reduce calories, increase activity, and change eating habits.

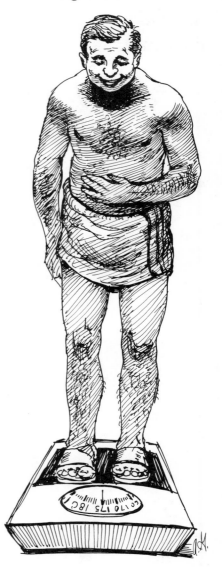

How does illness affect food needs?

Diabetes can get rapidly out of control during illness. Fever, dehydration (loss of body fluid), infection and stress of illness can all trigger the release of "stress" hormones (glucagon, epinephrine and nor-epinephrine, cortisol, growth hormone) that raise blood glucose levels. As a result of this, the body requires additional insulin.

Insulin helps keep blood glucose in the normal range. Insulin also prevents the uncontrolled breakdown of fat, which leads to ketoacidosis. When there is not enough insulin to allow blood glucose to be used as the body's energy source, the body then starts using fat for energy. When too much fat is burned, ketones are produced rapidly and in larger quantities than the body can use. When the body does not have the help of adequate amounts of insulin, the ketones build up in the blood and then are filtered into the urine so the body can get rid of them. When present in large amounts in the blood, ketones cause ketoacidosis. If untreated, ketoacidosis can lead to coma and even death.

People with insulin-dependent (Type I) diabetes **must** have insulin throughout illness to prevent ketoacidosis. People with non-insulin-dependent diabetes (Type II) who take insulin or diabetes pills to help control blood glucose also must continue taking their medication. Even people with Type II diabetes who are not taking insulin or diabetes pills may temporarily need insulin to control blood glucose during times of illness.

During brief illness you can manage your food and insulin balance by following the guidelines explained on the next page. These guidelines apply to mild, one-day illnesses.

Insulin requirements may increase during illness, even though food intake is decreased

Guidelines for Managing a Brief Illness

1. It is very important when you are ill to take your usual dose of insulin or diabetes pill. Your need for insulin continues or increases during illness. Never omit your insulin.

2. Blood glucose monitoring and urine testing for ketones (see Chapter 4) should be done at least four times a day—before each meal and at bedtime—and they may need to be done more frequently. Even with blood glucose monitoring you still need to test urine for ketones. If your blood glucose reading is higher than 240 mg/dl, it is especially important to test a urine sample for ketones. The combination of high blood glucose and moderate to large ketones in the urine is a danger signal. Call your health care provider if this happens.

3. If you can't eat your regular foods, replace them with carbohydrates in the form of liquids or soft foods (see next page for "Foods to Replace Meals During Brief Illness"). Eat at least 50 grams of carbohydrates every three to four hours, especially if blood glucose level is 240 mg/dl or less. This will provide some readily available sugar so the body won't have to burn fat for energy, which produces ketones. It will also prevent blood glucose from dropping too rapidly. Because the simple carbohydrate foods used during illness are absorbed very rapidly, it is important to consume them in small, frequent feedings.

If your blood glucose levels are higher than 240 mg/dl, don't be too concerned if you are unable to consume the entire 50 grams of carbohydrate. However, be sure to continue drinking fluids, especially fluids that do not contain calories, such as water, broth, diet pop, tea, etc.

4. Drink a large glass of one of the above liquids every hour. During illness body fluids and minerals are lost rapidly and must be replaced to prevent dehydration. This is especially true if you have a fever, diarrhea, or vomiting. If you are feeling nauseated or are vomiting, take small sips of liquids—one or two tablespoons every 15 to 30 minutes—and call your health care provider.

5. Call your health care provider if you need help. These guidelines apply to mild, short-term, one-day illnesses only. If you are unable to eat regular foods for more than one day, or if you are vomiting or having diarrhea, call your health care provider.

6. When illness subsides you can return to your regular meal plan (and regular insulin dosage if your doctor has increased it during the illness). Call or visit your health care provider if you think continued insulin adjustment might be necessary.

Call your health care provider if you have high blood glucose and moderate or large ketones.

Foods to Replace Meals During Brief Illness

The following foods contain concentrated sugar and are easily tolerated by most individuals during periods of illness. To replace 10 grams or 15 grams of carbohydrate, use any of the following foods in the amount indicated.

Foods Containing 10 Grams Carbohydrate

	Quantity
Carbonated beverage containing sugar (gingerale, cola)	1/2 cup (4 oz.)
Popsicle	1/2 twin bar
Corn syrup or honey	2 tsp.
Granulated sugar	2½ tsp. or 5 small cubes
Sweetened gelatin (Jello)	1/4 cup
Coke syrup	1 Tbsp. (½ oz.)

Foods Containing 15 Grams Carbohydrate

	Quantity
Orange juice, grapefruit juice	1/2 cup
Grape juice	1/3 cup
Ice cream	1/2 cup
Cooked cereal	1/2 cup
Sherbet	1/4 cup
Jello	1/3 cup
Broth-based soups, reconstituted with water	1 cup
Cream soups	1 cup
Carbonated beverages containing sugar (gingerale, cola)	3/4 cup (6 oz.)
Milkshake	1/4 cup
Milk	1½ cups (10 oz.)
Eggnog, commercial	1/2 cup
Tapioca pudding	1/3 cup
Custard	1/2 cup
Yogurt, plain	1 cup
Toast	1 slice
Saltine crackers	6

For More Information on Nutrition

There are many other situations in which information about nutrition can make diabetes management easier and eating more fun. Chapter 27 (and chapters 15 and 16 in *Exchanges for All Occasions*) will give you more information about eating out in restaurants. Chapter 17 in *Exchanges* contains useful tips for meal planning while traveling. Chapter 27 (chapter 20 in *Exchanges*) contain ideas for holiday menus. Food labeling and information on alternative sweeteners are discussed in Chapter 27 (chapters 24, 25, and 26 in *Exchanges*). Chapter 30 and 31 in *Exchanges* will give you information on how to modify your own recipes to lower fat and calories and increase fiber.

The *International Diabetes Center* publishes several other sources of nutrition information which can make meal planning and dining more convenient and healthy for everyone. *Convenience Food Facts* contains nutrient values for more than 1,500 name-brand processed food products. The nutrient tables list the product name; serving size; number of calories; grams of carbohydrate, protein and fat; milligrams of sodium; and exchange value. Fast Food Facts includes the same nutrient information for menu items from popular fast-food restaurants. *Opening the Door to Good Nutrition* is a step-by-step guide for anyone wishing to make changes in eating habits and improve nutrition to lower the risks for various diseases. *The Joy of Snacks* is a new cookbook designed to help you prepare easy, nutritious snacks that make eating fun. (See Appendix for ordering information.)

Armed with the information from this manual and other nutrition publications, meal planning can be enjoyable. It can help control blood glucose and blood fat levels, provide healthy and nutritious meals, and at the same time taste good. After all, "the proof of the pudding is in the eating!"

Short-Term Complications can result in high or low levels of blood glucose.

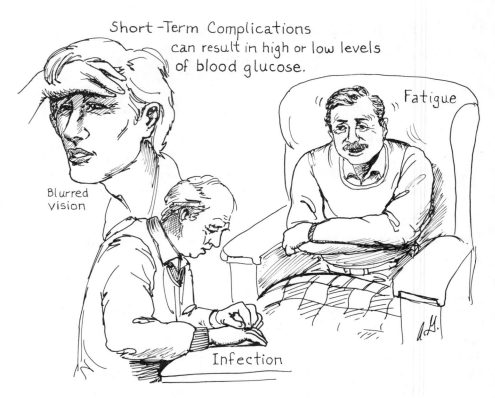

Fatigue

Blurred vision

Infection

Intermediate Complications can affect growth, development and pregnancy.

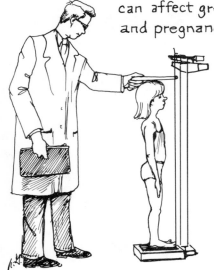

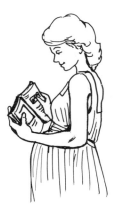

Long-term complications

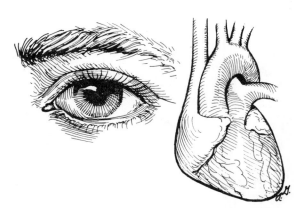

Chapter 11
What You Need to Know About the Possible Complications of Insulin-Dependent (Type I) Diabetes

Richard M. Bergenstal, M.D.

Like many other diseases, diabetes affects more than just one system in the body. Much has been learned in recent decades about the total effects, or complications, of diabetes. This knowledge about diabetes complications was made possible because people with diabetes began to live longer after the discovery of insulin in the late 1920s. Since that time, doctors and researchers have been learning more about how to help people with diabetes live long, healthy, productive lives. Much of this challenge has involved recognizing, treating, and looking for ways to prevent complications of diabetes.

A major change in health care philosophy has occurred as a result of experience with chronic diseases such as diabetes. We now know that the individual and family members can play a major role in staying healthy and living well. This is especially true for diabetes because it demands close attention every day, which only the individual and family can provide. Studies are beginning to show that besides improving everyday health and wellbeing, well-informed and strongly motivated individuals can reduce their risks of developing complications of diabetes. This chapter will explain the different types of short-term, intermediate, and long-term complications that can occur, and it will refer you to other chapters for more information about each complication and specific steps you can take to reduce your risks.

What is meant by short-term, intermediate, and long-term complications?

Complications associated with diabetes can be divided into three groups. First, those that are short-term, meaning they can develop in minutes to days and are usually completely reversible if recognized early and treated appropriately. The second group, intermediate complications, can become a concern over months to years, but problems can usually be prevented with proper treatment. The third group, long-term complications, usually develop gradually over years to decades, and treatment is aimed at slowing the progression of the problem or learning the best way to cope with it, as opposed to completely reversing the complication.

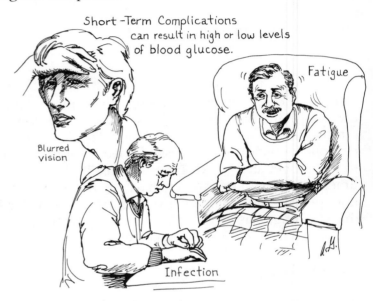

Short-Term Complications can result in high or low levels of blood glucose.

Fatigue

Blurred vision

Infection

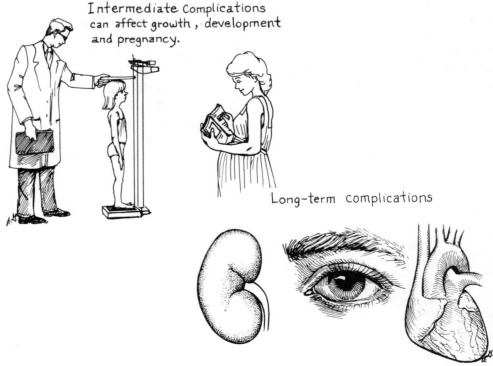

Intermediate Complications can affect growth, development and pregnancy.

Long-term complications

SHORT-TERM COMPLICATIONS

Symptoms of a High or Low Level of Glucose in the Blood

Anything that causes the blood glucose to rise for a period of time (fever, stress, underactivity, overeating, not enough insulin) may lead to the development of the same symptoms (feelings) that often occur when diabetes first develops. These include increased thirst, excessive urination, weight loss, fatigue and other symptoms discussed in previous chapters. These uncomfortable feelings are short-term complications because with correction of the cause leading to the high blood glucose the symptoms will go away.

Low blood glucose (hypoglycemia) can develop within minutes, causing shakiness, sweating, dizziness, headaches, or confusion. These symptoms disappear just as quickly with prompt treatment.

Diabetic Ketoacidosis and Severe Hypoglycemia

Developing extremely high blood glucose levels (diabetic ketoacidosis) or unconsciousness from low blood glucose levels (hypoglycemic coma) are possible complications that can develop in just a few hours or days. These problems were discussed in detail in Chapter 8.

Blurry Vision

Blurry vision is also a short-term complication or side-effect of diabetes due to high blood glucose. A high level of glucose in the blood also increases the level of glucose in the lens of the eye, which causes the lens to swell. Since the lens of the eye is important in focusing the incoming images, any swelling of the lens will result in blurry vision, as if one were wearing glasses with the wrong prescription. This blurring is due to the increased glucose level, and will go away when the blood glucose level is corrected. It does not cause permanent damage to the eyes.

Infections

Individuals with diabetes are often told they are at increased risk of developing infections. In a general sense this is true, but increased risk for infections appears to be linked at least in part to high blood glucose levels. The most common infections involve the skin (especially the feet), the kidney or bladder, the vaginal area, the ears, and the lungs (bronchitis or pneumonia). Often one of these infections may be present at the time diabetes is diagnosed.

A high level of glucose in the blood leads to an increased amount of glucose in body tissues, especially in the bladder, kidney and vagina. This high glucose environment is ideal for allowing bacteria to multiply and cause an infection. High blood glucose levels have also been shown to paralyze one of the body's defenses against infection, the white blood cells.

Ask your health care provider about the following infection-related topics:

- **Flu Shot:** Recommended yearly (in the fall) for older people with diabetes. This shot helps prevent or minimize types of flu or virus called influenza. This type of flu often results in a long illness, during which it is difficult to control one's diabetes. It also raises the risk of developing pneumonia. A flu shot does not prevent common colds.
- **Pneumonia Shot (Pneumovax):** This is given once in an individual's lifetime. It prevents the most common type of bacterial pneumonia (Pneumonococcal pneumonia), often called walking pneumonia. This shot is recommended for some people at high risk of developing infections, including some people with diabetes.
- **Use of an Intrauterine Contraceptive Device (IUD):** There is some concern that this form of birth control may lead to an increased risk of pelvic infections, especially if glucose control is poor. This should be discussed with a woman's gynecologist.

INTERMEDIATE COMPLICATIONS

Growth and Development

Poor blood glucose control can upset the way the body changes food into energy for current needs and for growth and development of sexual characteristics. This is why children and adolescents with diabetes should have regular height and weight measurements made and recorded on a growth chart (see Chapter 10). This is discussed under intermediate complications because there can be a dramatic improvement in delayed growth and physical development if blood glucose is brought under good control and an appropriate meal plan is followed.

Pregnancy

Excellent blood glucose control must be maintained before and during pregnancy.

Diabetes and pregnancy is discussed in detail in Chapter 17. In the months before and during pregnancy special attention must be given to achieving excellent blood glucose control in order to avoid possible complications for the mother and baby. It is important that diabetes is in good control before a woman becomes pregnant, because poor blood glucose control can affect the baby's health even before the woman knows she is pregnant. With proper pre-pregnancy planning and close follow-up throughout the pregnancy a healthy baby can be expected. No longer is diabetes a reason not to have a family.

174

LONG-TERM COMPLICATIONS

Which parts of the body are affected?

Diabetes can sometimes cause gradual damage to various organs in the body, including the eyes, kidneys, and heart, and can also damage body systems such as the nervous system and the blood vessel system. These gradual types of problems are referred to as long-term complications. Diabetes greatly increases the risk of gradual damage to blood vessels. Different parts of the body can be affected depending on the size of the damaged blood vessels. For instance, small blood vessel (microvascular) damage is primarily responsible for long-term problems in the eyes and kidneys. Large blood vessel (macrovascular) damage can cause complications such as heart attacks, strokes, or poor blood circulation to the arms and legs.

Diabetes can also affect the nervous system throughout the body. This can result in reduced sensitivity to touch, temperature, and pain, especially in the feet and hands. The function of nerves in any part of the body may be affected. Certain areas of the body are more likely than others to be affected by a combination of blood vessel and nerve problems. One example is the need for special care of the feet, because they depend on a combination of healthy large blood vessels, small blood vessels, and nerves.

Microvascular
Eyes & Kidneys

Macrovascular
Heart attacks, strokes, poor blood circulation in arms & legs.

What causes long-term complications?

Enormous efforts are being put into finding the causes of the long-term complications of diabetes. These efforts have identified certain factors that are likely to play an important role.

High blood glucose (hyperglycemia) and the changes it causes in the way the body functions appear to have a major influence on the development of long-term complications. This evidence has led to efforts to obtain "tight control" of blood glucose levels in the hope of preventing or slowing the development of long-term complications. Most diabetes experts agree that good blood glucose control appears to slow the development of complications. Yet experts admit that the perfect study to prove whether maintaining normal blood glucose levels will prevent complications in man has not yet been done. It is also realized that there are other factors besides blood glucose levels that are also important.

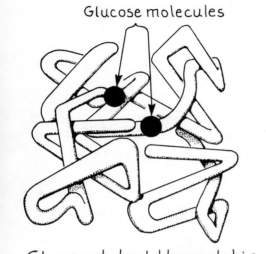

Glucose molecules

Glycosylated Hemoglobin

IF the glucose level is high, more glucose than normal attaches to hemoglobin in red blood cells.

How does high blood glucose cause damage?

There are several ways high blood glucose levels appear to damage various systems in the body:

1. Thickening of small blood vessels

High blood glucose levels and other related factors appear to lead to a thickening of the lining (basement membrane) of small blood vessels (capillaries). This appears to damage the small blood vessels by making them leak and unable to supply needed nutrients. This is most evident in the eyes and kidneys.

2. Attaching onto body proteins

As glucose circulates in the bloodstream it attaches to many proteins, including the protein in the red blood cell called hemoglobin. By measuring how much glucose attaches to the hemoglobin protein we get a fairly good estimate of the average blood glucose for the individual during the preceeding four to eight weeks, which is how long a red blood cell lives. This has become a helpful test to look at how well the blood glucose has been controlled over a long period of time. This test is called a **glycosylated** (which means to attach glucose onto) **hemoglobin** or **hemoglobin A1C** test (see Chapter 4). Results of this test vary depending on the procedure used, but the International Diabetes Center standards are to keep the A1C level below 6.8%.

When glucose levels are high, excess glucose attaches not only to hemoglobin but also to other proteins. This may be responsible for some complications. For example, glucose attaching to protein in the lens of the eye may lead to cataracts. And glucose attaching to proteins in the tissue of the hands or the joints may lead to stiff hands or a type of arthritis.

3. Accumulating in body tissues

Certain tissues have the ability to change the glucose that passes through them into an alcohol form of sugar called sorbitol. The higher the blood glucose the more sorbitol accumulates; this appears to disrupt the normal functioning of these tissues. If sorbitol accumulates in nerves it appears to be partly responsible for the nerve damage sometimes experienced by people with diabetes. It may also build up in the kidneys and the eyes. Drugs are now being tested that prevent glucose from being changed into sorbitol (Aldose Reductase Inhibitors).

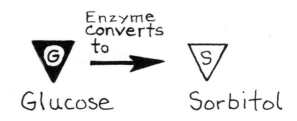

Enzyme converts to

Glucose   Sorbitol

What factors other than high blood glucose contribute to long-term complications?

Hormone Imbalances

Insulin is the hormone that is most important in regulating blood glucose levels. But there are other hormones that can influence blood glucose levels. Examples are epinephrine, cortisol, glucagon, growth hormone and thyroid hormone. These hormones must also be kept in balance to maintain normal blood glucose levels.

High Blood Pressure (Hypertension)

It is now clear that high blood pressure can greatly increase the damage caused by high blood glucose levels. The kidneys, eyes, and heart are very sensitive to high blood pressure, particularly if high blood glucose levels have already caused some weakening of the tissues. Acceptable blood pressures vary somewhat with age but in general should not be above 140/90. The top figure (systolic) is the pressure on blood vessels when blood is being pumped through them by the heart, and the bottom figure (diastolic) is the pressure when the heart is resting.

There are many medications and other methods used to control high blood pressure. Medications should be selected carefully for the individual with diabetes because some of them may increase blood glucose levels or have other undesirable effects. Some can increase levels of fats in the blood or make it difficult to recognize an insulin reaction (hypoglycemia).

High Levels of Cholesterol and Triglycerides in the Blood

The two major fats (lipids) carried by the blood—cholesterol and triglycerides—have been shown to increase the risk for the development of heart and blood vessel disease (cardiovascular disease). These fats may be high because of a genetic trait passed on in the family, excessive amounts of fat in the diet, and/or high blood glucose levels. Whatever the cause of the high level of fats in the blood, it is important to attempt to lower it into the normal range. The average American range for blood fat levels is too high, so ask your health care provider to test your blood for these fats and if necessary help you reduce them to healthy levels (see Chapter 2).

Smoking

Smoking is another factor that can greatly increase the risk of developing heart and blood vessel disease. Smoking is especially harmful in anyone with another risk factor for heart and blood vessel disease, which includes everyone with diabetes, high blood pressure, and high blood fat levels. The risk of heart disease is reduced promptly and greatly when an individual becomes a nonsmoker (see Chapters 16 and 19).

Obesity

Being overweight increases one's risk of developing high blood pressure, Type II diabetes, and high blood fat levels. Since all of these factors are also known to increase the risk for cardiovascular disease, it makes sense to avoid obesity as a preventive measure, especially when one has diabetes.

Alcohol

As discussed in Chapter 2, alcohol has certain effects that must be understood and planned for if alcoholic beverages are consumed by persons with diabetes. Consuming large amounts of alcohol can damage nerves and/or increase nerve problems already present because of diabetes. Impotence and numbness in the feet are especially common when a person with diabetes regularly drinks large amounts of alcohol.

Prevention

Major positive steps include good blood glucose control, normal blood pressure and blood lipids, not smoking, maintaining a healthy weight, and limiting alcohol intake.

While there is now a great deal of emphasis being placed on controlling blood glucose levels in order to slow or prevent the development of long-term complications, the person with diabetes and the health care team must not overlook the other risk factors mentioned above. As we continue to learn more about the precise causes of the long-term complications we will discover new steps to take in preventing and treating them. At the moment there are some very positive steps that can be taken, including improving the control of blood glucose, blood pressure and blood lipids; not smoking; maintaining a healthy weight; and limiting alcohol consumption. These steps are major objectives leading to the goal of a healthy and enjoyable lifestyle.

We have briefly mentioned that many body systems can be affected by the long-term complications of diabetes and that there are many factors contributing to the risk of damage to these tissues. We will now look at the major organs involved and describe how you and your health care providers can lower your risks, monitor whether or not these complications are developing, and treat them appropriately. This will be just a brief overview, and each organ system will be discussed in much greater detail in Section Four.

The Eyes

Diabetes is the leading cause of new cases of blindness in people between the ages of 24 and 70. Partial or total loss of vision can result from damage to the retina, the light-sensing tissue in the back of the eye. Vision loss can also be due to glaucoma (increased pressure in the eye), or cataracts (cloudiness in the lens of the eye). Retinal damage, glaucoma, and cataracts are all much more common in individuals with diabetes than in the general population.

Changes in the eyes can be caused by Type I or Type II diabetes. In Type I diabetes, eye damage is rare in the first 5 years, but the risk increases the longer one has the disease. However, in Type II diabetes, eye changes may be present at the time of diagnosis, since the diabetes may have gone undetected for a number of years. Also, people with Type II diabetes are more likely to have additional risk factors such as high blood pressure at the time of diagnosis. It is important to achieve good blood glucose control and normal blood pressure to reduce the risk of eye damage.

Your eyes should be checked at least once a year for changes related to diabetes.

Important advances have been made in preventing minor eye changes from becoming major problems. For example, laser therapy for retinal changes has been effective when used early and in the proper situations. Also, the use of special eye drops to treat glaucoma will decrease the pressure in the eye and decrease the chance of loss of vision. Cataracts can often be surgically removed and vision improved, and good blood glucose control appears to decrease the occurrence of cataracts.

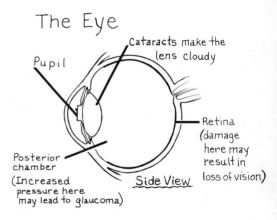

Individuals with diabetes must have regular eye examinations with the pupils dilated (drops put in) at least yearly, even if one's vision is normal. The eye is the only place in the body one can directly see the small blood vessels which can be affected by diabetes. An ophthalmologist (a doctor specializing in diseases of the eye, not an optician who prescribes glasses) or a diabetes specialist should check your eyes at least once a year if you have had Type I diabetes for more than five years.

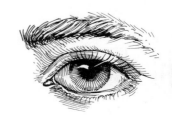

The Kidneys

The kidneys contain many small blood vessels which act as filters to remove waste products from the bloodstream. Urine is then formed to carry the waste out of the body. One fourth of all new cases of kidney failure occur in people with diabetes. Since one cannot directly see the small blood vessels in the kidney like you can in the eye, we need other tests to see if the kidney is healthy. The best test for kidney function is to check a urine sample for protein. Protein in the urine is the earliest sign that there is some irritation of the small blood vessels in the kidney. It can be found even before there is actual damage to kidney function. If protein is present in the urine, regular blood tests should be done to monitor the function of the kidneys. Recent studies have shown that this condition can be reversed with good control. The most common blood tests are blood urea nitrogen (BUN), and creatinine (Cr.), which are measurements of the amounts of waste products in the blood.

People with diabetes should be checked regularly for high blood pressure and kidney infections, and if necessary, should be treated promptly and vigorously, since both may hurt kidney function. Certain medications may also be damaging to the kidney and should be used cautiously in individuals with diabetes.

If extensive damage to the kidneys does occur, an artificial kidney machine can be used to filter the blood (dialysis). A kidney transplant (replacing the kidney) is another option that can help maintain or restore kidney function. However, both dialysis and kidney transplants are extreme measures that require great amounts of time, energy, and money.

Protein in the urine indicates a need for further kidney evaluation.

Kidneys filter blood from the heart and empty wastes into the bladder

The Heart and Blood Vessels

Whereas damage to the eyes and kidneys involves small blood vessels (microvascular disease), individuals with diabetes are also at risk for accelerated large blood vessel disease (macrovascular disease). Damage to large blood vessels can result in hardening of the arteries (atherosclerosis), heart attacks or heart failure, strokes, cramps in the legs due to a lack of blood supply to the muscles (claudication), or foot infections. Besides diabetes the risk factors of high blood pressure, high level of blood fats, and smoking all contribute to one's risk of cardiovascular disease.

The Nerves

As mentioned earlier, diabetes can damage any part of the nervous system. It appears that high blood glucose levels can damage the nerves. Since the nerves to the toes and fingers are the longest nerves in the body, they have a longer path over which to be affected and are often the first nerves to show damage due to diabetes. This nerve damage may cause pain, a sensation of pins and needles, numbness, and/or loss of feeling in the feet and hands.

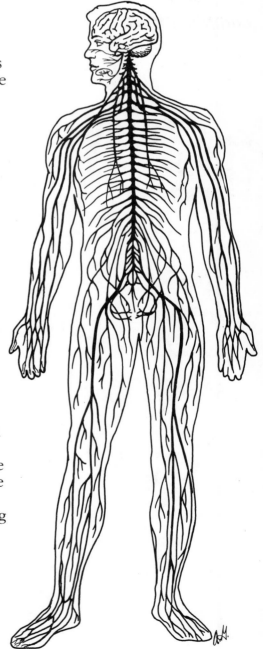

The nerves to the organs (autonomic nerves) may also be damaged. Signs of damage to these nerves may be:
- Delayed emptying of the stomach causing bloating
- Changes in bowel habits (constipation or diarrhea)
- Increased heart rate
- Drop in blood pressure and dizziness when first standing up
- In men, changes in the ability to have or maintain an erection (impotence)

Your doctor can monitor your nervous system by asking you about various symptoms and by directly measuring the nerve function. Measurements might include testing your ability to feel a light touch or a pin prick, testing your reflexes, or measuring your heart rate and blood pressure while you are sitting and then standing. Sometimes more sophisticated testing by a neurologist may be needed. A test called a nerve conductor velocity (NCV) and another called an electromylogram (EMG) can measure how nerve impulses have been disrupted. Nerve pain (neuropathy) often goes away when blood glucose control is improved. If blood glucose control does not relieve the pain, there are some medications that your doctor might prescribe (Tegretol, Elavil, Prolixin, Dilantin). These must be used under close medical supervision. New medications for nerve impairment are being tested.

*Blood glucose control,
early recognition and
prompt treatment can
minimize the risk of
long-term
complications.*

Summary

Considerable progress has been made toward understanding the causes and consequences of many of the short-term, intermediate, and long-term complications of diabetes. We have emphasized positive steps that can be taken to reduce the risk of developing these problems, and we have discussed signs and symptoms to watch for in monitoring the onset or progress of these complications. We have also outlined some of the effective treatment measures currently available.

However, there are many answers we do not yet have about complications. That is why the International Diabetes Center and 20 other centers across the country are involved in a research study called the Diabetes Control and Complications Trial (DCCT), which is supported by the National Institutes of Health. This study will attempt to measure more precisely than previous studies whether good blood glucose control prevents or slows the development of long-term complications. See Chapter 25 for more information on this major research effort.

There has already been encouraging evidence found to support the value of efforts to improve the health and quality of life for people with diabetes. A recent study compared individuals whose diabetes was diagnosed in the 1950s to those who were diagnosed in the 1970s. Although diabetes was still associated with an increase in complications compared to the general population, the rate of development of problems was lower for the people diagnosed in recent years. This implies that as we learn more about the causes of complications and ways to treat them, and if people with diabetes and their health care providers are willing to make a commitment to work toward applying what is learned, we can expect the frequency and severity of complications to continue to diminish.

Section III

Information for People
With Non-Insulin-Dependent
(Type II) Diabetes

Your Health Care Plan
Nutrition
Diabetes Pills
Possible Complications

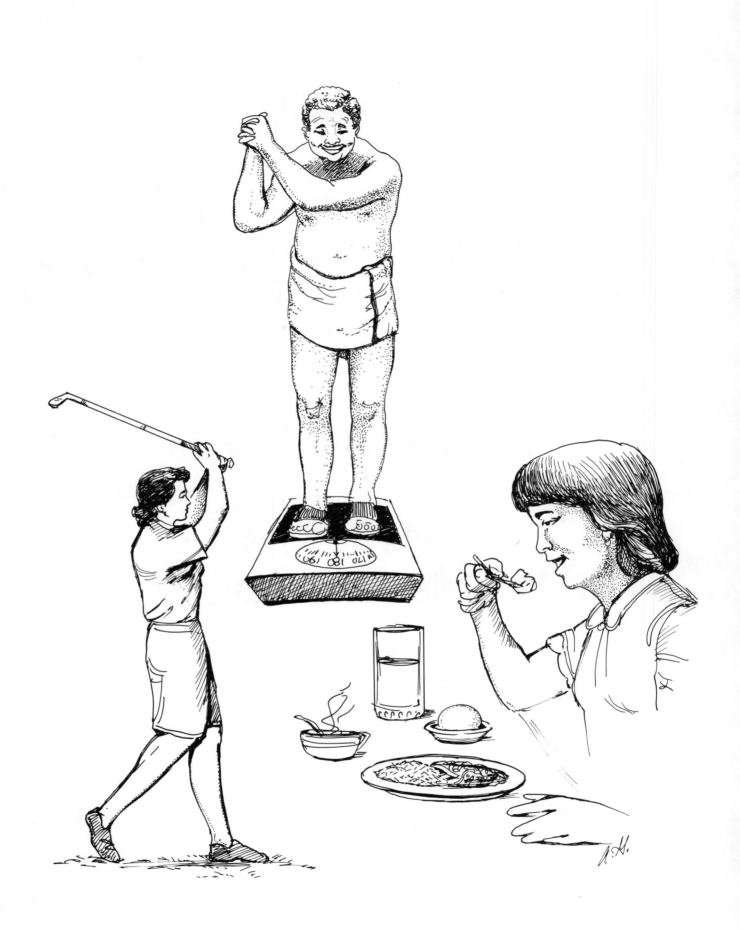

Chapter 12
Your Health Care Plan for Management of Non-Insulin-Dependent (Type II) Diabetes

Priscilla Hollander, M.D.

Diabetes can appear at any age, but as you learned in Chapter 1, the type of diabetes that usually appears in childhood (Type I) is quite different from the type of diabetes that usually appears in adulthood (Type II). Type I diabetes is often called insulin-dependent diabetes because insulin is the key to management. Type II diabetes is often called non-insulin-dependent diabetes, but it would be more helpful if it were called "meal planning-and-exercise-dependent diabetes." Nutritional guidance and exercise advice are always the first medicines given to people diagnosed as having Type II diabetes. However, if a program of meal planning, exercise, and weight loss (if necessary) does not lead to blood glucose (sugar) control, diabetes pills (oral agents) or insulin injections may be added to the health care plan.

In the past, Type II diabetes was sometimes referred to as "adult-onset," "nonketosis-prone," or "stable" diabetes. These descriptions and the general approach to Type II diabetes made it seem like a less serious form of the disease than Type I diabetes. We now know that although there are not likely to be sudden problems (ketoacidosis and hypoglycemia) if a person with Type II diabetes is not using insulin, Type II diabetes can cause serious medical problems if left undiagnosed or is poorly treated. The large blood vessels are affected by Type II diabetes, increasing by two to four times the normal chance of suffering a heart attack or stroke. Small blood vessel problems may also occur, and diabetic eye disease (retinopathy) is seen in many people with Type II diabetes. Blood circulation problems in the extremities can lead to foot infections and possibly amputation. Damage to nerves in various parts of the body is very common and can result in loss of feeling and impaired function in affected areas. Prevention and treatment of Type II diabetes complications are discussed in Chapter 15.

Many individuals with Type II diabetes and their health care providers have not appreciated the need to care for this form of the disease. We hope that this chapter will assist you in caring for your Type II diabetes just as aggressively as if it were Type I diabetes. The methods are a little different, but the goals are the same: a healthy today and many healthy tomorrows.

How is Type II diabetes different from Type I diabetes?

In Type II diabetes the individual's cells are usually resistant to the action of insulin.

Type II is by far the most common of the two types of diabetes. It affects 85 to 90 percent of all Americans known to have diabetes, or about five and one half million people. It is estimated that an additional five million people have Type II diabetes that has not yet been diagnosed. In the general U.S. population, one out of five people over the age of 65 and one out of four people over the age of 85 have Type II diabetes. If this trend continues, by the year 2000 almost 15 million Americans over the age of 40 will have this disease.

Both Type I and Type II diabetes are characterized by high blood glucose levels. The difference between the two types of diabetes is the importance of injected insulin for treatment. The role of insulin is to help move glucose from the blood into the body cells, where it can be used for energy. Insulin acts like a key, "unlocking" areas on the outside of the cell wall, allowing glucose to pass into the cell. These areas on the cell wall where insulin attaches are called **insulin receptor sites**.

In the person with Type I diabetes, the pancreas produces little or no insulin, so it is difficult for glucose to enter body cells. Body fat must then be relied on for energy, and this produces too many ketones. The person is in danger from ketoacidosis and cannot survive without insulin injections.

The situation is quite different for the person with Type II diabetes, because the pancreas is capable of producing at least some insulin. The problem is that either not enough insulin is produced, or the insulin is not effective enough to keep the blood glucose at a normal level. The reason the insulin is not effective is because of changes in the receptor sites and within the cells.

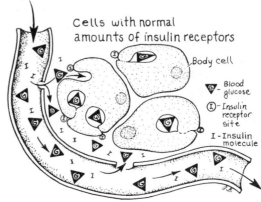

Cells with normal amounts of insulin receptors

Body cell

🔻 - Blood glucose

① - Insulin receptor site

I - Insulin molecule

Type II diabetes may cause a decrease in the number of receptor sites, so the cells become less effective at using insulin. The cells also seem to change the way they use insulin in the process of burning glucose for energy.The decrease in receptor sites and changes within the cell reduce the ability of the person with Type II diabetes to remove glucose from the blood. This problem is commonly called insulin resistance.

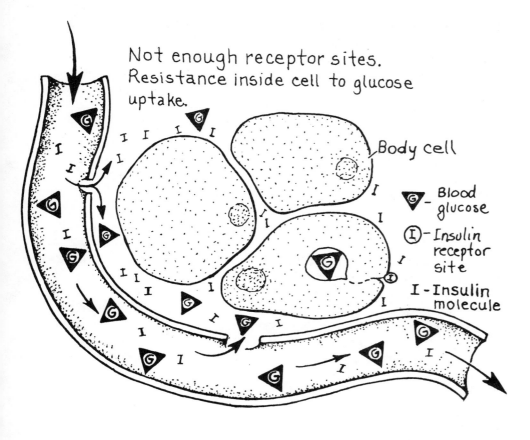

Not enough receptor sites. Resistance inside cell to glucose uptake.

Body cell

▼ - Blood glucose

ⓘ - Insulin receptor site

I - Insulin molecule

Enough insulin is present in Type II diabetes, however, so that the person's blood glucose can often be controlled by meal planning and exercise, sometimes with the addition of a diabetes pill (oral agent). (See Chapter 14 for a discussion of oral agents.) A person with Type II diabetes is very rarely at risk of developing ketoacidosis and does not need injected insulin to prevent this life-threatening problem. Your doctor may ask you to start injecting insulin if meal planning, exercise, and oral agents do not bring your Type II diabetes under control. But you do not need this insulin in the same way the person with Type I diabetes needs it to survive. Later in this chapter we'll discuss why insulin might be used to help treat Type II diabetes.

Members of families with a history of Type II diabetes should avoid obesity and be checked annually for diabetes when over age 40.

Two important factors in determining who develops Type II diabetes are heredity and obesity. Heredity plays a greater role in the appearance of Type II diabetes than Type I. Some families have a genetic make-up that makes them more likely to develop the problems of insulin inefficiency that result in Type II diabetes. There are many families in which Type II diabetes develops in one or more members of each generation. People who are members of such families are more likely to develop diabetes than are people who do not have such family backgrounds. It is important for members of families with a strong history of diabetes to be checked regularly for diabetes, especially after they reach the age of 40. It is very important that they maintain a normal weight. (More information about inheritance of Type I and Type II diabetes can be found in Chapter 24.)

Obesity is another key factor in the development of Type II diabetes. Almost 80 percent of all people with Type II diabetes are obese. People with Type I diabetes are more likely to be lean when diagnosed, because their lack of insulin makes them unable to use carbohydrates as fuel, which leads to the burning of stored fat.

Obesity is related to the appearance of Type II diabetes because it causes insulin resistance (the decreased number of receptor sites and changes within cells which result in poor use of insulin). Insulin does not function well in people who are obese, whether or not they have diabetes. However, obese people who do not have an inherited tendency to develop diabetes can overcome insulin resistance by releasing extra insulin from their pancreas. In overweight people who have an inherited tendency to develop diabetes, the pancreas cannot produce extra insulin needed to control blood glucose levels, and Type II diabetes develops.

In a person with Type II diabetes who is not overweight, meal planning and exercise still play a major role in treatment. Caloric intake is set at a level that will meet daily needs, and a healthy distribution of carbohydrates, protein, and fat are planned to maintain good blood glucose and blood fat levels. If these steps are not successful in controlling diabetes, the next step would be either an oral agent or insulin therapy.

Both Type I and Type II diabetes are diagnosed on the basis of elevated blood glucose levels. Normal fasting blood glucose levels are between 60 and 120 mg/dl. Fasting blood glucose levels that are higher than 140 mg/dl on two occasions, or fasting blood glucose below 140 but 200 or higher two hours after a 75-gram glucose tolerance test would be considered abnormal and would result in a diagnosis of diabetes.

Type I diabetes usually occurs rapidly, with the person's fasting blood glucose going from normal to high values such as 300-400 mg/dl in a matter of days or weeks. This is not true for Type II diabetes, in which increases in blood glucose may occur very slowly over many months or even years. A person with Type II diabetes may have an average fasting blood glucose of 110 mg/dl one year, 130 mg/dl the next year, and 150 mg/dl the following year. In fact, it may take several years until this person's blood glucose gets high enough to cause the kidneys to filter glucose into the urine so that it can be detected by routine urine tests in a visit to the doctor. The blood glucose level at which glucose begins to spill into the urine is called the **renal threshold**. When average blood glucose levels exceed the renal threshold, the symptoms of diabetes begin to appear, such as frequent urination and extreme thirst. In most people, the renal threshold is between 180 and 200 mg/dl.

In Type II diabetes, increases in blood glucose levels may occur slowly over months or years before diabetes is diagnosed.

In the past, two other methods—urine testing and oral glucose tolerance tests—were commonly used for the diagnosis of diabetes. Neither of these methods is as useful for diagnosis as is the abnormal fasting blood glucose level. Urine testing is inadequate because the urine does not become positive for glucose until the blood glucose has reached the renal threshold. This may take several years in some people with Type II diabetes, so their disease would be undiagnosed for several years. This is why it is thought that five million people have Type II diabetes that has not yet been detected.

Is Type II diabetes treated the same as Type I diabetes?

The goals of treatment in Type II diabetes are really quite similar to the goals of treatment in Type I diabetes. The first goal is to help the person achieve a general sense of wellbeing, so that he or she feels well from day to day. The second and equally important goal is to help the person maintain good blood glucose control. Good blood glucose control means keeping blood glucose levels as close to normal as is possible for that particular person. Specific goals are:

Before meals—80 to 120 mg/dl
After meals—below 200 mg/dl

Most studies now support the conclusion that development and severity of long-term diabetic complications are closely associated with the average level of blood glucose. A third goal is to help the person achieve and maintain healthy levels of blood fats. High levels of cholesterol and triglycerides also have been closely associated with development of blood vessel and heart disease.

What should be done in routine care of Type II diabetes?

As a person with Type II diabetes, you should have certain expectations about your health care. Routine visits to your health care providers are important. The key to successful management of your diabetes is to involve yourself as part of the health care team and be aware of your current health and blood glucose control.

Routine health care visits for diabetes should take place three or four times a year, with one of the visits being a complete physical exam.

Routine visits should probably take place three to four times a year, and more frequently if you have other health problems. At each visit certain key aspects of your health should be checked, including weight, blood pressure, pulses, heart sounds, eye exam, and foot exam (paying particular attention to nerve responses). The doctor should review your blood glucose monitoring records with you and recommend changes if levels are often over your goals. A glycosylated hemoglobin test can also be done at each visit to evaluate your average blood glucose over the past six to eight weeks (see Chapter 4 for an explanation of this test). Your health care team can use your daily blood glucose test results and the glycosylated hemoglobin test to decide which if any changes need to be made in your health care plan.

Once a year a thorough physical examination should be completed. Special attention should be paid to cholesterol and triglyceride levels. Ideally, cholesterol levels should be below 200 milligrams and triglyceride levels below 150 milligrams. An EKG (electrical tracing of heart activity), chest x-ray, and other diagnostic tests may be done to evaluate long-term complications. Your eyes should be thoroughly examined once a year by a diabetes specialist or ophthalmologist. Your kidneys should be checked through a urine and blood test. An in-depth evaluation of your blood pressure should be made, with the pressures taken several different times. If your blood pressure is over 140/90 your doctor should work with you in an aggressive program to bring it down to the more ideal level of 120/80. Your doctor can also listen to pulse sounds in arteries in different parts of your body to determine if you are developing blood circulation problems. In other words, it is important that you receive an in-depth annual evaluation of your total health.

The Health Care Plan

When Type II diabetes is diagnosed, a health care plan is developed to control blood glucose levels. The focus of this health care plan is to decrease insulin resistance. Unlike Type I diabetes, in which insulin treatment is always necessary, many people with Type II diabetes can at first be treated with meal planning and exercise. There are three main objectives of this treatment: to cut daily caloric intake, increase physical activity, and achieve weight loss if necessary. All three of these changes have been shown to be successful in decreasing insulin resistance and lowering blood glucose.

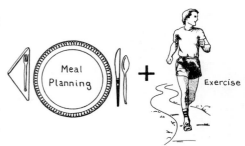

Weight loss is a key factor in treatment of most people with Type II diabetes, because as we explained earlier, obesity causes insulin resistance. If a person can lose weight, insulin resistance will decrease, making the person's own insulin more effective in lowering blood glucose. Meal planning and exercise should not be expected to work instantly, because it takes time to lose weight safely. The ability to lose weight varies from person to person, but safe weight loss should not exceed one to two pounds per week. At least three to six months may be allowed for the meal planning and exercise to take effect.

Nutritional strategy in Type II diabetes is discussed in Chapter 13. Exercise for people with Type II diabetes was discussed in the last half of Chapter 3. When the use of diet and exercise does not result in normal blood glucose levels, oral agents may be prescribed to help keep blood glucose within normal limits. Sometimes the pills are mistakenly called oral insulin, but they are not insulin and they do not work like insulin. In fact, they are not effective unless the person's pancreas is producing some insulin. Oral agents increase the effectiveness of the person's own insulin. They have been found to be effective in controlling blood glucose in about 60 percent of the individuals for whom they are prescribed. However, after several years the oral agents may lose their effectiveness, and they are usually not much help after five years of therapy.

If meal planning, exercise, and oral agents do not succeed in keeping a person's blood glucose near the normal range, he or she may need to stop using oral agents and begin injecting insulin. There are several reasons a doctor may decide to use insulin therapy in a person with Type II diabetes. One possibility would be the obese person who is not successful in losing weight. Insulin resistance from the weight may be so high that even with a meal plan, more activity, and the use of an oral agent, blood glucose will remain high and insulin injections will be needed to keep it in the normal range.

Another possibility would be a person who started out with Type II diabetes and as the years go by, his or her pancreas makes less and less insulin. This person has moved closer to Type I diabetes and needs insulin to help keep blood glucose in the normal range.

Occasionally, people with Type II diabetes will need insulin therapy for short periods of time when under stress, or during an illness such as a serious infection, a heart attack, or surgery. These situations may require more insulin than the person's pancreas is presently producing. Meal planning and/or oral agents may not meet the increased need for a short period. Once the stressful period is over, the need for extra insulin usually disappears.

If your doctor has prescribed insulin injections to help control your blood glucose, it is important that you read the section on Type I diabetes, which starts on page 129. This information will help you avoid problems, such as insulin reactions, which can occur when insulin injections are part of the health care plan.

Blood Glucose Testing

Blood glucose testing can play an important role in monitoring Type II diabetes.

A key factor in evaluating the success of the health care plan in both Type II and Type I diabetes is blood glucose monitoring. Urine glucose testing will not provide the level of control needed to achieve blood glucose levels in the normal range.

If you are injecting insulin as part of your health care plan, it is best to test blood glucose three to four times a day; before meals and at bedtime. If you are using meal planning, exercise, and/or an oral agent, test before breakfast and before and one hour after your largest meal of the day; do this two or three days a week as long as your blood glucose levels stay in the normal range.

No matter how often you test, it is important to record the results and discuss them with your health care providers. In this way you can do everything possible to feel good every day and prevent long-term health problems.

Summary

Type II diabetes is a serious disease. It affects millions of people in our society, and it has enormous social, medical, and economic consequences. In the past, individuals with Type II diabetes and their doctors did not always give the disease the attention it deserves. We now know that this was unfortunate, because the consequences of poor control and the development of long-term complications are as great in Type II diabetes as they are in Type I. This outlook is rapidly changing, however, as the importance of good blood glucose control in all people with diabetes becomes more apparent.

NOTES

Chapter 13
Type II Diabetes Nutrition: In Search of Desirable Weight

Marion Franz, R.D., M.S. and Arlene Monk, R.D., B.S.

Changes in lifestyle, including nutrition and eating behaviors, exercise, and mental wellbeing, are major goals for everyone, but especially if you have Type II diabetes. Most individuals who develop Type II diabetes are overweight at the time of diagnosis. Obesity can cause high blood pressure, increased levels of blood fats (cholesterol and triglycerides), and other health problems. This is why the nutrition goal of Type II diabetes is to help the person reach and maintain a desirable weight while keeping blood glucose and blood fat levels in the normal range.

Why are obesity and Type II diabetes related?

With obesity, the body cells become resistant to the action of insulin. On the outside wall of each cell there are places called receptor sites whose job it is to help insulin move glucose into the cell. Obesity seems to cause the number of these receptor sites to decrease, so the cells become less effective at using insulin. Obesity also seems to cause changes within the cells which make them less effective at using insulin in the process of burning glucose for energy.

Type II diabetes can often be controlled if a person is successful in changing food intake and activity patterns. However, as was explained in Chapter 12, if weight loss and meal planning are unsuccessful a diabetes pill or insulin injections may be required to return blood glucose to the normal range. The person must still follow a meal and exercise plan and test to make sure blood glucose stays in the normal range. If this person succeeds in losing weight, the pills or insulin may be reduced in dosage or even discontinued.

Because heart disease and high blood pressure (hypertension) are associated with diabetes, it is important to change nutritional factors that affect all three conditions. One way is to reduce the total amount of fat in the diet, especially saturated fats and cholesterol. Diets high in fat are associated with high levels of cholesterol, which is a risk factor for heart disease. Foods high in fat are also high in calories, so they make a major contribution to obesity, and therefore to diabetes and heart disease. See Chapter 2 for a discussion of types of fats and how to reduce fat in the diet.

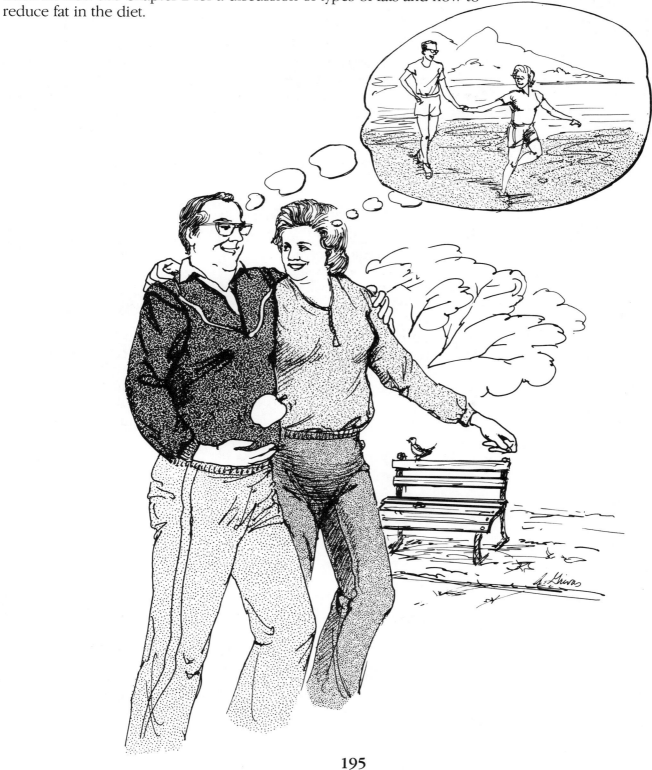

High sodium intake increases the risk of high blood pressure in susceptible individuals.

Another important nutritional change is to reduce the amount of salt eaten. More and more scientific studies are showing that the amount of sodium in the average American diet is one of the contributing causes of high blood pressure in people who are genetically susceptible. Since people with diabetes appear to be especially susceptible to high blood pressure, and high blood pressure greatly increases the severity of diabetic complications, weight loss and sodium reduction are crucial. Together they can often bring high blood pressure into the normal range.

Table salt is a common source of sodium, because salt is 40 percent sodium. The average American consumes 8 to 12 grams of salt a day, but it is recommended that salt intake be limited to no more than 5 grams a day, which is about one teaspoon. Processed foods (soups and other canned or packaged foods) and food served in fast-food restaurants are also major sources of sodium. Sodium content is sometimes listed on food packages as the number of milligrams of sodium. One teaspoon of salt is equal to about 2,300 milligrams of sodium.

To help reduce sodium:

- Experiment with herbs and spices as alternatives to salt used in cooking and salt-based condiments such as soy sauce, steak sauce, catsup, and seasoned salts.
- Cook with only a small amount of added salt.
- Be aware of sodium content of processed foods such as regular canned soups and frozen entrees and dinners.
- Add little or no salt to foods at the table. Taste foods before salting to let yourself appreciate their natural flavors, which are often obscured by salt.
- Avoid snack foods and other foods that contain visible salt.
- Limit intake of salty foods such as pickles, sauerkraut, and cured or smoked meat products such as ham, bacon, and lunch meats.

Reduce daily salt intake to:

 or or

1 teaspoon   5 grams   2300 milligrams
of sodium

From all sources

What is involved in reaching desirable body weight?

To reach and maintain desirable body weight, you must first find out what weight is desirable for your height and body frame size (muscles and bones). The best way to do this is to work with a professional who is knowledgeable and skilled in the methods of measuring what percentage of total body weight is fat. Several methods are available, but the most commonly used is called skinfold measurement. This involves the use of an instrument called a skinfold caliper, which is used to measure the thickness of fat that can be pinched on several sites on the body. These measurements are then inserted into equations that have been developed based on detailed studies of the amount of fat on men, women, and children. The resulting estimate of your percentage of body fat can be used to set goals for weight loss. Repeating the skinfold measurements every two or three months will show if you are making progress toward reaching your weight goal.

The percentage of fat that is desirable differs among individuals and between sexes. The average fat content for men is 15 to 19 percent, and for women it is 22 to 25 percent. It is thought that a more ideal percentage is between 10 and 17 percent for men, with 25 percent considered obesity; and between 20 and 22 percent for women, with greater than 30 percent considered obesity. Higher percentages are thought to contribute to high blood pressure, heart disease, and diabetes.

After you have set goals for weight loss, a health professional such as a registered dietitian can help you design a meal plan with a total caloric intake that will help you lose weight gradually. It is also important that you examine eating behaviors that may be contributing to your weight problem. The third important factor in reaching and maintaining desirable weight is increasing your activity level through a safe and moderate program of regular exercise.

Exercise can help you: burn calories, control appetite, decrease body fat, increase the amount of calories your body burns at rest, and replace stress eating. See Chapter 3 for more information about exercise and Type II diabetes.

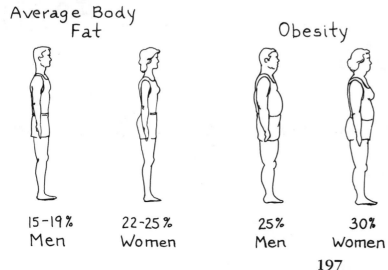

Average Body Fat

Obesity

| 15-19% Men | 22-25% Women | 25% Men | 30% Women |

197

Caloric Level

For safe and effective weight reduction, the meal plan should be nutritionally adequate for the individual, but total daily calories should be restricted. Unless the meal plan calls for fewer than 1,000 to 1,200 calories, vitamin and mineral supplements will not be necessary. Meal plans at or slightly above this caloric level can be nutritionally adequate but should be evaluated and/or designed by a dietitian.

Calories that are consumed in excess of your body's needs are stored as energy reserves—fat. Fat is a very efficient means of storage, and the body has an almost limitless capacity to accumulate fatty tissues. To lose fat, you must reverse the process by which you gained it—you must consume fewer calories than your body needs for energy. Since each pound of fat contains about 3,500 calories, to lose a pound of fat you must cut back your food by 3,500 calories or increase your energy level by 3,500 calories. Actually, the best way to lose weight is to combine calorie restriction and increased exercise.

Most people find that a level of calorie restriction that is not too hard to maintain is 500 calories per day less than the number of calories needed to stay at their present weight. By adding 250 to 300 calories of exercise per day, you can have a negative energy balance of 750 calories per day (but because of the effect of exercise, you will feel like you have more energy). This will result in a reduction of 5,250 calories in a week, which will be one and a half pounds less fat. Again, please see Chapter 3 for specific information on how to burn calories through exercise.

250 calories
Daily Exercise
       +
500 calories
Food Reduction

$\times$ 7 days = 5250 Calories

How to lose 1½ lbs. per week

Eating Habits

It is important to remember that it is not only how much and what we eat that is important, but also when and how we eat our food. For individuals whose Type II diabetes is treated with insulin or diabetes pills, regular meal times and adjusting food intake for exercise will be necessary, just as they are for individuals with Type I diabetes (see Chapter 10 for this information).

Timing of meals and adjusting food for exercise are not as crucial for individuals whose Type II diabetes is treated with meal planning and exercise alone. However, these individuals usually do better when they divide their daily food into several meals and perhaps snacks. Well-planned breakfasts and lunches are especially important to control appetite throughout the day. Also, the body of a person with Type II diabetes seems to be better able to handle food when it is divided into smaller meals and snacks. This is because the pancreas is still making insulin, but this insulin is not effective in keeping blood glucose normal. The insulin may be effective if food is eaten in smaller amounts spread over the day.

There are many other factors besides timing of meals that can contribute to obesity. The next section will discuss some specific examples of ways you can identify and change these habits.

The amount of food eaten is what is crucial in Type II diabetes.

Changing Eating Habits

Maybe you have lost weight before—maybe several times. It is not uncommon for people to lose weight and then regain the lost weight plus more. These people may feel that they are not motivated enough, but if this were so they wouldn't keep trying to lose weight. They are simply not getting to the root of their overeating problem.

There are many ways to lose weight. Diets that tell you exactly what to eat and how much to eat will produce weight loss. So will a rigid limit of calories per day, or many of the gimmicky weight-loss programs. One problem with these methods is that they are often not nutritionally balanced, so the person does not feel well while on the diet. But the larger problem is that these diets come to an end and the person goes right back to old eating habits that led to obesity in the first place. So of course the weight comes back.

There are many reasons you may be overweight. Some may be habits you developed during early childhood, while others may have resulted from change of lifestyle or occupation. The important thing to remember is that you have developed these habits over your lifetime, and you cannot expect to change them overnight. But no matter what is the cause of your obesity, with the proper mix of activity and planned eating behavior you can gradually lose weight and keep it off.

The goal is to eliminate habits that have contributed to your obesity and replace them with habits more suited to weight loss and maintaining desirable weight. Again, this will be a gradual process of unlearning reactions to food that have been learned over a lifetime. But with effort and perseverance you can change habits and reach desirable weight—and with far less pain than the fad diets ask of a person!

There are four major strategies to use in changing eating patterns. The first strategy is to become aware of your eating habits. Although you may feel you know all about your eating behavior, it is indeed rare to find someone who is aware of all the eating patterns and variables that influence eating. To become aware of your eating habits, keep a record of your food and beverage intake.

1. *Become aware of your eating habits.*

1. Record everything you eat and drink except water.
2. Record how long it takes to eat each meal and snack.
3. Record where you are eating and with whom.
4. Record what else you were doing while eating.
5. Record how hungry you were.

If you keep records honestly for a week or two, you will discover things about yourself that you never before realized. When you review your records, patterns will emerge. And you will no longer be able to fool yourself into thinking you have consumed less than you actually have. This self monitoring will develop the awareness, skills and attitudes that will be the foundation of any change you make in your eating habits.

Many behavior techniques evolve when you simply become more aware of a certain behavior. For example, eating slower while sitting in one place and not doing other things will keep you aware of the eating process. Continue to keep records throughout the behavior changing process.

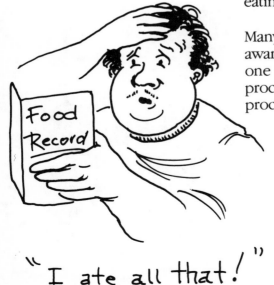

"I ate all that!"

The second strategy is to look at ways to avoid situations in which problem eating occurs. People in our society usually eat not because of physical hunger but because certain times, places and even people become associated with food and eating. For example, if you are accustomed to reading the newspaper in the kitchen and nibbling because food is close at hand, you may have to find a different place to read the newspaper. Keeping food out of sight keeps it out of mind. It will be helpful to keep food out of rooms other than the kitchen, limit food intake to one specific place in your home, change your route if a particular store or vending machine is a problem, and clear the table immediately after finishing eating.

While it is best to change your exposure to problem eating situations, it is not always possible to do so. In this case, a third strategy can be used, which is to plan how to change your susceptibility to the causes of problem eating. For example, grocery shopping may be a necessity for you, but shopping on a full stomach and with a firm shopping list can reduce the chances of impulse buying. Planning daily menus helps reduce indecision at meal times. Proper planning can also reduce the tendency to overeat at parties or restaurants. Do not try to go without food all day so that you "can eat as much as I want" later. You will be so hungry when you arrive that you will eat far more than you feel you should or even want to. By avoiding long periods without food you can arrive in a frame of mind to enjoy yourself but stick to your meal plan.

The fourth strategy is to learn to respond differently to situations you know cause your eating problems. For example, social occasions such as business lunches and parties often create eating problems. Especially if you regularly socialize, you must learn to respond to the waiter, hostess and the abundance of attractive foods in ways that allow you to enjoy yourself without overeating. Try leaving a bit of food on your plate without feeling guilty, and practice responding politely but firmly to people who try to encourage you to eat more than you intended.

In the process of changing eating habits, remember that perfection is not demanded. Most diets are followed in the all-or-nothing fashion; you are either on the diet or off it. To expect such perfection in the face of all the pressures to eat in our society is to set yourself up for failure. No one is ever totally in control or out of control. By allowing yourself some leeway and looking for gradual and permanent changes, you will avoid the pitfalls of "dieting." Set realistic goals for yourself and view your weight loss as a series of small accomplishments, each one an important step toward the results you want for yourself.

2. *Look for ways to avoid situations in which problem eating occurs.*

3. *Plan how you can change your susceptibility to the causes of problem eating.*

4. *Learn to respond differently to situations which cause your eating problems.*

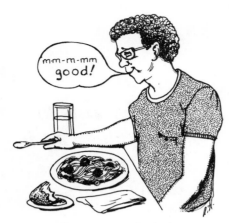

Savor each bite

The following specific tips have helped others like you make permanent changes in eating habits and lose weight:

1. **Slow down your eating speed.** By eating slower you are less likely to finish off a second helping before your body has had a chance to tell you it was satisfied with the first.

- To slow down the pace of eating, try to take 30 minutes for meals and 15 minutes for snacks.
- Put down your utensil between bites. Savor each bite. Do not put it back into food until you have swallowed what is in your mouth.
- Count your chews per bite. Try to take at least 15 chews per bite.
- When 3/4 of the meal is finished, stop eating for five minutes. At the end of this time, if you feel like eating more, continue. If you don't feel like finishing, stop and congratulate yourself.
- If you want to take a second helping, wait 10 minutes before serving yourself seconds.

2. **Eat in one location and set a full place setting for any food or beverage you take.** This reduces the number of locations you associate with food and makes it difficult to "eat on the run." Make eating a special occurrence, and take time to enjoy it.

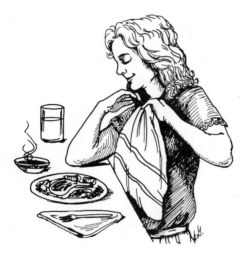

Make eating special

- Do not participate in other activities while eating. No television, radio, telephone, or reading while eating. Without these distractions, you will feel like you are getting more out of each mouthful.
- Use a smaller plate or dessert plate for your meal rather than a full dinner plate. It will seem like you are getting more food than you really are.
- Become aware of portion sizes. Use a scale and measuring cups as you begin and until you feel comfortable "eyeballing" your correct portion.
- Do not serve food family style. Instead serve your plate from the pots and pans in which it was cooked. You will be better able to resist taking seconds with this technique.
- Have someone else in the family clear the plates and put away leftovers. This reduces the temptation to nibble after you have finished your meal.

3. **Store food out of sight and out of reach.**

- Do not leave any food on the counter or table in plain view—this tests willpower too much. Use containers you can't see through.
- Store food, especially problem foods, in an inconvenient place.
- Spend less time in places or situations where you are surrounded by food.
- Avoid purchasing food that you tend to overeat, especially high calorie foods. You will be less likely to snack if it requires a walk to the grocery store rather than a walk to the kitchen.

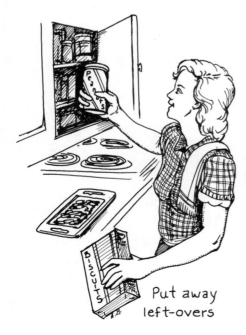

Put away left-overs

4. Change purchasing and preparation habits.

- Cut down the amount of food available to you at meals by preparing smaller portions. Prepare only one serving per person.
- Avoid buying food that you tend to overeat. Write out a shopping list before you go to the supermarket. Stick to the list and don't buy extra items.
- Avoid shopping for groceries while you are hungry. You are less likely to be attracted to foods not on your list when you shop with a full stomach.
- If eating while preparing a meal is a problem, prepare the evening meal immediately after lunch or prepare the next evening's meal immediately after supper. Then, re-heat before the meal. This will reduce the temptation to nibble.

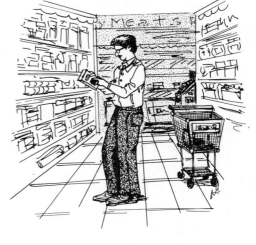

5. Make specific plans to change eating habits.

- Keep a written food diary of eating patterns. Does any pattern of overeating emerge that you could change? Set aside time each day to think ahead and plan your food intake for the next day.
- Develop the habit of eating three or more balanced meals daily. Never skip a meal. This could be dangerous if you take insulin. Besides, most people find if they skip one meal, they just overeat at the next meal.
- Try leaving a little bit of food on your plate without feeling guilty. Many people feel compelled to finish everything on their plate because of childhood "clean plate" training. This technique is especially important when eating in restaurants.
- Try drinking a glass of water, tomato or vegetable juice or a cup of broth before meals to help curb your appetite.
- Keep a supply of low calorie foods on hand—diet gelatin, raw vegetables, or diet pop.
- Don't feel compelled to eat because of social pressure. At the dinner table or at a party, you can converse without eating.
- Reward yourself (non-food related) for small units of weight loss.
- Keep a written record of weekly weights. Don't weigh yourself too often. It is easy to become discouraged if you don't see results on the scale each day.

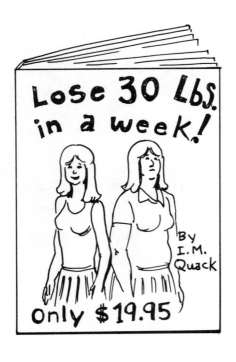

6. Set goals to gradually increase your energy expenditure. Keep written records of your exercise.

7. Avoid fad diets. New and supposedly miraculous ways of losing weight are publicized almost every day. They are popular because they promise ways that weight can be lost effortlessly and quickly. Some of the characteristics of fad diets are:

Temporary—a new fad diet seems to appear every week.

Irrational—most fad diets distort or ignore principles of good nutrition and defy the laws of nature. They may overemphasize one food or food group, assigning almost magical powers to it. They are often medically dangerous.

Something for nothing—beware of the "calories don't count" type of diet.

Limited variety—they often provide few food choices and are difficult to stick to for any length of time.

Off target—fad diets often cause loss of muscle and body water instead of fat. The water is quickly replaced and the muscle tissue loss causes loss of body tone.

Expensive!—there is usually some "special" product or food or book necessary for the "success" of the diet.

Summary

For weight loss to be successful and permanent the following guidelines should be followed:

1. Consume 500 to 1,000 calories per day less than usual in a nutritionally balanced meal plan.

2. Participate in a regular exercise program to burn additional calories and increase mental and physical well-being.

3. Identify problem eating behaviors and make gradual changes.

4. Maintain a gradual weight loss of 1 or 2 pounds per week until you reach your desirable body weight.

5. When you reach your goal weight, continue to make healthy eating habits and regular exercise a permanent part of your lifestyle. Enjoy the new you!

Chapter 14
Diabetes Pills: Giving Natural Insulin a Boost

Wayne Leebaw, M.D.

Ever since the discovery of insulin, scientists have been trying to find a diabetes medicine that does not have to be injected. Unfortunately, no way has been found to give insulin by mouth and still preserve its ability to lower blood glucose (sugar). However, in 1955, pills were developed that increase the effectiveness of the body's insulin. These pills are often called **oral agents**, or more accurately **oral hypoglycemic agents**. They are not "oral insulin" and should not be thought of as a substitute for insulin. This chapter will discuss oral agents and will help you understand when and why they are used, and how they differ from insulin.

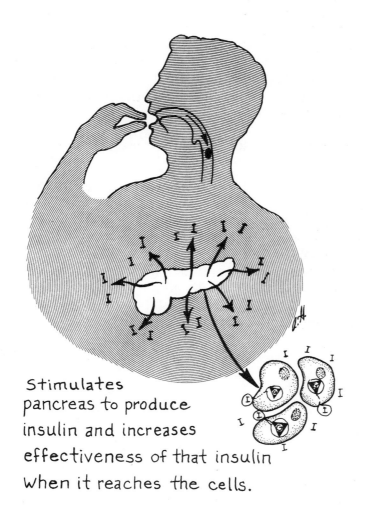

Stimulates pancreas to produce insulin and increases effectiveness of that insulin when it reaches the cells.

Why are oral agents only useful in Type II diabetes?

Despite more than 30 years of research, scientists do not completely understand how oral agents lower blood glucose. They do know, however, that some natural insulin must be present for oral agents to work. This is why they are only useful in Type II diabetes. In Type I diabetes the body stops producing insulin, so there is nothing for the oral agents to act with. Oral agents are clearly not a substitute for insulin.

It is thought that when a person with Type II diabetes first uses oral agents, the pills may stimulate the pancreas to release more insulin. But in the long run, the pills do not seem to cause an increase in insulin levels. Recent studies have shown that oral agents help lower blood glucose by increasing the effectiveness of insulin when it reaches the cells.

Diabetes specialists disagree about how to decide if a person with Type II diabetes might benefit from the use of oral agents. Most experts agree, however, that oral agents should NOT be used in Type I diabetes or by a pregnant or breast-feeding woman. They should also not be used if the person has liver or kidney disease, because the body would not be able to dispose of them and severe hypoglycemia would result as they build up in the blood. Doctors also agree that nutrition and weight control are the primary methods for controlling Type II diabetes, and that oral agents should only be used when dietary management has been unsuccessful. If the oral agents do not result in good blood glucose control after a trial period (about 3 to 6 months), their use should be stopped.

Commonly accepted guidelines for the use of oral agents are as follows:

1. Only people with Type II diabetes and who are over the age of 40 are given oral agents.
2. Oral agents are tried after meal planning and attempts at regular exercise and weight loss have been unsuccessful in providing reasonable blood glucose control.
3. Use of oral agents is continued if blood glucose levels are reasonably controlled (usually under 120 mg/dl fasting and 180 mg/dl one to two hours after eating). If high blood glucose persists despite a maximum oral agent dose, the person with Type II diabetes should be started on insulin. (See Chapter 12 for an explanation of how and why insulin is used in Type II diabetes.)

Some natural insulin must be present for oral agents to be effective.

Can any problems occur when using oral agents?

Side effects from the use of oral agents are uncommon. But as with any medication, an allergic reaction can occur if you are using oral agents. Upset stomach, loss of appetite and rashes are the most common problems. Oral agents can also cause facial flushing or other unpleasant reactions when alcohol is used.

Because they have a blood glucose lowering effect, oral agents can cause problems similar to an insulin reaction. These reactions are usually not as frequent nor as severe as insulin reactions can be, but in rare cases they may be severe enough to require hospitalization.

The most controversial problem related to the use of oral agents is their possible connection to an increased risk of heart disease. An eight-year study by a group of 12 universities, which was published in 1970, reported this possible increased risk. However, recent studies have failed to find the same increased risk of heart disease in people using oral agents. The 1970 study also has been criticized for the way it was designed and the way its conclusions were reached.

It is not likely that the controversy about oral agents will be settled in the near future. But the discussion of their use has helped doctors concentrate more heavily on trying to control Type II diabetes with meal planning, exercise and weight loss before prescribing oral agents. It also has pointed out the possible danger of continuing the use of oral agents when they do not seem to be helping blood glucose control. The accepted practice in these cases is to place the person with Type II diabetes on an insulin injection program.

Are there different kinds of oral agents?

All oral agents are produced from sulfa drugs which are commonly used by doctors to fight infections. The scientific name for oral agents is "sulfonylurea agents." Four oral agents have long been available in the United States: Orinase, Dymelor, Tolinase, and Diabinese. Two other oral agents that are 100 to 200 times as potent as the ones named above have recently been marketed in the United States: Diabeta/Micronase, and Glucotrol. Their superior strength makes it possible to give them in smaller doses.

Like insulin, the different kinds of oral agents are given in different daily doses. They also act for different periods of time, as does insulin. The usual daily dose and action times for the six oral agents now available are given in the table below:

Oral Hypoglycemic Agents

Generic Name	Trade Name	Size	Usual Daily Dose	Duration of Action (hours)
Tolbutamide	Orinase	500 mg.	500 to 3000 mg. (divided doses)	6-12
Acetohexamide	Dymelor	250 mg. 500 mg.	250 to 1500 mg. (divided doses)	12-24
Tolazamide	Tolinase	100 mg. 250 mg.	100 to 1000 mg. (divided doses)	10-18
Chlorpropamide	Diabinese	100 mg. 250 mg.	100 to 500 mg. (once daily)	24-60
Glyburide	Diabeta Micronase	1.5 mg., 2.5 mg. 5 mg.	2.5 to 30 mg. (once daily)	Up to 24
Glipizide	Glucotrol	5 mg., 10 mg.	3 to 40 mg. (once daily)	12-24

Chapter 15
What You Need to Know About the Possible Complications of Non-Insulin-Dependent (Type II) Diabetes

Priscilla Hollander, M.D.

As the focus of our society has turned to maintaining wellness throughout a full and productive life—including the senior citizen years—we are finally paying more attention to the long-term complications of diabetes. It used to be thought that Type II diabetes did not cause as many or as severe long-term health problems as Type I diabetes. Recent statistics tell us that this is definitely not true. It is just as important for people with Type II diabetes to do everything possible to control the disease in order to avoid or reduce the severity of its serious and life-threatening complications.

This chapter will introduce the types of long-term complications that can affect people with Type II diabetes. It will also discuss the differences and similarities between the types of complications faced by people with Type II diabetes compared to those with Type I diabetes. Specific complications and preventive measures will be discussed in more detail in Section IV.

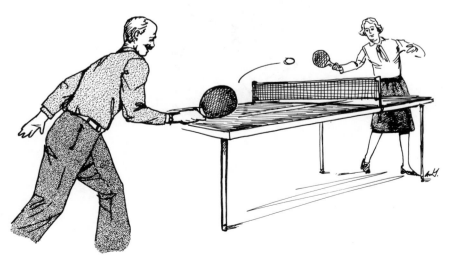

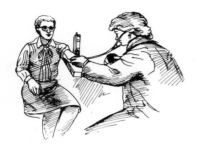

What causes long-term complications of diabetes?

Earlier chapters have discussed the role of high blood glucose in the development of long-term complications. However, other factors, including obesity, high blood fats, high blood pressure, and inheritance also appear to contribute to complications.

The use of "long-term" to describe diabetes complications means that it usually takes eight to ten years before the first signs of the problem appear. This is not always true, however. Some problems may be obvious when Type II diabetes is diagnosed, especially if blood glucose levels have been slowly increasing for several years before diagnosis.

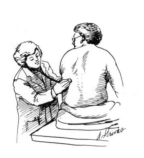

The long-term complications of diabetes develop mainly because of damage to blood vessels. Diabetes may cause damage to any blood vessel in the body, but certain blood vessels seem to be more at risk than others. The problems caused by blood vessel damage are related to the size of the blood vessels in the area of the body in which problems develop. Problems that occur in the eyes, kidneys, and nerves are due to damage to the small blood vessels which supply those areas (microvascular disease). Problems that occur in the heart, feet, and brain are due to damage to the large blood vessels which supply those areas (macrovascular disease).

In general, people with Type II diabetes are more likely to develop complications of the large blood vessels, while people with Type I diabetes have a greater risk of complications caused by small blood vessel disease. But it is important to be aware of all possible complications and preventive measures whether you have Type I or Type II diabetes.

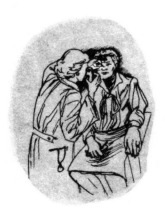

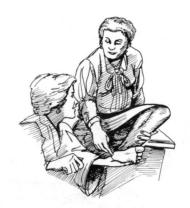

Large Blood Vessel Complications

One of the most important areas of the body that can be affected by damage to large blood vessels is the heart. The blood vessels which supply blood to the heart (arteries) can become clogged and brittle, causing heart disease (coronary artery disease). Heart disease is the most common cause of death among people with diabetes. Heart disease can occur in both Type I and Type II diabetes; people with diabetes have a two to four times higher risk than those without diabetes.

The large blood vessels which supply the brain may also be affected by diabetes. When these blood vessels become blocked, parts of the brain do not receive oxygen and nutrients. This is called a stroke, and it can have permanent effects on body function, depending on which sections of the brain are affected and for how long. People with diabetes have about two to four times the risk of suffering a stroke compared to those without diabetes.

Damage to the large blood vessels can be greatly increased when high blood pressure is present. As we discussed in Chapter 13, it is important to control not only high blood glucose, but also to control high blood pressure and high blood fats and to reach and maintain desirable body weight. All are important in reducing the risk of long-term complications.

Normal blood glucose, blood pressure, blood fats, and weight are all important in reducing risks of long-term complications.

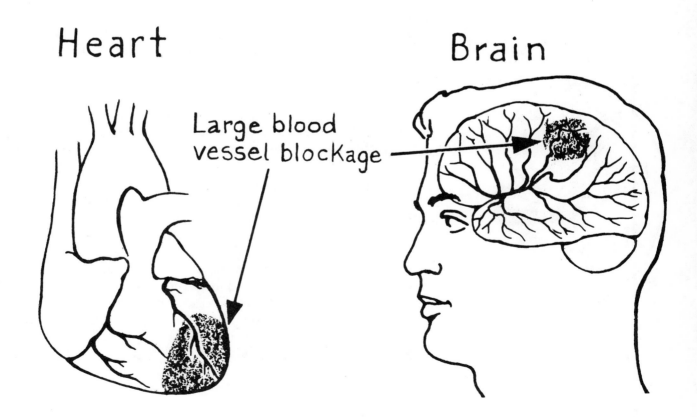

Heart

Brain

Large blood vessel blockage

Small Blood Vessel Complications

The most common small blood vessel problem involves changes in and damage to the small blood vessels in the back of the eye, which is called the **retina**. This type of eye problem is called **retinopathy**. Early mild blood vessel changes which do not cause any symptoms are called **background retinopathy**. Statistics show that after 15 years with either Type I or Type II diabetes, 80 percent of all people with diabetes will have these mild blood vessel changes. These common changes usually do not get any worse.

But in some people with diabetes, blood vessel damage worsens. New, inferior blood vessels may form which may rupture and bleed into the eye, affecting vision. When eye disease reaches this stage it is called **proliferative retinopathy**, and it can lead to blindness. This problem is much less likely to occur in Type II diabetes than in Type I diabetes. However, people with Type II diabetes can have other diabetes-related eye problems such as cataracts, glaucoma, and swelling in the back of the eye (**macular edema**). All these problems can affect vision, and when they are all taken into account, the risk of blindness is about the same for people with Type II diabetes as it is for those with Type I diabetes. Statistics show that about 5 percent of all people with diabetes develop blindness. See Chapter 20 for more information on how to protect your eyesight.

The kidneys can also be affected by damage to small blood vessels. Diabetic disease of the kidneys is called "diabetic nephropathy," and it is seen much less commonly in Type II diabetes than in Type I diabetes. About 5-10 percent of people with Type II diabetes develop kidney disease, compared to 30-40 percent of people with Type I diabetes.

The first sign of diabetic kidney disease is usually protein in the urine. This is a sign that the kidneys are beginning to lose their ability to keep valuable proteins in the blood. If the body loses too much protein, fluid balance is upset, often resulting in swelling of the ankles and fluid in the lungs. Advanced diabetic kidney disease is usually accompanied by high blood pressure. Control of high blood pressure is a key to prevention of diabetic kidney disease, as well as a method of treatment.

Diabetic kidney disease can eventually destroy the ability of the kidneys to filter waste and fluid from the body. This results in serious illness caused by the buildup of poisonous wastes in the blood. This can be treated by placing the person on an artificial kidney machine which cleans the blood, or by transplanting a healthy kidney into the person's body. More information on kidney disease can be found in Chapter 21.

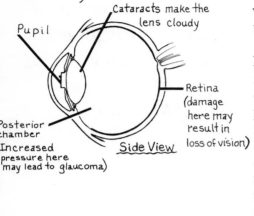

The Eye

Pupil

Cataracts make the lens cloudy

Posterior chamber (Increased pressure here may lead to glaucoma)

Side View

Retina (damage here may result in loss of vision)

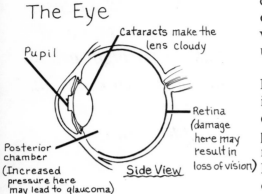

Damage to small vessels here.

The Kidney

A third type of long-term complication that is related to small blood vessel damage involves the nerves—the body's telegraph system. Nerves carry messages from the brain to various parts of the body and from those parts back to the brain. The nerves are supplied with oxygen and nutrients by a network of small blood vessels which surround them. When these blood vessels become damaged by high levels of blood glucose, the nerves in the area of the damaged blood vessels do not receive the nutrients they need to function properly. They begin to have trouble carrying messages of touch, temperature, pain, and other sensations. This can cause numbness or tingling or pain in the affected area. It can also cause the affected body part to fail to function properly.

Nerve damage is called **neuropathy**, and it is the least understood of all the long-term complications of diabetes. This is surprising, because it is one of the most commonly occurring complications. Neuropathy occurs at about the same rate in people with Type II diabetes as in those with Type I diabetes. However, it seems to appear earlier in people with Type II diabetes. In fact, it may be the first sign that a person has Type II diabetes.

Neuropathy can affect almost any nerve in the body, but it appears more commonly in certain areas of the body. The feet and lower legs are the area in which neuropathy is most commonly seen. This may be because the nerves which carry messages between the brain and the feet are the longest nerves in the body, so there is more opportunity for them to be affected by blood vessel damage. Another commonly affected area in men is the penis, and damage to the nerves in this area can cause impotence in as many as 50 percent of men with diabetes (see Chapter 18). Neuropathy can also affect the nerves to the intestines, causing constipation or diarrhea. See Chapter 22 for information about preventing and detecting nerve damage.

Combination of Small and Large Blood Vessel Complications

The long-term damage to small and large blood vessels can result in complications involving the extremities of the body, especially the feet. If the large blood vessels which supply the lower legs and feet become damaged, and the nerves between the feet and brain are affected by damage to small blood vessels, this can set the stage for serious problems in the feet.

Nerve damage can lead to loss of sensation in the feet, which makes it more likely that the person will suffer an injury or infection without being aware of the problem. The nerve damage together with the poor blood circulation hurts the body's ability to heal the foot injury. If not treated promptly and properly, the area can become severely infected and can lead to "gangrene," which means "death of tissue" in Greek. The gangrene can spread throughout the foot and leg, requiring amputation. People with diabetes are 15 to 20 times more likely to require amputation of a limb than are people without diabetes. Chapter 23 describes how you can take care of your feet daily and be on the watch for problems which could lead to serious infection.

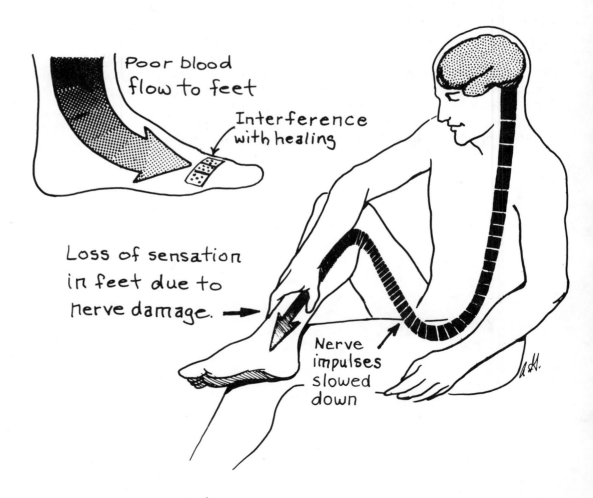

Poor blood flow to feet

Interference with healing

Loss of sensation in feet due to nerve damage. →

Nerve impulses slowed down

214

Reducing Your Risks for Complications

It is useless to know about how and why diabetic complications occur unless you make changes to reduce your risks of developing these problems. The list below includes specific goals that you can work toward with the help of your health care providers.

1. **Do not smoke.** Smoking greatly increases the risk of both small and large blood vessel disease.

2. **Avoid obesity.** Work with your doctor and a dietitian to determine your desirable body weight and then work to maintain your weight within 10 pounds of that goal. Work with your health care providers to design a safe and effective individual exercise program. This will help you maintain weight, normal blood glucose levels, and overall health and well-being.

3. **If you drink alcohol, do so in moderation.** Heavy drinking can contribute to obesity, poor blood glucose control, and kidney and liver disease.

4. **Avoid high blood pressure.** If repeated blood pressure tests show readings higher than 140/90, work with your doctor in an aggressive program to bring your blood pressure down to more normal values of 120/80 or lower. High blood pressure can help cause and/or greatly worsen all diabetic complications.

5. **Avoid high blood fat levels.** Total blood cholesterol values should be below 180 to 200 milligrams and triglycerides below 150 milligrams.

6. **Maintain blood glucose levels below 200 mg/dl.** Use regular blood testing records and glycosylated hemoglobin test results to work with your health care providers to make changes in your health care plan if necessary.

7. **Schedule regular visits to your health care providers to evaluate and discuss your diabetes control, risk of complications, and general health.**

Conclusion

It is discouraging to read about the risks of long-term complications of diabetes. But it must be remembered that the percentages of people with diabetes who have developed problems in the past are probably high because those individuals did not have the information and skills which could have helped prevent the complications. Today there is a great deal of awareness of how these problems can be prevented or treated promptly before they become serious. The key is for you to do everything possible to help yourself enjoy a life free of diabetic complications.

Today there is greater awareness of how complications can be prevented or treated before they become serious.

NOTES

Section IV
Special Topics of Interest to People With Diabetes and Their Families

Healthy Habits
Pregnancy
Sexual Concerns
Heart Health
Eye Health
Kidney Health
Nerve Health
Foot Health
Genetics
Research
Meal Flexibility
Sports

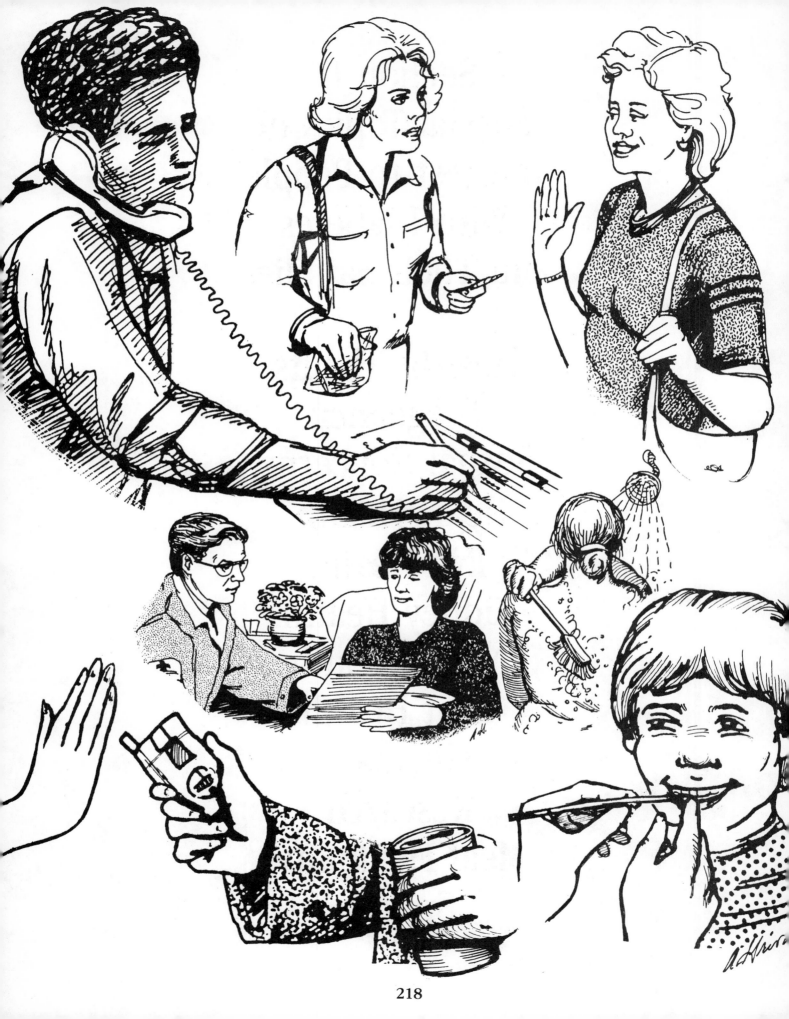

Chapter 16
Healthy Habits for Living Well

Helen R. Bowlin, R.N., B.S.N.Ed.

As you strive to make the lifestyle changes necessary to control diabetes, don't forget about the general health habits that are important for everyone. Your desire to live well with diabetes may be just the motivation you need to make positive decisions about your health that are often ignored by people who do not have diabetes. This chapter and several of the other chapters in this section will make recommendations about how you can best maintain good health.

Maintaining Good Health

Dental Care

Care of your teeth and mouth is a very important part of personal health and can prevent tooth decay and mouth infections. Gum disease is more likely to occur if your blood glucose is not well controlled. All of us have germs in our mouths. If they are not regularly removed by brushing and flossing, they can eat away at the protective enamel on the teeth and cause cavities.

Brushing after meals and flossing daily will also prevent the buildup of plaque on the teeth. If plaque is not removed, it will harden to form calculus, which can grow underneath the teeth and into the gums, causing inflammation and infection.

Other helpful daily habits are to use a water-spraying device designed to flush food and bacteria from around the teeth, and to gently massage and nudge back the gums at the roots of your teeth.

Think of your dentist as a member of your health care team.

This manual stresses the importance of team health care for diabetes, and your dentist should be thought of as part of this team. Your dentist needs to know that you have diabetes and should contact your doctor whenever questions arise about your inability to eat after dental work, especially after oral surgery. Your doctor and dentist can work together to time the dental work and adjust your medication if necessary.

Your dental history chart should include the fact that you have diabetes, but remind your dentist at each appointment. Try to time appointments so that they will not interrupt your meal schedule. Blood glucose monitoring before and after a visit is helpful in making sure your blood glucose does not get too low. Also remember that dental work can be a source of stress that could increase your blood glucose level. Again, make sure that both your dentist and doctor are working together and with you to prevent problems.

Healthy Dental Habits

1. Brush after eating, using a soft toothbrush and fluoride toothpaste.

2. Floss daily, gently moving the floss back and forth until it works its way between the teeth.

3. Ask your dentist for advice and instructions about other preventive habits you can follow.

4. See your dentist at least twice a year to make sure any problems are caught early.

5. Carefully plan for your dental visits to avoid an insulin reaction, and make sure your dentist knows you have diabetes and is familiar with treatment of an insulin reaction.

6. Make sure your doctor and dentist are working together, especially when anesthesia is needed for dental work or oral surgery. If you are taking insulin or a diabetes pill and can't eat your regular meal plan because of dental work, consult your health care provider.

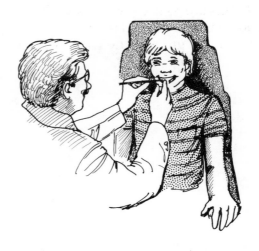

Preventing Infections

It is especially important for people with diabetes to avoid infections. Infections tend to change the rate at which the body breaks down food for energy. If an infection is present, your body will need more energy to fight the infection. This may cause you to require more insulin. Call your health care provider for help.

Keeping your blood glucose under control will help you avoid infections. High levels of glucose decrease your resistance to infection. Testing often for ketones when blood glucose is high will give you early warning of the possible development of ketoacidosis.

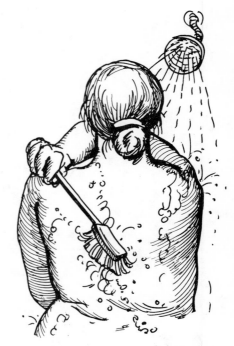

Skin infections may be avoided by following some good health practices:

1. Take a daily bath or shower, using a lanolin lotion to lubricate your skin if it is dry. If you are obese, carefully dry all areas of overlapping skin and powder with a substance such as cornstarch.

2. Promptly treat all cuts or broken skin. Wash with soap and water, cover with a clean bandage, and watch carefully for warmth, soreness, swelling, or redness until the area has healed.

3. Use caution while shaving, being careful not to break the skin. Use an electric razor if you shave your legs. A sharp-edged razor is more likely to cause cuts, which may become infected. Other hair-removing methods, such as chemicals, waxing, and electrolysis may also irritate the skin.

4. If pimples show excessive redness, swelling, or warmth, or become painful, a boil or carbuncle may be developing. If this occurs, contact your doctor. You may need an antibiotic or other medical treatment.

5. Urinary tract or bladder infections may also be a problem for people with diabetes. The symptoms of a urinary tract infection are frequent urination, a constant feeling of having to urinate, a burning sensation, blood in the urine, and/or back pain. If symptoms of a urinary infection occur, contact your doctor for treatment.

   Prevention of urinary tract infections includes:
   • For females, careful daily washing around the rectum and vagina. Wipe from front to back.
   • Wearing cotton underwear to absorb moisture.
   • Drinking a lot of fluids and urinating every three to four hours. This helps to wash away any bacteria.

Making Decisions About the Use of Mood-Altering Substances

A crucial part of a healthy lifestyle is making intelligent decisions about the many tempting but dangerous substances in our society. These can range from the use of legal substances such as alcohol and tobacco, to the abuse of prescribed drugs such as tranquilizers, sedatives, and "diet" pills, to involvement with illegal drugs such as marijuana, cocaine, amphetamines and other "street" drugs.

No one can make these decisions for you. It is important, however, that you be aware of and think about the information that is available on the health effects and dangers of these substances. Ask your health care provider for reliable sources of up-to-date information. It is also necessary to be aware of how specific substances could affect your diabetes control. The rest of this chapter will report what is known about each drug's possible effects when used by a person with diabetes.

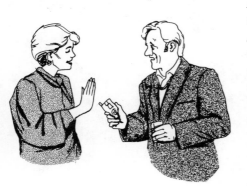

Alcohol and Tobacco

Alcohol was discussed in detail in Chapter 2, but in summary, under certain circumstances it can cause hypoglycemia in Type I diabetes. Alcohol contributes to obesity in Type II diabetes as well as possibly causing unpleasant reactions if you take diabetes pills. Individuals with diabetes should discuss their possible use of alcohol with their health care provider.

After more than 20 years of intensive research, medical experts are now unanimous in confirming the relationship of tobacco use to major health hazards, especially lung cancer. In addition, smoking has been found to cause damage to blood vessels, both large and small, adding to the already high risk of these problems among people with diabetes.

The nicotine in tobacco interacts with the walls of blood vessels, contributing to "hardening of the arteries," or arteriosclerosis. In large blood vessels the nicotine can contribute to the formation of plaque from high blood fat levels. This can narrow and even block arteries, reducing blood flow to the rest of the body and endangering the heart or brain. In small blood vessels, the nicotine causes them to become inflexible and narrowed or blocked. This contributes to the development of retinopathy, kidney disease, nerve damage, and increases the risk of foot problems.

Recent studies have raised concern that there are health hazards involved from inhaling other people's smoke (passive smoking). It seems especially prudent for people with diabetes to avoid exposure to tobacco smoke at any time. This is even more important for pregnant women. If you are concerned about being exposed to smoke at work or in other controlled situations, ask your doctor to write a letter informing your supervisor or other officials of the danger of this exposure.

Be sensible in deciding not to use tobacco, and be assertive in your right to breathe clean air!

Prescription and Non-Prescription Medications

Everyone who takes any kind of medication should be aware of why, how, and when to take it and what are its intended effect and possible side-effects. It is also very important to know what NOT to do while taking medication, such as not drinking alcohol, not taking with food or on an empty stomach, etc. The best source of this information is your pharmacist.

Your pharmacist is a good source of information about medications.

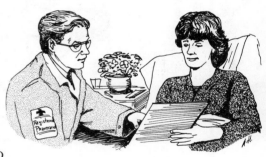

Another reason you need to know how a medication is supposed to affect you is because you need to be able to tell if you are allergic to the medication. Any individual can be allergic or have an unusual response to a specific medication. If you detect a rash, pain, or any other unusual symptoms after taking a medication, tell your doctor.

If you have diabetes, it is especially important that you be very careful when taking medication. Many prescription medications and even some non-prescription medications can interact with diabetes medications to reduce or increase their effects or cause side-effects. Some medications can raise blood glucose levels, while others tend to lower blood glucose. Some medications can cause shakiness, light-headedness, or confusion, which may lead you to think you are having an insulin reaction. In other words, there are many possible effects—some desirable and some definitely not desirable—that can occur when you take a medication. This is especially true when you are taking more than one medication.

It is hard to list non-prescription medications which may cause specific undesirable effects, because the strength, manufacturer, changes in ingredients, or just your individual response to a specific medication must be taken into account. In general, though, be careful when taking large amounts of aspirin, cold remedies, or diet pills because these types of medications tend to affect blood glucose. Even though they contain sugar, medications such as cough syrups and throat lozenges will have very little effect on blood glucose levels if they are taken according to directions. When taking a medication, you may wish to record it in your diabetes record book. This may help you detect if the medication causes undesirable effects or if it affects blood glucose levels.

There are many types, manufacturers, and strengths of prescription medications. To avoid problems, ALWAYS ask your pharmacist or doctor to tell you about the effects and cautions regarding any prescribed medicine. Write down all the information you will need to use the medication correctly.

Street Drugs

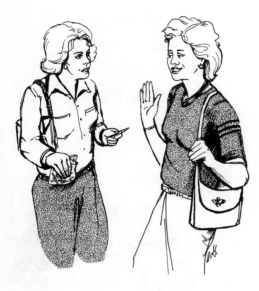

Many experiments are being conducted on drugs such as marijuana, hashish, cocaine, "uppers," "downers," "angel dust," LSD, and heroin. The trouble is, most of these experiments are being done by people who use their own bodies as laboratories. The devastating long-term effects of drugs such as heroin are well known, but research scientists have not been studying most street drugs long enough to detect long-term problems.

The short-term effects of street drugs are fairly well known, but when purchased on the street it is almost impossible to tell if the drug is actually what the seller says it is, what its strength is, and what other chemicals might have been used to prepare it or mixed with it. Unfortunately, most of this type of information is gathered by emergency rooms and drug clinics when it is too late to help the victim.

A person with diabetes is as vulnerable as anyone else to the peer pressure, curiosity, or emotional problems which lead many people in our society to use street drugs. However, as a person with diabetes you are already working very hard to control the physical and emotional processes which can promote a healthy and productive life. Street drugs can very definitely jeopardize your ability to make decisions about your diabetes, as well as being a threat to your overall emotional and physical health. When under the influence of drugs it is hard to recognize and treat an insulin reaction, which could lead to unconsciousness and death. It is very dangerous to consume alcohol or use street drugs while taking medication, so don't take chances.

Each individual must make his or her own choice about street drugs, and hopefully your ability to control diabetes will give you the strength to decide not to risk your healthy future.

Families must deal openly with the very real presence of drug abuse in our society. This includes not only street drugs but alcohol, tobacco, and abuse of prescription or non-prescription medications. Parents who abuse any of these substances can't expect their children to avoid the same pattern of abuse, perhaps with a different drug.

New information about the effects of street drugs is appearing constantly, but much of it is the product of emotion rather than factual information. Your health care team can help you sort out the facts. Take advantage of their help to remain free of chemical abuse rather than waiting until that abuse has threatened your health and happiness. A family counselor can be an especially helpful source of an outsider's perspective into present or possible problems.

Tips for Interacting with Your Health Care Team

As a person with diabetes, you are the most important part of the health care team. Nurses, doctors, dietitians, counselors and other health care professionals need your input to help you stay in good health. You are the person who knows just how you feel, physically and emotionally. You know what is possible to fit into your lifestyle to help you lead a happy and productive life.

Be assertive when discussing problems with your health care provider. If answers or directions are not clear, ask that they be repeated or explained. Here are several suggestions for making health care discussions more rewarding:

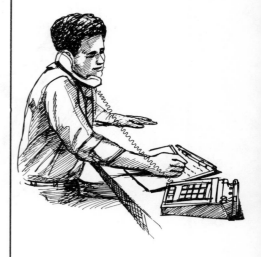

1. Before phoning or visiting your health care provider, collect all the information you might need. Have your diabetes record book in front of you so that you can share important information in case adjustments in your diabetes management plan are needed.

2. Have a written list of questions so that you will not forget any important items.

3. If you are not feeling well, take your temperature and record it.

4. List symptoms in the order they have happened. Think about your symptoms so you can describe them accurately.

5. Know what medications you take, how much, and how often. If medications are new to you, be sure that you understand why you are taking them and what side-effects might occur, especially when used in combination with other medications or alcohol.

6. Report any situations of stress that might lead to changes in blood glucose and poor control.

7. Make sure you understand everything the health care provider is saying. Repeat your instructions and write them down, and if you do not understand a medical term, ask that it be explained in words you understand.

Again, you are the most important member of the team. With the proper information, you can make intelligent decisions about your own state of health. Use your best judgment to make good health decisions, using your health care providers as important resources and partners.

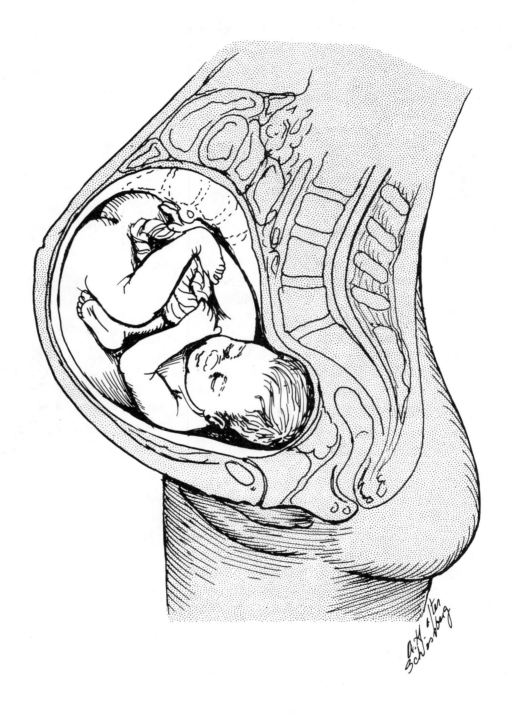

Chapter 17
Pregnancy and Diabetes: Careful Planning and Control

Priscilla Hollander, M.D. and Leslie Pratt, M.D.

The decision to have a child is a major step for any woman, but for a woman with diabetes it takes on special significance. In the not too distant past the chances for a successful pregnancy were poor. However, during the past ten years the importance of strict blood glucose control before and during pregnancy has been recognized.

Recent developments such as blood glucose monitoring and new techniques in obstetrical care have helped to greatly enhance the ability of a woman with diabetes to have a safe pregnancy and a healthy baby. In fact, the chances for a woman with diabetes to have a safe pregnancy are now within one or two percentage points of the rate in the general population.

This chapter will help you understand the importance of careful pre-pregnancy planning and strict diabetes control and will discuss how you can work with your health care team to protect your health and that of your baby.

Why is a planned pregnancy important?

For a number of reasons, pregnancy for a woman with diabetes must be given careful consideration and planning by both prospective parents. It is important to realize that a pregnancy complicated by diabetes will require more time, effort, and expense. Extra costs may include blood glucose monitoring equipment, frequent physician visits, and more laboratory tests. If a problem develops during pregnancy, hospitalization may be necessary. Occasionally a prospective mother may be asked to be less active during the last months of her pregnancy. She may need help with housekeeping and child care. If she is working outside of the home, she may have to take extra time away from her work.

Strict blood glucose control before and during pregnancy is the key to having a healthy baby.

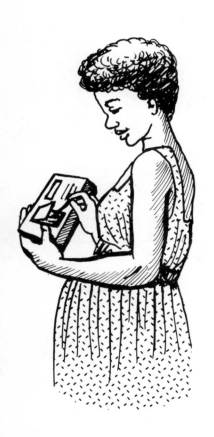

Once you have made the decision to have a child it is essential to understand the need for strict blood glucose control **both before and during pregnancy**. Although the chances of a successful pregnancy are good, the incidence of birth defects is still higher for infants of mothers with diabetes than the general population. Most birth defects originate during the first month of pregnancy, so it is essential to have tight blood glucose control during this period. Most women do not yet know that they are pregnant during the first month, so strict blood glucose control must be maintained whenever there is a chance that you might become pregnant.

For this reason, it is important that women with diabetes who are sexually active but not desiring pregnancy receive advice on contraception methods from their doctor. There is no *one* best method of contraception for every woman, so the choice should be made carefully with your doctor. Contraception is discussed in the next chapter, which covers sexual concerns for men and women with diabetes.

A successful pregnancy depends on the ability of the woman to achieve and maintain strict blood glucose control prior to the time of conception, during the first month of pregnancy, and throughout the remainder of her pregnancy. This requires a very close working relationship with a health care team that is knowledgeable about diabetes and pregnancy. You are the most important member of this team, which should also include a diabetes specialist, obstetrician, pediatrician, dietitian, and nurse practitioner. Each has an important role in caring for you and your child, both before and after your baby is born.

The achievement of strict blood glucose control during pregnancy depends on several factors. Perhaps the most important one is the use of blood glucose monitoring. The ability to reliably check one's blood glucose level at any time has transformed care of the pregnant woman with diabetes. A standard blood glucose testing schedule for people with diabetes who use insulin includes checking the blood glucose level at least four times a day: before breakfast, lunch, dinner, and bedtime. Additional tests may be done at other times depending on whether the individual is having problems with control.

However, frequent blood glucose testing is not enough to ensure strict control. Another key factor is that your health care team works with you to set up and evaluate an individualized insulin schedule and meal plan. You should be given guidelines and taught to make certain insulin adjustments independently and immediately at home on the basis of your blood glucose findings. Your diabetes control should be evaluated at each health care visit. Blood glucose testing records are only one way to accomplish this. In addition, a glycosylated hemoglobin laboratory blood test should be done at two week to monthly intervals to help monitor overall blood glucose control. See Chapter 4 for information on this test.

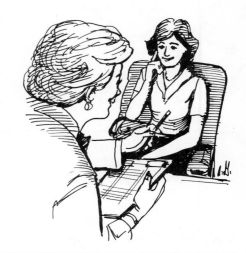

Nutrition During Pregnancy

The meal plan for a pregnant woman must take into account not only her nutritional needs but also those of the developing baby. An individualized meal plan also plays a crucial role in helping the woman to keep her blood glucose levels under strict control.

A total weight gain of 24 to 30 pounds is recommended, with a gradual pattern of weight gain being more important than the total amount gained. Pregnancy is not a time for weight reduction.

The caloric requirements of pregnancy can usually be met by the addition of 300 calories per day to the pre-pregnancy meal plan. This is done at the beginning of the second trimester (fourth month). The additional calories should be supplied by eating an additional 50 grams of carbohydrate (two bread and/or fruit exchanges), two additional glasses of skim milk, and 30 additional grams of protein (2 ounces of meat, fish, or poultry; plus the 16 grams of protein in the skim milk) daily. The meal plan should contain approximately 1,800 to 2,500 calories a day.

Pregnancy is not a time for weight reduction.

Caloric needs may drop from the pre-pregnancy level during the first three months of pregnancy due to a decrease in appetite and nausea. Insulin needs may also drop slightly during this time. As appetite improves, usually toward the beginning of the second trimester, caloric needs and insulin requirements should be reevaluated.

The importance of maintaining a regular schedule of meals and snacks during pregnancy cannot be overemphasized. The daily caloric intake should be divided into three meals and two to three snacks. The bedtime snack is particularly essential to prevent hypoglycemia during the night. The baby continues to feed continuously 24 hours a day even when the woman is sleeping. Some women even find they need to drink an extra glass of milk and eat some crackers in the middle of the night to prevent hypoglycemia.

Frequent appointments with your health care team will help you to continually modify your insulin schedule and meal plan as needed throughout your pregnancy. You should have telephone access to your team at all times in case you have a problem or question.

Questions Women with Diabetes Have about Pregnancy

Will my diabetes be more difficult to manage before and/or after my pregnancy?

There are many questions women with diabetes have asked and should ask about pregnancy. One of the most basic questions is "Will my diabetes be more difficult to manage during and/or after my pregnancy?" Pregnancy is a form of stress to any woman's body. For a woman with diabetes, this stress can increase the need for insulin. One reason for this is the effect of hormones secreted by the placenta. The presence of these hormones in the blood tends to make it more difficult for insulin to do its work (insulin resistance).

Another factor which increases insulin needs is the increase in body weight which occurs during pregnancy. This added weight may come from several sources, including the increasing weight of the fetus and the placenta, plus the additional weight that the mother may gain during the pregnancy. By the end of the pregnancy a woman's insulin requirements may actually have doubled or even tripled. This does not mean that your pregnancy has made your diabetes worse. Once pregnancy is over, insulin requirements will generally return to what they were prior to pregnancy.

Will pregnancy increase my risk of diabetic complications?

Perhaps the second most frequently asked question is "Will pregnancy increase my risk of developing diabetic complications such as eye disease?"; or, if they have already developed, "Will pregnancy make diabetic complications worse?" Studies have found that pregnancy does not appear to promote the development of complications nor make existing complications worse. Most studies indicate that if eye problems do develop during pregnancy, they would probably have occurred anyway even if the woman had not been pregnant. Women with eye, nerve, or mild kidney damage can all accomplish successful pregnancies. Pregnancy is not advised if a woman has uncontrolled high blood pressure, advanced kidney failure, and/or heart problems. These problems make pregnancy dangerous for the mother and baby.

A third question asked by women with diabetes is a very important one: "What effect does low blood glucose or ketoacidosis have on my baby?" Ketoacidosis may be harmful to the survival of the baby, as well as being a danger to the mother. Ketoacidosis is more likely to occur when blood glucose control is poor. It could, however, occur in any pregnant woman if problems develop which put extra stress on her body and increase her insulin needs. The best examples would be an illness such as the flu, or a bladder infection. Both will cause increased insulin needs and could lead to ketoacidosis. It is crucial that a pregnant woman with diabetes be aware of the problems that infections can pose and be familiar with how to manage diabetes during illness. She should also not hesitate to call her health care team as soon as an illness or infection is suspected. Early treatment of these problems can reduce their effect on diabetes control and prevent ketoacidosis.

Mild hypoglycemia may occur occasionally whenever people with diabetes have strict blood glucose control. Studies have indicated that mild hypoglycemia does not appear to hurt the chances for the success of the pregnancy or the health of the baby. That is not to say that hypoglycemia is encouraged. It is important to try to avoid the rare severe episode of hypoglycemia. However, the dangers to the success of pregnancy come more from high blood glucose levels and ketones than from the occasional episode of mild or moderate low blood glucose. Ideally blood glucose control will be stable during the pregnancy, with no prolonged periods of high or low blood glucose.

Another question frequently asked by women with diabetes is "Will diabetes affect my ability to become pregnant?" Most women with diabetes have no difficulty becoming pregnant. This is true whether or not the woman's diabetes is well controlled. However, women who are in very poor control with frequent bouts of ketoacidosis may have some difficulties in conceiving a child, which is good because with poor control the pregnancy would probably not be successful. Before the introduction of insulin, it was very rare for a woman with insulin-dependent diabetes to become pregnant.

One final concern often expressed by women with diabetes is, "How likely is it that my child will have diabetes?" The risk is really fairly low; about five percent greater than that of the general population. The inheritance of diabetes is discussed in Chapter 24.

What effect does hypoglycemia or ketoacidosis have on my baby?

Will diabetes affect my ability to become pregnant?

Will my baby have diabetes?

Gestational Diabetes

Approximately 1 to 3 percent of all women who become pregnant develop a type of diabetes during pregnancy. This type of diabetes is called gestational (during pregnancy) diabetes. The stress of pregnancy increases insulin needs even for women who do not have diabetes. Some women may have a pancreas which cannot meet the increased need for insulin during pregnancy. The result will be high blood glucose levels, usually beginning the 24th to 26th week of pregnancy. Often, treatment with a prescribed meal plan and mild exercise may be enough to control the blood glucose in this type of diabetes.

Some women who develop gestational diabetes require insulin to maintain strict blood glucose control during the remainder of their pregnancy. After delivery, the blood glucose levels will usually go back to normal. Having had gestational diabetes, however, increases the woman's risk for the development of diabetes in the future. Approximately 50 percent of women who have had gestational diabetes will develop diabetes later in life.

A number of factors have been identified which increase a woman's risk for the development of gestational diabetes:

1. A family history of diabetes in a relative such as the mother, father, brother, or sister.
2. A pregnancy in the past with delivery of an infant who weighed 10 pounds or more.
3. A history of glucose in the urine in a previous or the present pregnancy.
4. Repeated miscarriages or spontaneous abortions in previous pregnancies.
5. Obesity.

The American Diabetes Association recommends that all pregnant women be tested for diabetes between the 24th and the 28th week of pregnancy. This testing involves more than the routine urine analyses done throughout pregnancy. Testing must be done and diabetes diagnosed early enough to have positive effects on the baby's health, but late enough so that diabetes can be detected if it is developing.

To test for gestational diabetes, a woman is asked to drink a liquid containing 50 grams of glucose. One hour later, a blood sample is drawn. It is not necessary to go without food before this test, but the test will be more accurate if a small meal rather than a large one has been eaten in the four hours before the test. If blood glucose is 140 mg/dl or higher, an additional test called the glucose tolerance test is done to confirm the diagnosis of gestational diabetes.

In gestational diabetes, blood glucose levels usually return to normal after delivery.

232

The woman taking the glucose tolerance test will be asked to eat a special diet high in carbohydrate for three days before the test. On the day of the test, the woman should not eat or drink anything except water from midnight the night before until the test is done. The test itself involves drinking a liquid containing 100 grams of glucose. Then, each hour for three hours afterward, a blood sample is drawn and tested for glucose amounts.

Diagnosis of Gestational Diabetes

(Two or more of the following values must be met or exceeded during a 100-gram oral glucose challenge.)

Plasma Glucose Level
(mg/dl)
- 105 .... Fasting
- 190 .... 1 hour
- 165 ... 2 hours
- 145 ... 3 hours

Obstetrical Care for Women with Diabetes

Your obstetrician and diabetes specialist will both want to see you before you become pregnant to discuss possible problems and cautions. Your initial pregnancy visits will allow the obstetrician to determine a due date, rule out medical problems other than diabetes, and do routine laboratory blood tests to determine your blood type, hemoglobin level, immunity to rubella (German measles), and evaluate your kidney function.

A schedule of routine visits will be set up for the rest of your pregnancy. Women with diabetes are usually seen every two weeks for the first 28 weeks, weekly from 28 to 34 weeks, and every three to seven days from 34 weeks to delivery.

Some of the obstetrical problems which may develop during the first half of pregnancy include:

- Infections, especially bladder infections. One in every five pregnant women with diabetes develop a bladder infection. Your urine will be checked for signs of a bladder infection at each visit.

- Miscarriage, although if blood glucose control is good the risk of miscarriage is no greater for women with diabetes than in the general population (about one in five pregnancies end in miscarriage).

In the second half of pregnancy, problems may arise with toxemia (a buildup of waste products in the blood). Other potential problems include premature labor, excessive weight gain by you or your baby, extra fluid in the placenta which can increase the risk of premature labor, and problems with the function of the placenta in delivering nutrients to your baby.

If you have blood vessel disease, which can occur as a result of diabetes, the blood vessels in the uterus and placenta may be affected. This may cause a decreased supply of nutrients to your baby and result in low birth weight. In extreme cases this may result in the baby dying in the uterus (stillbirth). In the past, there was a much higher rate of stillbirth among women with diabetes, but with improved blood glucose control and close monitoring of the fetus in the last two months of pregnancy, the stillbirth rate is now close to that of pregnancies in the general population.

Several tests and procedures have been developed that greatly increase doctors' and nurses' ability to closely monitor the fetus during the last two months of pregnancy:
- Nonstress test, which involves using a fetal monitor to compare the movement of the baby with the baby's heart rate. This is usually begun at 30 weeks and at weekly intervals thereafter.
- Stress test, which involves injecting a medication into a vein to cause mild contractions. This allows the function of the placenta to be evaluated by watching a fetal heart-rate monitor to see how the baby reacts to the contractions.
- Ultrasound, which uses very low frequency sound waves to measure the size and rate of the baby's growth and its movements within the uterus.

Delivery

The best time to deliver the baby is decided by the results of the above tests, the maturity of the baby (especially the lungs), and the mother's condition. Premature babies may have severe problems with breathing, which is called respiratory distress syndrome (RDS). RDS occurs more frequently in babies born to mothers with diabetes. A test called an amniocentesis, which involves withdrawing and examining fluid from around the baby, can be done to determine the maturity of the baby's lungs and allow a decision to be made on when to deliver the baby.

Pregnant women with diabetes are not allowed to go past their due date.

In the last month of your pregnancy, if all of the tests are normal and your pregnancy is preceeding normally, deciding on a time for delivery may mean simply waiting for your labor to begin. If early delivery is necessary, the amniocentesis will help to evaluate the risk to your baby.

Women with diabetes are not allowed to go beyond their due date, because the function of the placenta decreases at this time and increases the risk of stillbirth. Approximately 50 percent of pregnant women who have diabetes are delivered by cesarean section. This is much higher than the general population rate of 15 percent. Reasons for a cesarean section include a large baby, toxemia, placental problems, and having had a previous cesarean section.

After Delivery

Breast feeding your baby is a healthy and gratifying experience. There is no reason why an otherwise healthy woman with diabetes should not breast feed her baby. In general, if you breast feed your baby, your insulin requirements will be less.

Before you leave the hospital, discuss with your doctor the type of birth control you will use. Breast feeding mothers cannot use birth control pills. Also discuss your diabetes control; adjustments in insulin and your meal plan will have to be made as your body adjusts to not being pregnant.

Stay in touch with your health care team after you go home, and feel free to ask for help with any of the concerns and adjustments that new parents have. Maintaining the good diabetes control you achieved during your pregnancy will prepare you for a full life as an active and proud parent!

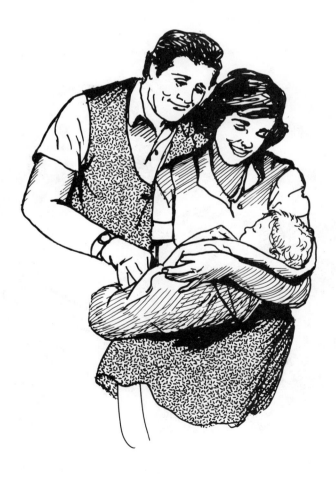

Chapter 18
Sexual Concerns for People With Diabetes

Priscilla Hollander, M.D.

A healthy sexual life is an important part of an overall healthy lifestyle, and people with diabetes are just as capable of enjoying this facet of life as is anyone else. Good diabetes control is important to allow normal functioning of the reproductive organs and to prevent long-term complications which may interfere with sexual functioning.

This chapter is divided into two sections, one for men and one for women, but as we emphasize in the title of the first section, sexual concerns are a matter for both partners to discuss, pursue answers, and if necessary seek professional help together.

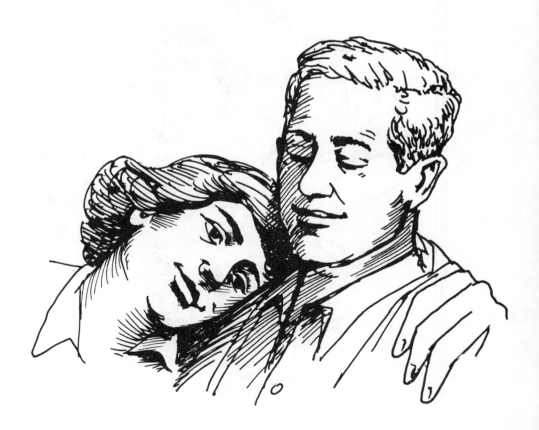

Diabetes and Impotence: A Concern for Couples

Sexual function is one area of concern among men with diabetes. This section will help you understand the possible problem of sexual impotence which can occur in men with diabetes. Such understanding will help you reduce your risk of developing impotence related to diabetes and will help prevent unfounded fears from creating problems.

What is impotence?

Impotence is defined as the inability to have an erection suitable to complete a successful act of sexual intercourse. Any man may have problems with impotence at one time or another in his life, but it occurs more frequently in men with diabetes. Studies indicate that up to 50 percent of men with diabetes eventually have problems with sexual dysfunction. However, medical advances are helping many men overcome this problem.

What causes impotence?

It is important to realize there are many causes of impotence and that the problem can range from an occasional nuisance to a permanent impairment. *Approximately 50 percent of the cases of impotence are caused by psychological problems.* For example, almost all men have occasional episodes of impotence when under extra physical or psychological stress. This chapter will not deal with these occasional episodes of impotence.

A more severe type of impotence can last for months or years and usually has a physiological (body function) cause. There are many such causes, including hormone imbalances, blood vessel and heart diseases, kidney problems, nervous system disorders, strokes, certain medications, surgery or injury to the pelvis, as well as diabetes.

To understand *how* diabetes can cause impotence, it is helpful to understand how the body produces an erection. A normal erection requires a complicated series of events. First, the man must be sexually excited. Then, a series of signals passes from the brain, along the nerves, to the blood vessels in the penis. This causes spongy tissue within the penis to fill with blood and expand. This expansion produces a shaft that is stiff enough to allow insertion into the vagina. The erection must be maintained until orgasm and ejaculation occur. Problems at any stage of this process can result in impotence.

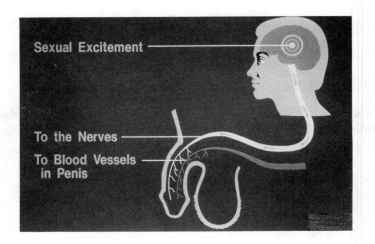

In some men, diabetes can cause damage to nerves that carry the signals to the blood vessels of the penis. If nerve signals are blocked, the penis does not expand and there is no erection. Impotence related to diabetes is usually a result of this nerve damage, which is called **diabetic neuropathy**. There is also a possibility that diabetes will damage some of the blood vessels important for penile erection. So, in some cases of impotence in men with diabetes, there may be problems with the nerves *and* blood vessels that work together to produce an erection.

Impotence related to diabetes is usually not reversible. It may develop slowly over many months or years. Erections may become softer and less frequent until there is a total inability to achieve or maintain an erection. This physical impotence need not mean the end of a pleasurable sex life. A man with impotence usually experiences a normal sexual drive, orgasm, and ejaculation. Some couples emphasize other facets of intimacy when physical impotence makes intercourse impossible. However, new methods of treatment have been developed which make erection and intercourse again possible.

How can impotence be diagnosed and treated?

If you experience impotence, you should first see your physician for a complete medical evaluation of the problem. Just because you have diabetes does *not* mean that it is the cause of your impotence. Any of the many other psychological and physical causes of impotence may be responsible.

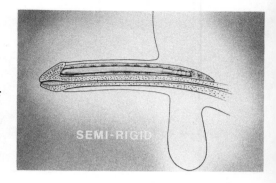

Over the last ten years, many advances have been made in diagnosis of impotence. There is a variety of tests available to determine the causes of impotence. Some of these can be performed in the privacy of your own home. Others require hospital admission. Your doctor can determine which of these tests are appropriate in your particular case. A proper diagnosis is essential before treatment can be undertaken.

Many types of treatment options are available, including surgery to implant a **penile prosthesis**. This is a device implanted into the penis to provide sufficient rigidity for intercourse. The devices do not interfere with urination or ejaculation.

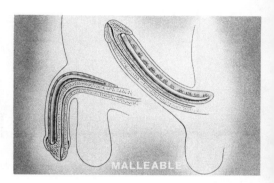

There are three types of penile prostheses now available: the **semi-rigid**, the **malleable**, and the **inflatable**. The semi-rigid prosthesis causes the penis to be permanently partially erect. The malleable prosthesis allows the man to position his penis either in the resting or erect position. The inflatable prosthesis allows the man to work an implanted fluid pump to change his penis from a relaxed state to a rigid erection. The choice of which prosthesis will be most appropriate for an individual depends on many factors which should be discussed with the man's physician and a urologist who is an expert in this type of surgery.

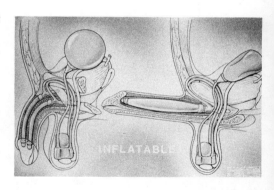

Studies of men who have been treated with an implant have revealed that more than 90 percent are satisfied with the device. Wives who were involved in the planning, and who agreed with the decision for surgery, are almost always satisfied with the results as well.

Marital counseling is recommended before surgical treatment of physical impotence, and is suggested as a source of support after the procedure.

Can impotence be prevented?

It is not yet known how or if the onset of diabetic impotence can be delayed or prevented. One of the confusing factors is that impotence may appear very early after the onset of diabetes or be present at the time of diagnosis in older men. This is unlike most other complications of diabetes, such as eye and kidney problems, which usually take eight to ten years to appear if they are going to develop.

Most physicians now believe, however, that good blood glucose control can delay the development of diabetic complications, including the damage to nerves and blood vessels which is at the root of most diabetic impotence. Recent studies of men with diabetes show that the incidence of impotence is lowest in men who:

- Maintain good blood glucose control
- Are not heavy drinkers of alcohol
- Do not smoke

These are positive steps you can take to help prevent or reduce the severity of diabetic impotence. With help from a physician knowledgeable in diagnosis and treatment of impotence, you can overcome the problem if it does occur—and regain a satisfying sexual lifestyle.

Sexual Concerns for Women with Diabetes

Because diabetes can affect so many aspects of one's well-being, many women have concerns about its possible effect on their sexual health. Many of these concerns arise from the knowledge that diabetes can cause impotence in men. Some common questions include: "Will diabetes inhibit my ability to enjoy sexual intimacy?" "Can diabetes affect my menstrual periods?" And, "Does diabetes affect my use of contraceptive methods?" These are legitimate concerns and should be discussed with your doctor. It is important that current information be sought to prevent unfounded fears from causing psychological problems. This chapter discusses recent information about frequently expressed sexual concerns.

Does diabetes affect a woman's enjoyment of sexual intimacy?

Research into how diabetes affects sexual response in women is somewhat limited. However, several recent studies have found no significant differences when sexual response in women with diabetes was compared to those without diabetes. No differences were found with regard to sexual interest, enjoyment of orgasm, or discomfort during intercourse.

It does not appear at this time that the diabetic neuropathy which can cause impotence in men has an equivalent effect in women with diabetes. However, if a woman has poor diabetes control which causes frequent urination, thirst, fatigue, and possibly ketoacidosis, obviously her sex life may not be the most enjoyable. Many women have problems with vaginitis, which is an inflammation of the vagina caused either by large amounts of yeast or bacteria. This appears to occur more often in women with diabetes and can decrease the pleasure of sexual intercourse. Therefore, as with all aspects of health, good diabetes control can help in maintaining a satisfying sexual lifestyle.

Can diabetes affect menstrual periods?

The menstrual cycle is an important part of all women's lives. Menses usually begin about the age of 10 and end for most women in their early 50s. The timing or character of one's menstrual cycle is sensitive to mental or physical stress such as illness. Variations in the menstrual cycle are not unusual for any woman. Sometimes menstrual periods are accompanied by severe cramps and heavy bleeding.

From our present knowledge, it does not appear that diabetes has an inherent effect on the menstrual cycle. Women who are in good control of their diabetes are no more likely to have variations in timing or symptoms related to the menstrual cycle. However, teenage girls with poor control of diabetes may not experience normal growth and development and as such may have a delay in the onset of the menstrual cycle. And in a woman of childbearing age who often has high blood glucose and experiences repeated bouts of ketoacidosis, the menstrual cycle may be irregular or absent.

Many women feel that blood glucose control is more difficult to maintain just before and during their periods. The nature of the problem varies among individual women; some women have problems with high glucose, others with low glucose, and many women have no control problems during this time. According to some older studies, women had more problems with ketoacidosis around the time of their menstrual periods, but more recent scientific studies have not supported this belief.

If you experience problems with diabetes control that seems to be related to your menstrual cycle, frequent blood glucose testing can help reveal a pattern. Work with your health care providers to determine if your insulin therapy could be adjusted to aid control during this time. Also ask for help or advice if depression or moodiness during your periods interferes with your ability to control diabetes and live an enjoyable lifestyle.

What birth control options exist for a woman with diabetes?

An important aspect of sexuality for any woman is the ability to feel secure in making the decision to have a baby. Many women with diabetes have concerns about the safety of various methods of contraception, the advantages and disadvantages of each, and whether one method is especially recommended.

Family planning is an important topic of concern for all women, but it takes on a special significance for women with diabetes. Choosing the most appropriate and safe time to have a child is one of the keys to a successful pregnancy for a woman with diabetes. As discussed in Chapter 17, "Diabetes and Pregnancy: Careful Planning and Control," the unplanned pregnancy at a time when diabetes control is not good may lead to problems for both the pregnant woman and her unborn child.

One of the most important aspects of family planning is choosing the right method of contraception. There are several methods of contraception available, and no one method is appropriate for all individuals. Each woman has special needs and considerations which may make one method better for her than another. The important point is that the method chosen should be reliable and effective. Unfortunately, not all methods used today can be said to offer the continued protection that is needed.

Perhaps the best known and one of the most frequently used methods of contraception is the oral contraceptive, known as "the pill." The greatest advantage of this method is its reliability; it is 99 percent effective when taken correctly. The pill contains a combination of estrogen and progesterone, two female hormones that are important for the menstrual cycle. If a woman takes the pill for 21 days out of the usual 28-day cycle, release of the egg cell (ovulation) will be prevented.

But since the pill was introduced in the early 1960s there has been controversy over its long-term side effects in regard to increased risk for heart problems, stroke, and blocking of the blood vessels in the lower legs. It is thought that large amounts of estrogen taken over many years may cause or accelerate blood vessel disease, leading to an increased incidence of heart problems or stroke. Because of these concerns, this question has been studied fairly extensively in the more than 20 years since the pill became available. It has been found that for most women the risk of taking the pill is far less than the risk of an unwanted pregnancy. However, for women who have personal or family histories of heart disease, stroke, or hypertension, or who are over 30 and smoke, the pill presents additional risks and cannot be recommended.

The question important to women with diabetes is: Does diabetes place a woman at a higher risk for problems with use of the pill? Many opinions exist in regard to this question, and research has been limited. But a recent study indicated that diabetes itself does not appear to create additional risk for women using the pill, as long as they do not fall into one of the above mentioned high risk groups. Because of general concerns about estrogen, it is probably best to use the oral contraceptive containing the lowest amount of estrogen effective for the individual.

One last word about the birth control pill is that it may cause an increase in blood glucose levels. In some women this increase can be handled by changing the insulin therapy to gain appropriate blood glucose control. However, if appropriate control cannot be maintained, it may be necessary to discontinue the pill.

Another effective method of birth control (98 percent) is the **IUD** (**intrauterine device**). This is a small, usually plastic device which is placed inside the uterus by a physician. Some IUDs contain metal such as copper, or a hormone implant such as progesterone, but it is not yet completely understood how the IUD prevents pregnancy. An IUD can be left in place for several years if no problems occur, but it is possible for it to come out of the vagina without the woman being aware that she is no longer protected from pregnancy.

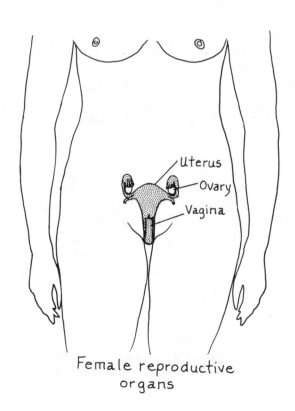

Female reproductive
organs

The problems with the IUD have included an increased incidence of infection of the reproductive organs, which can lead to sterility. IUDs also seem to cause increased cramping and bleeding during the menstrual period in women who have not previously been pregnant. Many gynecologists recommend that IUD users have had at least one previous pregnancy. The IUD is not generally recommended for women with diabetes.

The **diaphragm** is a method of contraception which can provide an excellent alternative to the pill or IUD. It is often recommended by physicians who feel uneasy about use of the pill by women with diabetes. The diaphragm is a rubber cap which the woman inserts in her vagina before intercourse. It fits over the cervix as a barrier to prevent sperm from entering the cervix and passing to the uterus, where they could fertilize the egg. For this reason the diaphragm is called a "barrier method" of birth control. When used correctly it can be up to 95 percent effective in preventing pregnancy.

Some women express the concern that a diaphragm is awkward and difficult to use. They feel it affects the spontaneity of their relationship. This need not be true, because the diaphragm can be inserted as much as one hour prior to intercourse. It is important for any woman who chooses this method to see her physician for proper fitting and instructions on how to use the diaphragm so that she feels comfortable and secure with the use of this technique.

Another barrier method is the **condom**, a thin membrane sheath which fits over the man's penis. It can be effective by itself but is even more effective when the woman uses a **sperm-killing foam or gel suppository**. Statistics indicate that the condom and foam or gel can be up to 85 percent effective in preventing pregnancy. The use of sperm-killing foam or gel alone is much less effective, and should not be relied upon by a woman with diabetes.

The newest barrier method is the **sponge**. This is a small porous sponge-like object which holds sperm-killing gel and is placed in the vagina before intercourse. It is not yet clear how effective this method is, although tests by the manufacturer have reported a fairly high rate of success. However, the sponge has been associated with an increased incidence of vaginal irritation and infection. More general experience is needed with this device before it can be recommended for women with diabetes.

Perhaps the major problem with barrier methods of contraception is that they do require some planning of intercourse. **They must be used every time intercourse occurs, and they must be used correctly.** If not, their effectiveness over time is drastically reduced.

The least effective method of contraception, which really cannot be recommended for the woman with diabetes, is the use of the **rhythm method**. The rhythm method is one of the oldest methods of contraception. Unfortunately it has a fairly low percentage of effectiveness. It requires the most motivation of all methods of contraception. It is based on avoiding intercourse over a three- to four-day period around the time of ovulation, which occurs during the middle of the menstrual cycle. Because menstrual cycles can be irregular, it may be very difficult to determine the exact time of ovulation. The best (but not foolproof) method of trying to determine this period is to measure one's rectal temperature daily in the early morning before getting out of bed. Body temperature increases slightly at the time of ovulation. A fair amount of planning is required to make the rhythm method even remotely successful, and it is not recommended for women with diabetes.

A variation of the rhythm method is to keep track of the type of secretions produced by the vagina. At the time of ovulation, a secretion is sometimes present. Again, as with the temperature rhythm method, this method is not suitable for a woman with diabetes.

Sterilization can be considered a form of contraception. Prior to the present era and the high rate of successful pregnancy in women with diabetes, women were often told not to attempt pregnancy because of its danger to them and their unborn child. In many cases sterilization was advised as a method of birth control. This is no longer good advice, because women with diabetes can have safe pregnancies, especially if they work closely with their health care team to control their diabetes very well before and during pregnancy.

The most common form of sterilization for women is a **tubal ligation**. This involves surgically blocking two tube-like structures through which the egg must pass from the ovaries to the uterus. If these tubes are blocked the egg cannot pass to the uterus and be fertilized. It may be possible to reverse a tubal ligation if a woman later wishes to attempt pregnancy, but this surgical procedure is not always successful.

Sterilization may be appropriate for women who choose not to have children or who feel they have completed their families, or for women who have serious diabetic complications such as kidney failure or heart disease. If a woman with severe complications of diabetes becomes pregnant, the pregnancy can pose a very serious threat to her life. In these cases, abortion may be a legitimate consideration for the woman.

An effective method of male contraception which may be an excellent choice for couples who choose not to have children or who have completed their family is a vasectomy. This is a minor surgical procedure which closes the tubes by which sperm travel to reach the semen. When these tubes are blocked, the semen will still be ejaculated, but it will not contain any sperm and therefore cannot cause pregnancy. Studies have found no long-term complications related to this procedure. Other methods of male contraception are currently being investigated. If male contraception is sufficiently reliable, it is an excellent alternative to the woman's using a method which may further increase her risks for health problems.

There are a number of new methods of contraception on the horizon which may be more helpful or safer for some individuals. Research continues actively in this area. Hopefully, women will soon be able to control their ability to reproduce by completely safe and effective methods.

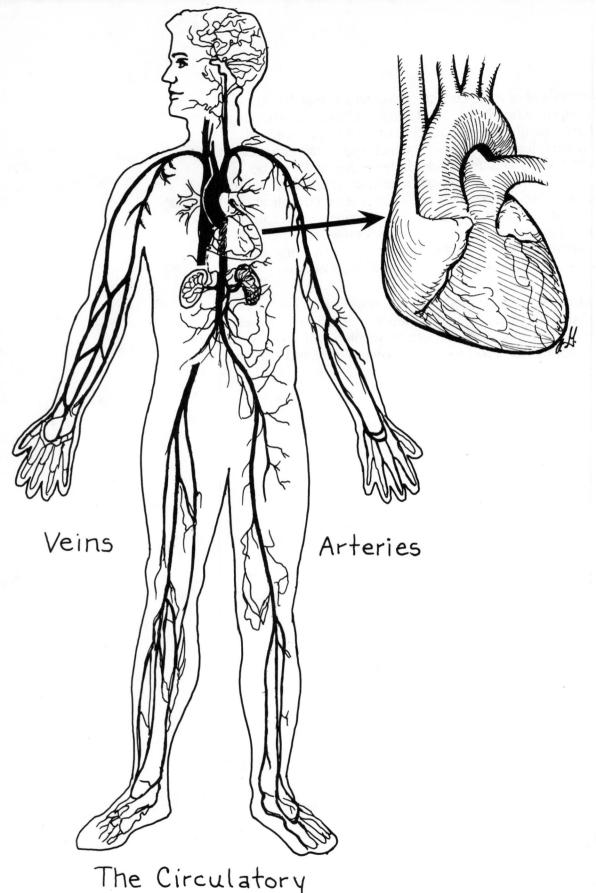

Veins

Arteries

The Circulatory
System
(Splenoportal system
not shown).

Chapter 19
Care and Maintenance of a Healthy Heart

Priscilla Hollander, M.D. and Leonard Nordstrom, M.D.

A great deal of current preventive medicine efforts are directed at ways to keep the heart and blood vessels healthy. Many parts of the body are crucial for the proper functioning of the whole body, but this is especially true of the heart, which supplies oxygen and nutrients to allow each part to do its job. If for some reason the heart becomes unable to pump enough blood throughout the body, or a blood vessel to a certain part of the body becomes blocked, the affected areas quickly lose their ability to function.

We now know there are several things a person can do to keep the heart and blood vessels—the **circulatory** or **cardiovascular system**—healthy and working efficiently. Research has led to the discovery of specific conditions which increase an individual's risk of developing circulatory problems. These conditions are called **risk factors**. Paying special attention to how these risk factors apply to you is the best way to make sure your heart and blood vessels remain healthy and continue providing vital nutrients and oxygen to your body over a long and active life.

This chapter will explain why heart disease is such a common problem in our society, especially for people with diabetes. Specific steps will be suggested to help you and your family identify and improve risk factors where possible. By supporting each other in these efforts, your family can take giant steps toward a life of vitality and fitness.

The essence of life is a healthy heart.

Proverbs 14:30

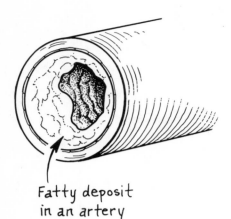

Fatty deposit
in an artery

How does heart disease develop?

Heart disease is the most common cause of death in the United States. It also is the number one cause of death among people with diabetes, who have two to four times as high a risk as the general public.

Heart disease, along with many other problems in the circulatory system such as high blood pressure (hypertension) and poor blood circulation to the extremities (peripheral vascular disease), appears to be caused by damage to large blood vessels. This damage is probably due to a process called atherosclerosis, or "hardening of the arteries," but the exact causes are not completely understood. It is thought that a high level of fat intake, especially foods containing large amounts of saturated fats and cholesterol, may be an important factor.

Atherosclerosis is a process which includes the gradual thickening and hardening of the walls of the blood vessels. This may occur in the large blood vessels as well as the small blood vessels. In some blood vessels this process may lead to actual blocking of the artery. If this happens, the tissue that was supplied by these blood vessels may die.

It appears that certain blood vessels in the body are more likely to be affected by atherosclerosis. One such group of blood vessels are those that supply the heart (the coronary arteries). If these blood vessels become narrowed or blocked, the heart muscle may be damaged and a heart attack may result.

As with most of the complications related to diabetes, damage to blood vessels appears to be the key factor in causing heart disease. Diabetes apparently causes an increased rate of atherosclerosis. Therefore, people with diabetes are at a higher risk of developing problems with parts of their circulatory system. These problems may include such things as a heart attack, hypertension, and peripheral vascular disease. The type of blood vessel damage that results in these problems can occur in anyone, but in people with diabetes it seems to occur at a faster rate. (This situation is different in the small blood vessel problems seen in the eyes and kidneys of some people with diabetes, as those type of blood vessel changes do not occur in people who do not have diabetes.)

Heart Disease

Heart disease can occur in individuals with insulin-dependent (Type I) diabetes or those with non-insulin-dependent (Type II) diabetes. Heart attacks may occur at an earlier age in people with diabetes than in the general population. Also, women in the general population tend to be protected from heart attacks until the time of menopause. The reasons for this protection are unclear, but this protection appears to be lost for women with diabetes and the rate of heart attack at all ages is the same for both men and women with diabetes.

The rate of heart attack at all ages is the same for men and women with diabetes.

Heart disease is characterized by chest pain called **angina**. As the vessels that supply the heart start to close off, the decreasing supply of oxygen and nutrients may cause chest pain because parts of the heart become damaged by the lack of nutrients. At first this pain usually occurs when the individual exercises or is active; in other words when the heart is working harder. However, as more of the heart muscle becomes affected, the chest pain can occur at any time. This does not mean the individual is having a heart attack, but it is a warning that there is a problem in the arteries which supply the heart. If the arteries go on to become completely blocked, the heart muscles supplied by these blood vessels may die and the person will be likely to experience a heart attack.

The blockage of the arteries that supply the heart can be reversed in a couple of ways. If a person experiences angina, a doctor should be seen immediately for an evaluation and cardiac testing. There are several types of medications available which may help to dilate (expand) the arteries to keep them open. Another possibility is an operation called a cardiac bypass, in which blood vessels are surgically implanted to bypass the blocked blood vessels.

Another form of heart disease which can affect anyone but is often seen in people with diabetes is called **cardiomyopathy**. This problem does not cause chest pain or a heart attack. Cardiomyopathy is the result of the small blood vessels which supply the heart becoming blocked by atherosclerosis. If these vessels are blocked long enough, the heart muscle becomes scarred and cannot expand and contract well enough to pump blood to all parts of the body.

If a large enough portion of the heart muscle loses this ability to pump blood, the heart will begin to fail. This leads to an accumulation of fluid in different areas of the body, especially in the lungs. The person will experience shortness of breath and heart failure may occur. This problem is difficult to treat although medications such as Lanoxin may make the heart muscle beat stronger and improve circulation. There are also medications called diuretics which can help remove fluid from the body. Both of these types of medications may be helpful to the person with cardiomyopathy.

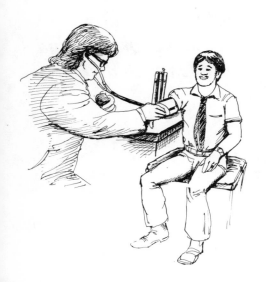

Hypertension, or high blood pressure, is a second area of concern in terms of maintaining a healthy circulatory system. Approximately two thirds of adults with diabetes have hypertension. It is a process which apparently also speeds the rate of atherosclerosis in large blood vessels and probably small blood vessels as well. Hypertension has been shown to increase the incidence of heart disease. Therefore, it is essential that everything possible be done to prevent high blood pressure. If it does develop, it is important to treat it early and aggressively.

The reason high blood pressure so often develops in people with diabetes is complex but probably has to do with kidney damage. Kidney damage can result from blocking of both the small and large blood vessels of the kidney. The kidney is an important organ in the regulation of blood pressure (see Chapter 21). Through a complex series of chemical reactions, the kidneys secrete a substance called renin. This raises the blood pressure if the kidney senses a drop in blood pressure. Damage to the large blood vessels leading to the kidney may cause an obstruction which decreases the amount of blood that can reach the kidney. Beyond this obstruction blood pressure will be low. This causes the kidney to believe that the blood pressure in the entire body is low, so it secretes renin to increase blood pressure throughout the body.

Small blood vessel damage may also cause the release of renin, again resulting in hypertension. Occasionally, surgical procedures can improve blood supply to the kidney by relieving the blockage in the large blood vessels. If this is not possible, then it is important that a person be treated promptly with appropriate medications to lower blood pressure.

There are many reasons good blood pressure control is essential for the person with diabetes. High blood pressure increases the risk of stroke, heart disease, and kidney disease and can worsen retinopathy. There are several medications available to treat high blood pressure. Your physician will work with you to determine the best treatment for you.

It is important to note that some blood pressure medications may interfere with diabetes control in people taking insulin. The group of medications most likely to cause problems are called beta blockers. These medications lower blood pressure by blocking the effects of adrenalin on the blood vessels. Adrenalin is a key agent in setting off the symptoms of an insulin reaction, and when its effects are blocked a person may not have the warning signs of low blood glucose and therefore may develop a severe reaction and lose consciousness. This side-effect does not happen in all people who take insulin and use beta blockers, and these medications can be very useful. If they are prescribed for a person using insulin, it is important to watch the patient closely at first to see if the medication is going to cause problems. If problems do occur, the beta blocker should be replaced by another medication for treating hypertension.

Poor Blood Circulation to the Extremities

A third concern in terms of circulation is poor blood circulation to the extremities, or peripheral vascular disease. This problem involves both the small and large blood vessels of the legs and feet and is very common in people with diabetes. When the large blood vessels to the legs become obstructed the person may have discomfort or pain in the thigh or calf muscles when standing, walking, or exercising. The extent of pain depends upon how much the blood vessels are obstructed. If they are only slightly clogged, the person may be able to walk a long distance before noticing pain. Usually when the person stops and rests for a minute the blood supply to that area is re-established and the pain and discomfort will go away. However, the pain usually returns after the person has performed the same amount of exercise.

How can atherosclerosis be slowed or prevented?

There are a number of circumstances—risk factors—which can accelerate the process of atherosclerosis. If these factors can be avoided or treated, it can help reduce the likelihood that an individual will develop serious problems with the large and small blood vessels which could result in a heart attack or peripheral vascular disease. Preventable risk factors include smoking, high levels of cholesterol and triglycerides in the blood, obesity, and hypertension.

Smoking is a very serious risk factor for both heart disease and peripheral vascular disease.

Smoking is a very serious risk factor in terms of both heart disease and peripheral vascular disease. People who smoke have two to four times the rate of heart attack experienced by nonsmokers. Smokers have approximately ten times the rate of peripheral vascular disease. Therefore, if you now smoke it is crucial that you do everything possible to quit. Of course, the best thing is not to start smoking at all, but unfortunately this is not a perfect world and some people do find themselves trapped by this particular addiction. It cannot be stressed enough how important it is to cut back or stop smoking. If you have tried to quit without success, ask your doctor for a referral to a reputable program that will help you succeed.

High blood levels of triglycerides and cholesterol have also been associated with increased incidence of atherosclerosis and heart attacks. This finding has been well supported by a number of different studies. It is interesting to look at the low rate of heart disease in a country such as Japan in which dietary fat intake is low, and compare it to the high rate of heart disease in countries such as the United States and Finland in which fat intake is quite high. There are also certain families who have a genetic tendency to develop high levels of triglycerides and cholesterol. Many of these people appear to be at great risk for heart disease at a relatively early age. They need to not only follow a healthy diet in terms of the amount of fat (see Chapter 2), but also may need special medications to help lower their cholesterol and triglyceride levels.

Prevention of high blood pressure is an important way to reduce the risk of heart disease.

Obesity is not always included as a risk factor for heart disease, but it does deserve mention. Obesity promotes hypertension and can lead to a worsening of diabetes, both of which increase a person's risk for the development of heart disease. For this reason obesity is indeed a risk factor for heart disease, but in an indirect way.

Prevention of high blood pressure is a very important part of reducing risk for heart disease. This includes keeping salt intake at recommended healthy levels (Chapter 2), exercising regularly (Chapter 3), avoiding obesity and losing weight if necessary (Chapter 10), and having blood pressure checked regularly to make sure hypertension can be treated promptly if it develops.

Diabetes is also considered a risk factor for heart disease. As we have already stated, people with diabetes have an increased rate of heart disease. The question asked is: Does good control of blood glucose play a role in preventing heart disease, as is the case with other complications associated with diabetes? This is not a well studied area. There have been some preliminary findings which indicate that improved blood glucose control may indeed lead to a slowing of the blockage of blood vessels in atherosclerosis and a lowering of blood pressure, and thus may reduce the risk of heart disease.

It is safe to say that good blood glucose control and good overall diabetes control are important parts of reducing the risk of heart disease. The other risk factors we have discussed must also be reduced if possible, and this is important not just for the person with diabetes but for everyone.

Summary

A healthy heart and blood vessels are obviously very important for continued good health. A healthy lifestyle with good control of diabetes, a nutritious meal plan, prevention or control of hypertension, no smoking, and regular exercise can lead not only to a healthy heart but to a healthy and long life as well.

What You Can Do

1. Do not smoke.
2. Reduce intake of foods high in saturated fats and cholesterol.
3. Reduce intake of foods high in sodium (salt).
4. Make moderate exercise a regular part of your lifestyle.
5. Maintain a healthy weight within the recommended healthy range for body fat.
6. Maintain good control of blood glucose levels.
7. See your health care providers regularly to monitor your success at caring for and maintaining a healthy heart.

What Your Health Care Providers Can Do

1. Refer you to a program to help you stop smoking.
2. Test your blood annually for levels of cholesterol and triglycerides and help you lower them if the cholesterol level is higher than 200 milligrams or the triglyceride level is higher than 150 milligrams.
3. Check your blood pressure at each visit and begin a treatment plan to lower it if it is higher than 140/90 on repeated tests.
4. Help you plan a safe and effective individual exercise program.
5. Help you lose body fat if necessary.
6. Review your blood glucose testing records and glycosylated hemoglobin and make changes in your management plan if your blood glucose levels have not remained in the desirable range.
7. Test your heart function and blood circulation to all parts of your body at least annually if you are over 30 or have had diabetes for more than ten years.

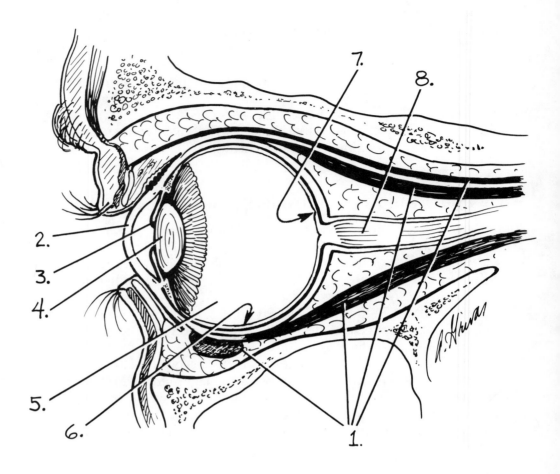

1. **Eye muscles:** turn the eyes in various directions to look at objects.
2. **Cornea:** clear window in front of eye which lets light enter.
3. **Iris:** colored part of eye, acts like the opening on a camera to adjust the amount of light entering the eye through the pupil.
4. **Lens:** focuses light onto the retina.
5. **Vitreous:** clear jelly-like substance that fills the inside of the eye and is loosely attached to the entire surface of the retina.
6. **Retina:** inner lining of back of eye, which through a chemical reaction develops a picture and sends it along the optic nerve to the brain for interpretation.
7. **Macula:** a small area at the center of the retina onto which light rays are focused.
8. **Optic nerve:** carries picture from the retina to the brain by means of electrical impulses.

Chapter 20
Diabetes and Eye Problems

William J. Mestrezat, M.D.

If you have Type I or Type II diabetes, it is very important that you follow a regular schedule of eye examinations. Eye problems can develop after about five years with Type I diabetes and at any time in Type II diabetes. Some physicians have been trained to detect changes in the eyes of people with diabetes and can check your eyes annually. Your physician may refer you to an ophthalmologist, who is a specialist in diseases of the eye. This doctor will set up a regular schedule of appointments and will advise you on how to prevent eye problems from developing.

Eye disease is one of the most serious and frightening complications of diabetes. Diabetes is a major cause of blindness in the United States. It is the most common cause of new blindness in people between the ages of 20 and 74. Fifty thousand Americans are legally blind due to diabetes. People with diabetes are 25 times more prone to blindness than is the normal population. Eighty percent of people who have had diabetes for more than 25 years have eye disease.

These statistics are frightening, but there is now hope that they can be improved by the newest methods of diabetes control and eye treatment. Remember, the above statistics include patients who have had diabetes for the last 20 to 30 years. These people did not until recently have the latest treatment methods available to them. This chapter will discuss and help you take advantage of the latest knowledge and treatment methods in diabetic eye disease.

How does diabetes affect the eyes?

The parts of the eye and their functions need to be understood before you can understand the effects of diabetes. Refer to the diagram on the opposite page as each part of the eye is discussed.

Five parts of the eye can be affected by diabetes. We will discuss separately the problems that can occur in the lens, eye muscles, cornea, vitreous, and retina.

The Lens: The Focuser of Images

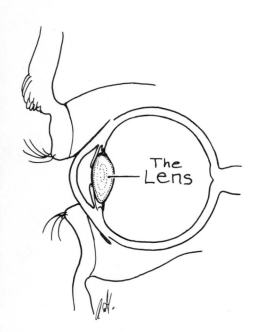

One of the most common diabetic eye complications is blurred vision that sometimes occurs with changes in blood glucose level, especially during times of poor control. The lens in the eye takes in glucose and water when the blood glucose rises, causing the lens to swell. The swelling causes light rays to no longer be focused on the retina, so the vision is blurry. After several weeks of high blood glucose, the lens will return to its normal shape and vision will improve. When blood glucose is abnormally low the lens will shrink, again blurring vision.

Blurred vision from lens changes will correct itself in two to six weeks. Treatment consists of controlling and stabilizing the blood glucose level. Glasses should not be prescribed during these episodes, because the new ones may not be needed when the lens stabilizes.

Cataracts are a more serious problem involving the lens. The lens is normally clear, allowing light rays to pass through it. Cataracts are areas in the lens that block or change the direction of light rays. This lens cloudiness blurs vision. Cataracts are more common and occur at an earlier age in people with diabetes.

The symptoms of cataracts are blurred vision and sometimes glare. Sometimes the very early diabetic cataracts are reversible with good blood glucose control. But if a cataract progresses to the point that vision is significantly impaired, cataract surgery is the only effective therapy.

Eye Muscles: Moving the Eyes

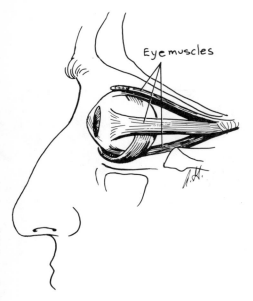

There are six eye muscles on each eye that work together to turn the eye in all directions. They are controlled by nerves coming directly from the brain. These nerves can be affected by diabetes just like any other nerve in the body (see Chapter 22). When this happens, the affected nerve stops turning the eye normally, and depending on which nerve or nerves are affected, different directions of gaze are lost.

The major symptom of eye muscle problems is double vision, especially when looking in certain directions. There may also be severe pain preceding the onset of double vision. People with this problem should have a complete neurological exam to make sure the double vision is caused by diabetes and not some other problem. If this exam is normal, then no treatment is needed. The double vision will almost always go away in four to eight weeks and usually does not recur. The individual can wear a patch over one eye until the problem clears.

The Cornea: Window of the Eye

In people who have had diabetes for many years, the cells on the front surface of the cornea are not as well attached to the underlying cells as they are normally. As a result, the surface cells can come off with minor force such as rubbing the eyes hard. Loss of these cells is called **corneal erosion**. People who have problems with corneal erosion could have great difficulty wearing contact lenses. This is seldom a problem for people who have had diabetes for only a few years.

Symptoms of corneal erosion include pain (usually severe), sensitivity to light, and excessive production of tears. The treatment consists of wearing a tight patch over the eye, use of antibiotic drops or ointments, and frequent follow-up visits to the eye doctor. Corneal erosion can heal slowly and can become infected.

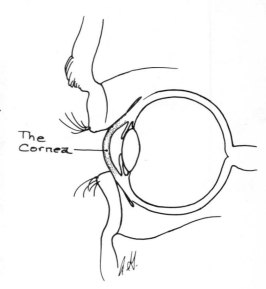

The Iris: Opener of the Pupils

The iris can be the site for formation of abnormal blood vessels as a result of diabetes. This can cause a severe form of glaucoma. There are no symptoms of this condition until it produces very high pressure in the eye, causing pain and blurry vision.

The abnormal iris blood vessels are often discovered before they can grow to the point of causing high pressure in the eye. They can then be treated using a laser method which will be described in the section about retinal problems. If glaucoma does develop, special eye drops and medications can be used to lower the eye pressure. Sometimes surgery is needed if the medications and laser treatments do not control the problem.

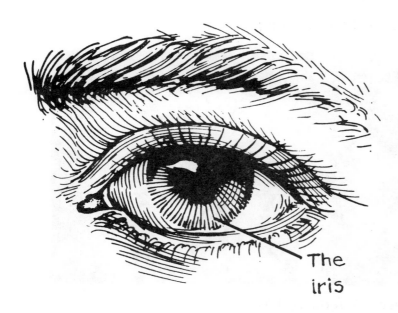

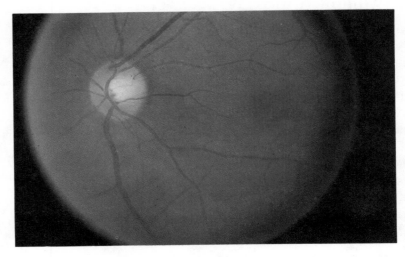

Normal anatomy of back of eye

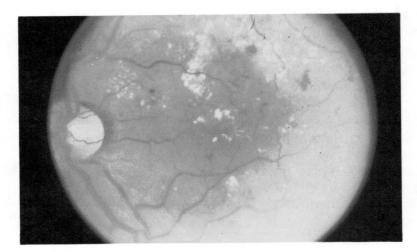

Background retinopathy

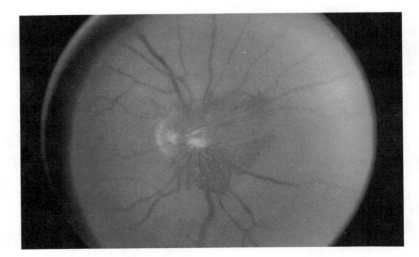

Proliferative retinopathy

The Retina: The 'Film' of the Eyes

Problems with the retina are referred to as **retinopathy** and are potentially the most serious diabetic eye complication. The first problem that usually occurs in the retina is the plugging of the smallest blood vessels, which are called capillaries. This causes other vessels to widen and to leak. Then abnormal blood vessels may begin to form.

Background diabetic retinopathy is a term used to describe loss of capillaries and leakage of other blood vessels within the retina. The vessels leak blood, fluids, and fats into the retina, causing it to become wet and hurting its ability to receive images. These changes can be seen in the eyes of 80 percent of people who have had either Type I or Type II diabetes for 25 years. These changes may not cause any symptoms and they may not get any worse.

Background retinopathy usually does not cause significant loss of vision unless there is leakage into the macula, the area of the retina used for detailed vision. This leakage can cause swelling of the macula, or **macular edema**. This is the most common cause of blurred vision from diabetic eye disease. It may go away when elevated blood glucose and/or blood pressure return to normal or may need to be treated with laser.

The diagnosis of background diabetic retinopathy is made by looking in the eyes with an ophthalmoscope. Occasionally it is necessary to take a special series of photographs called a **fluorescein angiogram**. This is the best way to study the blood vessels of the retina and show the exact location of leakage (if there is any) from the retinal blood vessels. The fluorescein angiogram is done by injecting a special dye into the patient's arm. The dye circulates up to the eye and a series of photographs is taken over a 15-minute period.

Treatment of diabetic retinopathy involves several factors. First, it is commonly felt that good diabetes control helps prevent retinal complications and, if they do occur, slows their progression. High blood pressure and kidney disease are known to make diabetic retinopathy worse, so their treatment is important for control of retinopathy.

Laser light can be used to seal leaking blood vessels in the eye, allowing the retina to dry and regain function.

If specific areas of retinal blood vessel leakage can be detected on the fluorescein angiogram, and if they are threatening significant loss of vision, laser treatments are indicated. The laser is a highly concentrated beam of light produced by electrically charging either argon or krypton gas. This produces a beam of light which is bounced back and forth between mirrors until it is extremely intense. This beam of laser light can be aimed by an ophthalmologist looking through a special microscope-like viewer. The doctor can release brief pulses of laser light to burn tiny areas of the blood vessel. This seals the blood vessel so the retina can dry itself and function normally. Laser treatments are usually done in the ophthalmologist's office. They take about 20 minutes after eye dilation and can usually be done with minimal if any eye discomfort.

If background retinopathy worsens and is not controlled, it can result in what is called **proliferative retinopathy**. This is the formation of abnormal blood vessels in the retina in response to the loss of capillaries. These abnormal blood vessels bleed easily and can cause large eye hemorrhages and severe loss of vision. This is usually seen in people who have had diabetes for more than 15 to 20 years. There are no symptoms of the abnormal blood vessels until they bleed.

Controlling medical problems such as high blood pressure and kidney disease is important for people who have proliferative retinopathy. Laser treatments need to be done in most of these patients because of the great risk of eye hemorrhage. The laser treatments destroy the areas of capillary loss, which reduces the formation of abnormal blood vessels. After laser treatment the abnormal blood vessels usually shrink or go away.

The Vitreous: A Clear Gel Filling the Eye

When abnormal retinal blood vessels bleed, they bleed into the vitreous. The symptoms of blood in the vitreous vary from dark floating spots in the visual field to almost total darkness, depending on the amount of bleeding.

Most vitreous hemorrhages will clear on their own, although it usually takes months. Limited activity is important so that the blood will settle to the bottom of the eye, where it will not affect vision. It is then absorbed gradually by the body. When the blood has cleared enough so the retina is visible, laser treatment is usually begun.

Surgery is usually performed after six months if the blood has not cleared enough to give good vision. In that eye, the blood and vitreous are removed with specially designed needles using an operating room microscope. This procedure is called a **vitrectomy**. The vitreous is replaced with a saltwater solution.

The vitreous is normally loosely attached to the retina. In people with diabetes, this adhesion can become strong. The vitreous can form scar-like bands that pull on the retina and cause it to detach. This is called **traction retinal detachment**. The detached part of the retina does not function, because it loses its blood supply. Blurry vision occurs when the macula is detached, but if the macula is not detached there will usually not be any symptoms.

Many patients who have traction retinal detachments also have vitreous hemorrhages. The blood in the vitreous makes it impossible to tell with an ophthalmoscope whether or not there is a traction retinal detachment. An ultrasound test, which sends sound waves through the blood in the eye, gives a picture of the back of the eye. It can show whether or not a traction retinal detachment is present behind the vitreous blood. The ultrasound is a painless, quick office procedure.

Traction retinal detachments are repaired by first doing a vitrectomy (replacing the vitreous). Special small scissors are then inserted into the eye and the traction bands are cut. When the traction is relieved the retina will reattach itself and usually will start to function again.

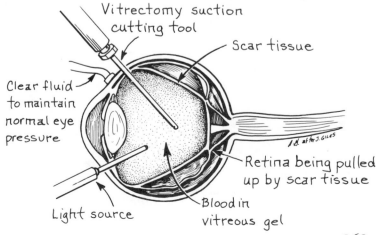

Vitrectomy suction cutting tool

Scar tissue

Clear fluid to maintain normal eye pressure

Retina being pulled up by scar tissue

Light source

Blood in vitreous gel

263

Summary

Diabetes can cause serious problems in all parts of the eye, but only a small percentage of people with diabetes develop serious complications. It is important to realize that minor vision problems can be caused by changes in blood glucose level or other temporary changes that **do not** progress to loss of vision.

It is hoped that good blood glucose control and control of other medical problems such as high blood pressure can prevent serious eye problems from developing. And if problems do develop, great progress is being made in successfully treating them, using laser therapy or microsurgery to save the person's vision. The key to prevention, early detection, and timely and effective treatment is to have your eyes examined regularly by a doctor who is trained to detect eye changes related to diabetes.

What You Can Do for Your Eyes

1. Carefully control the amount of glucose in your blood, testing your blood several times a day to make sure it is as close to normal as possible. Contact your doctor if blood glucose levels are high or low and you cannot control them.
2. See your health care providers often. Four visits per year—or more often if problems occur—will help you work as a team with the various health professionals.
3. Have your vision checked and your eyes dilated and examined at least once a year by a doctor trained to detect diabetic eye changes.
4. See an ophthalmologist promptly if eye changes are detected.

Remember, YOU are the most important person caring for your diabetes. Your actions and those of your doctor may save your vision.

What Your Doctor Can Do for Your Eyes

1. Ask you if you have any vision problems at each visit.
2. Put drops in your eyes and examine them in a dark room at least once a year.
3. Have you read an eye chart at least once a year.
4. Check your blood pressure at each visit and if it is high, start treatment right away.
5. If your doctor is not trained to detect diabetic eye changes, he or she should have you see an ophthalmologist at least once a year if you have had Type I diabetes for more than five years or if you have Type II diabetes.
6. If changes are found in your eyes, have you see an ophthalmologist who is experienced in detecting and treating diabetic retinopathy.

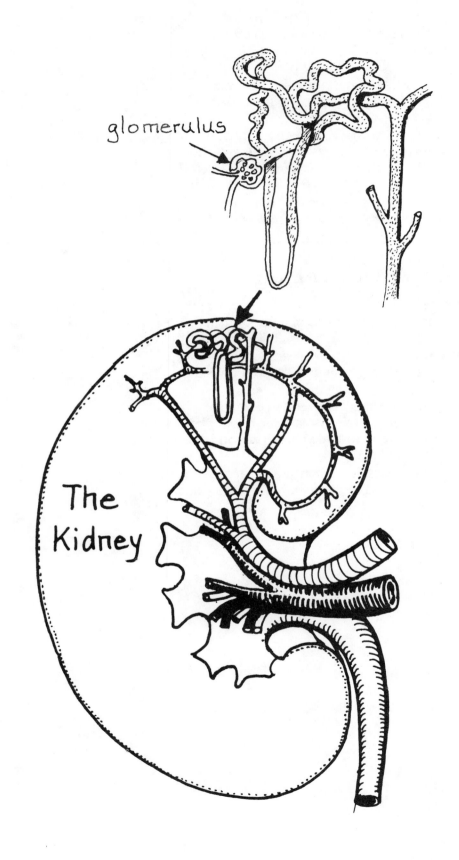

glomerulus

The Kidney

Chapter 21
Kidney Problems In Diabetes

Donald Duncan, M.D.

Kidney disease due to diabetes is a very serious problem. Past statistics show that between 45 and 50 percent of the people whose diabetes was diagnosed before the age of 20 eventually developed kidney failure. About 6 percent of people with Type II diabetes developed kidney failure. Between 20 and 25 percent of patients in kidney support programs in the United States today are there because of diabetic kidney disease.

Fortunately a great deal of research is underway and progress has been made toward finding the causes and improving prevention and treatment of kidney disease. Hopefully this will result in a much lower incidence of kidney problems in people who now have diabetes.

How does kidney damage occur in diabetes?

The kidneys are two organs in the lower back area near the spine. They are each filled with about one million tiny clumps of very closely packed small blood vessels. These clumps of capillary blood vessels are called glomeruli. It is their job to filter waste products from the blood and make urine. In diabetic kidney disease hardening and narrowing of the arteries (arteriosclerosis) which supply the kidneys, and damage to the glomeruli combine to reduce kidney function. The glomeruli become scarred and blocked and can no longer effectively filter the blood. When these filters are destroyed the waste products remain in the blood, causing uremia. Uremia means "urine in the blood."

There is considerable evidence that high blood glucose plays a significant role in damaging the glomeruli. However, it is not known why some people with diabetes are more susceptible than others to kidney damage as a result of high blood glucose.

The kidneys' filtering system can become damaged as a result of many years of high blood glucose.

Symptoms and Signs of Kidney Disease

The development of kidney damage is a very gradual process which, if it is going to occur, usually takes 15 to 20 years after the diagnosis of diabetes. If symptoms are detected early enough, problems can be reversed in some cases. If this is not possible, it will take another several years before kidney failure occurs. These large amounts of time can be used to do everything possible to reverse or reduce the extent of kidney damage, and it is necessary to work with a specialist in kidney disease to achieve the best results.

Usually the first indication of diabetic kidney disease is the appearance of protein (mostly albumin) in the urine. The protein, which we all carry in our blood, leaks through the damaged glomeruli and appears in the urine. It is detected when your doctor performs a routine urine test. The presence of albumin in the urine produces no discomfort and the person is not aware of its presence unless the urine is tested.

The first sign of kidney damage is protein in the urine (proteinuria).

As the amount of albumin lost into the urine increases, the level of albumin in the blood falls below the normal range of 3.5 to 5.0 grams/ 100 milliliters. Then some of the water in the blood vessels seeps out into the skin to produce a swelling called edema (your grandparents called it dropsy). After a person has been lying down all night, the eyes, face, and hands become swollen. After being in an upright position all day, the fluid moves downward to cause swelling of the legs and feet. Other diseases, such as heart disease, also can produce edema.

The combination of 1) loss of much protein in the urine, 2) low albumin in the blood, 3) edema, and 4) an associated increase in blood fat levels is characteristic of the kidney disorder known as nephrosis. Diabetic kidney disease is but one of several types of kidney disease that can cause nephrosis.

As damage to the glomeruli continues to progress, uremia develops. The first symptoms of uremia are weakness, loss of appetite, nausea, and then vomiting. The diagnosis of uremia is made by drawing a blood sample and finding that waste products which the kidney normally gets rid of are now present in large amounts in the blood. The two waste products usually measured are urea (often expressed as BUN or blood urea nitrogen) and creatinine. Normal values for BUN are 5-25 mg/100ml of serum and for creatinine are 0.5-1.5 mg/100 ml of serum.

As the uremia progresses, other symptoms occur. These include itching, easy bleeding, and mental confusion. When over 95 percent of both kidneys are destroyed, death will occur unless the patient is treated with an artificial kidney machine or receives a kidney transplant.

The development of high blood pressure (hypertension) is a major problem that contributes to and complicates diabetic kidney disease. At first it produces no symptoms to make the person aware of its presence, but it may be detected during a physical examination. Usually it occurs about the time protein appears in the urine. Only when blood pressure is very high does it cause symptoms such as headache, shortness of breath, visual disturbances, or even a stroke.

The combination of narrowed arteries and blocked glomeruli causes high blood pressure in a great majority of people with diabetic kidney disease. The high blood pressure in turn causes more damage to the smallest arteries (arterioles) in the kidneys. This accelerates the loss of kidney function.

Another contributing factor to diabetic kidney disease is infection. The bladder and kidneys of people with diabetes seem to be more prone to invasion by bacteria than those of people who do not have diabetes. A bladder infection usually produces an urge to urinate frequently. Often this is every 15 to 30 minutes. Urination may be painful, and sometimes the urine is bloody. An infection of one or both kidneys produces back pain near the lowest ribs, chills, high fever, and often cloudy urine.

High blood pressure contributes to and complicates kidney disease.

Prevention and Treatment

Considerable research evidence in recent years suggests that good blood glucose control prevents or at least slows the development of diabetic kidney disease. This is understandable since much of the damage to the glomeruli appears to be the result of the excessive glucose in the blood attaching to the protein-containing structures in the glomeruli. Several studies have indicated that good blood glucose control can reverse the very earliest stages of proteinuria (albumin in the urine). Once kidney disease becomes more evident with development of greater proteinuria and uremia, it is unfortunately too late for good blood glucose control to reverse the process. The best we can hope for then is that better control will at least slow down the progression of the kidney disease. There is no specific drug available to heal diabetic kidney disease.

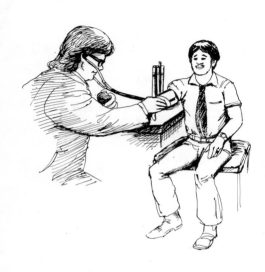

Prevention or control of high blood pressure very definitely decreases the damage to the small arteries in the kidneys. Today there are many excellent drugs available for the treatment of high blood pressure. Also, control of kidney infections through the use of antibiotics or sulfa preparations will preserve kidney function.

As kidney disease progresses, certain dietary changes become necessary. Restriction of salt (sodium chloride) in the diet both lowers blood pressure and reduces the amount of fluid retained by the body. Drugs that increase urination (diuretics) can be used to help eliminate excess fluid from the body.

When large amounts of protein are being lost in the urine and the level of albumin in the blood is low, the eating of high protein foods such as lean meats, skim milk, and egg whites is encouraged. This replaces some of the protein lost in the urine.

However, when the kidney disease progresses to the stage of uremia with weakness, nausea, and vomiting and the waste products in the blood rise to about three times their normal level, it is necessary to switch from a high to a low protein intake. Most people eat 80 to 100 grams of protein daily. In the presence of kidney failure, the protein intake is reduced to about 40 grams per day. The reduced protein intake decreases the formation of waste products such as urea that accumulate in the blood when the diseased kidneys cannot get rid of them. Reducing the level of waste products in the blood decreases the person's nausea, vomiting, and weakness. Also, studies suggest that a low protein diet actually slows the progression of the kidney disease itself.

Generally the daily insulin dose decreases as kidney failure develops. This is due both to weight loss as a result of a poor appetite and a prolonging of insulin action time which occurs with uremia.

Dialysis

Dialysis, the artificial filtration of waste products from the blood, becomes necessary when approximately 90 percent of kidney function is lost. Dialysis does not cure the kidney disease but does prevent death from uremia. Two methods of dialysis are available: hemodialysis (use of an artificial kidney machine), or peritoneal dialysis (filtering through a tube inserted into the abdomen).

In hemodialysis blood flows from the patient's arm through a plastic tube to a filtering device called the dialyzer. The dialyzer removes the waste products from the blood. The "cleaned" blood then returns to the patient. Most patients undergo hemodialysis treatments for four to five hours three times each week.

Peritoneal dialysis is accomplished by surgically inserting a plastic tube (catheter) through the abdominal wall into the peritoneal cavity. The peritoneal cavity is the space lined by the peritoneum, a thin membrane that lines the abdominal wall and intestinal tract. The peritoneum then acts as a filtering surface through which waste products in the blood can pass. A procedure often used today is CAPD (continuous ambulatory peritoneal dialysis). The patient runs two liters of a specially-prepared salt solution (dialysate) into the abdominal cavity, leaves the solution in for six hours, then drains it out. This is done four times a day, seven days a week.

Whether hemodialysis or peritoneal dialysis is used is a matter of physician and patient preference. Both methods accomplish the same purpose, which is to remove the waste products of uremia from the blood.

It is usually recommended that dialysis be started when the remaining kidney function is about 10 percent of normal. Waiting until less than 10 percent of kidney function remains increases the risk of advanced diabetic eye disease, which is often associated with advanced kidney failure.

Transplantation

Replacement of the diseased kidneys with a healthy human kidney by means of transplantation is the most satisfactory approach today to the treatment of end-stage diabetic kidney failure. This is especially true for the person who loses kidney function before the age of 60. Older individuals often do better staying on dialysis. Most patients are first treated with dialysis. Then, after their condition has been stabilized they are considered for a transplant.

Unless the patient's own diseased kidneys are seriously infected or are causing such severe hypertension that it cannot be controlled with drugs, they usually are left in place. The transplanted kidney is added as a third kidney. It is placed in the lower abdomen on one side of the urinary bladder.

The patient is less likely to reject the kidney if it comes from a living family member (related donor transplant) than if it comes from a deceased unrelated donor (cadaver transplant). However, recent figures from the University of Minnesota indicate that even when the kidney is received from an unrelated donor, 80 percent of patients still have their new kidney functioning well two years later. The likelihood of rejection of the transplanted kidney decreases considerably after the first two years. Some transplant patients now have kept their transplanted kidneys for more than ten years and continue to do well.

Fortunately, if a transplanted kidney is rejected, the patient can return to dialysis and then receive a second or even a third transplant. Anti-rejection drugs must be taken for the remainder of the patient's life.

Unfortunately, a transplanted kidney may after many years develop the same disease that destroyed the person's original kidneys. Pancreas transplants appear to be one answer to this problem (see Chapter 25). Although still quite experimental, their success rate is improving rapidly. There already is evidence that a successful pancreas transplant can keep the blood glucose normal and thereby prevent recurrence of damage in the newly transplanted kidney.

Conclusion

In conclusion, it is very important that people with diabetes do everything possible to control high blood glucose and prevent high blood pressure so as to reduce the risk of kidney disease. Considerable progress has been made in helping people with diabetes prevent kidney disease, and in treating it if it does develop. Present day research will result in even more progress in the very near future.

What You Can Do to Prevent Kidney Disease

1. Work with your health care providers to control your diabetes and keep blood glucose levels as close to normal as possible.

2. Guard against high blood pressure by lowering salt intake, maintaining a healthy weight, and exercising regularly. Have high blood pressure treated right away if repeated measurements show pressures 140/90 or higher.

3. Be on the lookout for kidney infections (constant urge to urinate or burning when urinating) and have them treated right away.

What Your Health Care Providers Can Do to Help

1. Talk to you about how diabetes and kidney damage are related.

2. Help you learn to test your blood glucose and keep it as close to normal as possible.

3. Check your blood pressure at each visit and suggest ways you can prevent or treat high blood pressure.

4. Check a urine sample at least once a year for early signs of kidney damage. A blood sample can be checked if signs of possible kidney damage are found.

5. Ask you about symptoms of kidney and urinary infections.

6. Refer you to a specialist if kidney damage develops.

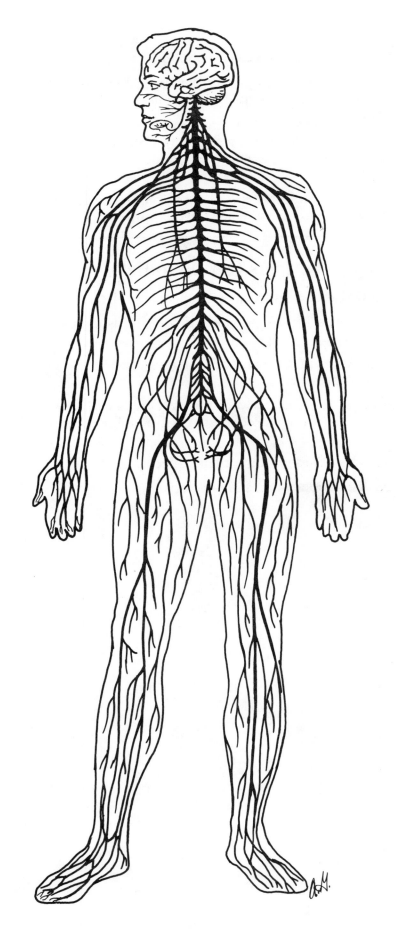

Chapter 22
Nerve Problems in Diabetes

Priscilla Hollander, M.D.

One of the most marvelous systems of our body is the nervous system. This network of nerves is the communication system of the body, much like a network of telephone lines allows communication throughout the United States. It allows the brain to send messages to other parts of the body and allows the rest of the body to send messages back to the brain. Some nerves carry messages of sensation such as pain, touch, or temperature. Other nerves carry instructions from the brain to the legs, feet, hands and internal organs. The nervous system is very extensive and its branches reach to every part of the body.

Damage to nerves—**neuropathy**— is very common in both insulin-dependent (Type I) and non-insulin-dependent (Type II) diabetes. In fact, studies indicate that 85 percent of all people with diabetes may at some time in their life develop damage to nerves. This damage can cause either distortion of messages travelling over certain nerves or not allow the messages to pass at all.

Neuropathy does not always cause obvious symptoms, but when it does, the individual may experience pain or loss of sensitivity or function. Symptoms of neuropathy tend to develop gradually and then increase in intensity. They may be severe for a while and then may disappear. Some symptoms may last for a few weeks to months, but in some cases the neuropathy may persist for months to years. Once in a while symptoms may appear suddenly—almost overnight—but they tend to disappear quickly.

How does diabetes cause damage to nerves?

We are beginning to understand how diabetes causes damage to nerves, but much is still not yet known. There is some evidence that diabetes affects small blood vessels which supply the nerves with oxygen and nutrients. If these supply lines are damaged, some nerves do not receive the oxygen and nutrients they need to maintain themselves and do their work of carrying messages.

Certain nerves tend to be affected more often by diabetes.

Another possible way nerves may be damaged by diabetes is through damage to the wall around the nerves. Nerves are insulated with a coat of fat. Like the insulation around a telephone wire, the fat protects the nerve from outside damage. Diabetes has been shown to cause a breaking down or even disappearance of the layer of fat around nerves. In a sense when this happens the nerve is "short circuited," in that messages passing along the nerve will be either distorted or blocked. In some cases the nerve may even transmit false messages.

The nervous system is divided into three main subsystems. The first is the **cranial nerves**, which go to the various areas of the head such as eyes, ears, face, and jaw. The second is the **autonomic nervous system**, which includes the nerves that go to the internal organs such as the heart, stomach, intestines, and blood vessels. The third subsystem is the **peripheral nervous system**, which includes the nerves to the extremities such as the arms, hands, legs, and feet as well as to the muscles in the abdomen and back.

Although in theory any nerve in the body can suffer damage from diabetes and cause symptoms of neuropathy, there are certain nerves in each of the above three subsystems that seem to be affected more often.

Cranial Nervous System

There are two sets of cranial nerves that seem to be most often affected by diabetic neuropathy. One of these sets is the group of nerves that go to the eye muscles. There are six eye muscles for each of your eyes. Their job is to move both eyes together so that you see only one image. If the eyes fail to move together, double vision results. This problem usually occurs suddenly. For instance, if one of the nerves to one of the muscles is damaged by diabetes, that muscle's action may be slowed or even stopped. Because of this problem the eyes will not be able to move in unison and double vision will usually result. Luckily this seems to be a temporary problem that usually disappears after several days or a few weeks. Until it clears, wearing a patch over one eye will help.

The other set of cranial nerves which may be affected are the right and left facial nerves. These nerves control the movement of the lower eyelids as well as the ability of the face to wrinkle, grimace, or smile. If there is a problem with a nerve on one side of the face, that side of the face may actually sag. The lower eyelid will droop and the outside of the person's smile will also droop. This problem is called Bell's palsy. It may occur in people who do not have diabetes but is much more common in people with diabetes. Fortunately, like the problem with the eye muscles, Bell's palsy is temporary. Neither of these problems leaves any permanent damage.

Problems with facial nerves are almost always temporary.

Autonomic Nervous System

One of the most common areas affected in the autonomic nervous system is the digestive system—the stomach and intestine. Diabetic nerve damage to the stomach usually causes it to empty more slowly than it should. This can lead to a feeling of fullness which may cause nausea and occasionally vomiting. This problem can be present all the time or may occur once in awhile. Often it seems to be worse in the early morning before or following breakfast. The medical name for this neuropathy is **gastroparesis**, which means "slow emptying" or "paralysis of the stomach." This condition can sometimes be difficult to diagnose, because there are a number of diseases which can cause the same symptoms. One of the best ways of evaluating someone for gastroparesis is by using an x-ray technique in which the person swallows a barium dye which outlines the stomach. A series of x-rays is then taken and used to evaluate whether there is a problem with the way food is passing through the stomach.

Digestive problems can be caused by neuropathy.

What can be done for gastroparesis? There are several approaches to the problem. One is to eat smaller meals. It is also important to evaluate the person's diabetes control to see if that is partly responsible for the problem. The third approach is to take a medication called Regalon, which works to actually speed up the rate of contraction of the stomach muscles to help digestion to occur at the normal rate.

Another problem area in the digestive system is the intestine. Diabetic neuropathy can affect the large and small intestines in two ways. It can lead to problems with diarrhea, or it can cause the opposite problem— constipation. The medical approach to both of these conditions is a well balanced diet plus the use of laxatives in people with problems with constipation. For people with diarrhea, medications such as Lomotil or Pepto Bismol may be used.

Another area where autonomic neuropathies may develop is in the genital-urinary system. Problems may occur with the ability to empty the bladder when it is full of urine. This occurs because of damage to the nerves which usually give a signal of pressure when it is time to urinate. Therefore the person may not urinate often enough, which can cause enlargement of the bladder and worsen the problem. The other genito-urinary problem that is common in people with diabetes involves problems with the function of the penis in men, causing an inability to have erections (see Chapter 18).

The final major problem area in the autonomic nervous system relates to nerves that go to the blood vessels. Neuropathy can result in low blood pressure in certain areas of the body, especially upon arising from a sitting or lying position. The amount of blood in the blood vessels must constantly be regulated to maintain a healthy blood pressure throughout the body. As we change from lying or sitting to a standing position, blood must be shifted so that the right amount is in the right place at the right time. Often when we jump up very quickly from a lying to standing position we experience a momentary twinge of dizziness. This is because it takes a little bit of time for your body to move some blood from your feet to your head.

Your body is able to shift blood by sending messages along various little nerves to the blood vessels telling them when to contract and when to expand. If these nerves are damaged they do not work as quickly and it takes longer to shift blood volume. Thus, when the person gets up suddenly, it may take so long to shift the blood from the feet to the head that the person gets quite dizzy and may even fall. This problem is called **postural hypotension**, which means that blood pressure is momentarily low because of a change in body posture. People with this problem can usually avoid dizziness by avoiding standing quickly after sitting or lying for some time. There are also medications that can assist the blood vessels in shifting blood.

Peripheral Nervous System

Two main types of neuropathy can occur in the peripheral nervous system, one involving a number of nerves at the same time (peripheral polyneuropathy), and the other in which only one nerve is affected (peripheral mononeuropathy).

Peripheral polyneuropathies are the most common of all neuropathies. They generally affect the feet and/or legs and occasionally the hands and/or arms. There are two main symptoms of this type of neuropathy. One is characterized by a "pins and needles" feeling, tingling, numbness, and/or burning. The symptoms are most noticeable at night and are usually found in both feet. When the problem occurs in both feet/legs or both hands/arms it is described as symmetrical (both sides of the body) neuropathy. The numbness from this problem can interfere with the person's ability to feel pain. This can be serious because the person may injure his or her foot or hand and not even notice it. If an infection occurs and is not treated, problems such as gangrene could result.

Symmetrical neuropathies can be quite painful. The pain is usually worse at night, and has been compared to an electric shock, a burning sensation, or even to a toothache. The painful neuropathy may come on very quickly or very slowly. Once it occurs it will usually last from 6 to 18 months and then will disappear. This is in contrast to the numbness and tingling which may go on for months or even years.

Occasionally an asymmetrical (one side of the body) painful neuropathy may develop. This usually occurs in one of the thighs and it may also cause loss of muscle and muscle weakness in the area. Again, this problem is usually temporary and will pass in three to six months. It is important to use specific exercises and other methods to help prevent loss of muscle strength in the affected area.

Specific exercises can prevent loss of muscle strength in areas affected by peripheral neuropathy.

When only one nerve is affected the problem is called mononeuropathy. This type of neuropathy most often affects a nerve in the chest or abdomen. Pain from the nerve may be confused with other medical problems such as appendicitis, kidney stones, or heart disease. This makes the problem difficult to diagnose. Like the other painful neuropathies, this type usually lasts from three to six months and then will usually disappear.

Peripheral neuropathies can be diagnosed and confirmed by the use of a test called an electromyogram or EMG. This test records the speed of nerve impulses as they move along a specific nerve. In diabetes the nerve impulse is usually slow and has other abnormal characteristics. An EMG is usually done by a neurologist (a specialist in the diseases of the nerves).

Treatment of Painful Neuropathies

Some methods of treating specific functional problems related to neuropathies have already been discussed. The focus in this section will be on methods of reducing the pain that sometimes accompanies neuropathy. Pain can vary from being quite mild to being very severe, and it may be continuous or sporadic. Several medications have been found to be useful in reducing or eliminating the pain of neuropathy. These medications were first developed to treat other conditions.

Several medications may be helpful in reducing pain from neuropathy.

One group of medications, Dilantin and Tegretol, were first developed to treat seizures, and then it was found that they could be very helpful in treating neuropathy pain. Elavil and Prolixin are another group of medications which were developed primarily to treat problems with depression. The combination of the two has been extraordinarily useful in helping some people with the pain of neuropathy. It is not yet known how these two groups of medications act to reduce pain in people with neuropathy.

Besides medication another important way to reduce the pain of neuropathy is to have strict diabetes control. As mentioned in the section on peripheral neuropathy, a test can be performed to measure the speed of electrical impulses as they move along the nerves. The speed of these impulses is slowed in people with diabetic neuropathy, but it has been shown that with improvement in blood glucose control the nerve impulses may regain their normal speed.

If, however, both good blood glucose control and the use of the above medications do not provide relief from pain, it may be necessary to use temporary pain killing medications. These pain killers may include such things as Tylenol or aspirin. It may be necessary to use one of the weaker narcotics such as codeine or even stronger narcotics for the most severe episodes of pain. These narcotics must be used under close physician supervision. Painful neuropathy may persist for months, but in most cases it will disappear.

Early Detection is Important

Your physician should check nerve function as part of routine care.

It is important for your physician to check the function of your nerves as part of routine diabetes care. This can be done by testing the reflexes in your upper and lower body, and checking your feet and hands for decreased sensation to pin prick and vibration. Your physician should ask if you have had any vision problems, trouble emptying your bladder, problems with impotence, or any numbness, tingling, or unusual pain in any area of your body. Some of these may be symptoms of neuropathies, but neuropathies can mimic almost any other pain.

New advances in the treatment of neuropathy may be near. There are several experimental drugs which may help to block the nerve damage caused by diabetes. These drugs fall into a category called **aldose reductase inhibitors**. They may actually block or reduce the effects of the chemical reactions in diabetes which may be damaging to nerves. It is hoped that these drugs may prevent the development of diabetic neuropathy and possibly help to repair damage that has already occurred.

What You Can Do

1. Maintain good blood glucose control.
2. Tell your doctor about any tingling, numbness, loss of feeling, muscle weakness, pain or other unusual sensations.
3. Ask your doctor to investigate any persistent digestive, urinary, or sexual problems.
4. If medications are prescribed, take them exactly as directed.
5. If you have loss of feeling in any part of your body be especially careful to avoid injury to that area, and check it daily for infections or other problems.

What Your Health Care Providers Can Do

1. Use glycosylated hemoglobin tests and your blood glucose testing records to help you maintain good blood glucose control.
2. Ask you regularly about symptoms of neuropathy.
3. Check the function of your nerves as part of routine care.
4. Refer you for diagnostic tests if symptoms occur.
5. Prescribe medication and pursue other methods of coping with painful neuropathy.
6. Teach you how to avoid problems which can occur with loss of sensitivity, muscle weakness, and other possible effects of neuropathy.

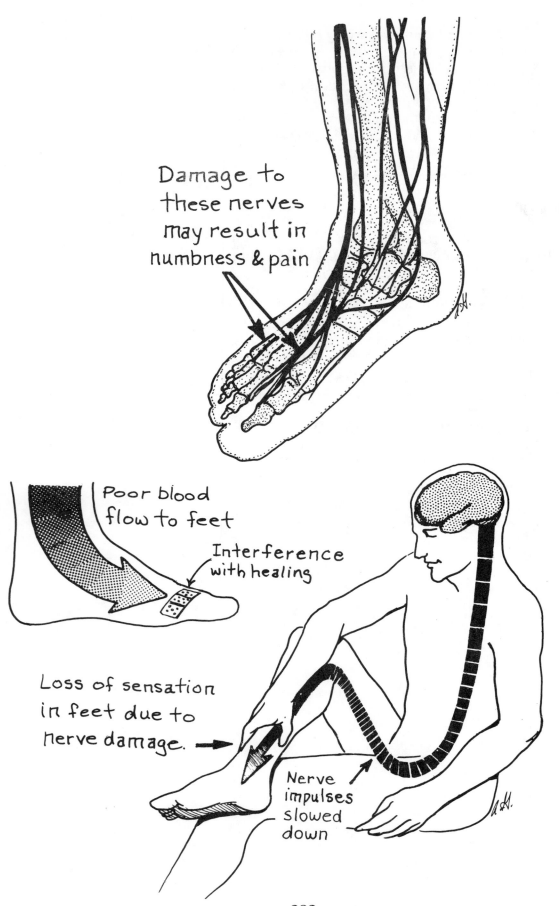

Damage to
these nerves
may result in
numbness & pain

Poor blood
flow to feet

Interference
with healing

Loss of sensation
in feet due to
nerve damage. →

Nerve
impulses
slowed
down

Chapter 23
Healthy FootSteps for People with Diabetes

Beth Olson, R.N., B.A.

People with diabetes have special reasons to make sure their feet are healthy and well cared for. Diabetes can cause foot problems which if not caught early and cared for promptly can cause serious damage and even require amputation. Experts estimate that proper care can prevent three-fourths of these serious problems.

You will gain much more from proper foot care than a reduced risk of amputation. Your feet will feel healthy, which will help you enjoy your daily activities. You have a special reason to avoid the sore and tired feet that are so common in our society.

This chapter will explain how diabetes increases the risk of foot problems and how you can prevent them with a few minutes of foot care each day.

How does diabetes increase the risk of foot problems?

Diabetes can affect your feet in two main ways:

1. Nerve damage
2. Blood vessel disease

Nerve Damage

Our nerves are the body's built-in telegraph line. They relay messages from different parts of the body to the brain, and from the brain to the rest of the body. Diabetes may cause **neuropathy**, which is a medical term for nerve damage. Neuropathy may result in part from many years of high blood glucose levels.

Having high blood glucose levels for a long time tends to slow the travel of nerve impulses and may lead to nerve damage. Nerve damage may result in tingling, numbness, and pain in the hands and feet. It may cause loss of feeling and difficulty with balance. The loss of feeling may mean that you could step on a tack and have it in your shoe all day without feeling any pain. Loss of feeling also makes it difficult for you to feel a blister forming when you've walked too far or too long. And hot water may feel warm instead of hot, so you could burn yourself without having pain.

Nerve damage may cause other problems. You may notice less sweating and more dryness of your feet. If not kept moistened with mild skin cream, the skin may crack and become infected. Sometimes nerve damage causes weakness of some of the muscles and shortening of the tendons in the feet. These problems can change the shape of your feet, making it very difficult to find shoes that fit properly.

Blood Vessel Disease

The other way diabetes can affect your feet is through the development of blood vessel disease. High levels of blood glucose can cause damage to blood vessels, resulting in poor blood flow which can interfere with your body's ability to heal an injury or fight an infection.

Healthy blood vessels have the ability to expand and contract. Blood vessels to your feet expand if you need extra blood or if your feet are warm. Blood vessels in your feet contract if your body is cold.

With blood vessel disease, there may be a loss of the ability of the blood vessels to expand and contract, because the walls of the blood vessels have become rigid. If your feet need extra blood to heal an injury or infection and your blood vessels aren't able to expand, the overall result is a decrease in the supply of blood to your feet, which will slow the healing process.

Something else happens to the blood vessels as a result of blood vessel disease. High levels of blood fats can cause a sticky substance called plaque to build up on the walls of the blood vessels. The inside area of the blood vessel then becomes narrow, which cuts down on the amount of blood that can flow through. This blood vessel blockage may result in poor blood flow to the feet. Your doctor may check the pulses in your feet to determine how good the blood flow is to your feet. It is very important to maintain normal levels of blood glucose and blood fats to prevent blood vessel disease.

Sometimes the blood flow through the large blood vessels is sufficient, but there is damage of the small (microscopic) blood vessels. These small blood vessels bring nutrients and oxygen to the cells in the feet. Sometimes diabetes causes the walls of the small blood vessels to become thickened or to leak fluid and nutrients. These changes reduce the amount of nutrients and oxygen that reach the cells. This may cause poor healing of an infection or injury, because the cells are not receiving enough nutrients and oxygen to repair the damage. So even though the blood flow to your feet may be okay, the blood flow within your feet may be poor, making it especially important that you prevent infections and injury and have them treated promptly if they occur.

The combination of nerve damage and blood vessel disease can lead to serious foot infections.

The combination of nerve damage and blood vessel disease can work together to cause serious foot problems. A minor injury or sore may not be treated because you may not feel it. The sore may not heal because of poor blood supply. It can then spread through the foot and even into the bone. The infected tissue kills healthy tissue around it, causing gangrene, which is a Greek word for "gnawing death of tissue." The gangrene is hard to treat, and it can spread up the leg, requiring amputation of the foot or lower leg. Approximately 20,000 amputations are needed annually by people with diabetes, but with good foot care amputations can be prevented.

Common Foot Problems

Some of these common foot problems may be more serious because of poor blood flow or loss of feeling in the feet:

Ingrown toenails—Ingrown toenails are usually caused by improper nail trimming or tightly fitting shoes. They occur when a sharp piece of nail irritates the skin. This causes an infection and should be treated promptly by a foot specialist or your doctor. Prevention includes trimming your toenails straight across and filing sharp edges, and wearing shoes with plenty of toe room. If you have an ingrown toenail, your doctor may decide surgery is necessary to remove part of the nail. This is usually a minor procedure which can be performed in the doctor's office. Antibiotics are often prescribed at this time to help prevent or treat a related infection.

Blisters—Blisters are formed when shoes rub and irritate the skin. Wash the area gently and protect it from further irritation. **Do not** try to pop or drain the blister; this would allow germs to enter and an infection could develop. If the blister seems to heal slowly or becomes inflamed, see your doctor promptly.

Plantar warts—Plantar warts are caused by viruses and may be very hard to get rid of. They occur on the bottom of the foot and may look like a circular callus. **Do not** use commercial wart removers to treat the wart unless instructed to do so by your health care team. Your doctor may prescribe a mild acid to apply directly to the wart. It is very important to wash off this acid every day before applying more medication. If the area around the wart becomes red or irritated, or if you notice a burning feeling, stop using the medication and contact your doctor.

Athlete's foot—Athlete's foot is a fungal infection that is usually found between the toes and may spread to the toenails. Cracking and peeling of the skin between the toes is the most common sign of a fungal infection. There may be pain, itching, and/or bleeding between the toes and thickening and crumbling of the toenails. Careful washing of the feet and drying between the toes can help prevent athlete's foot. Your doctor may prescribe a lotion or powder to heal the infection.

Calluses and corns—Sometimes a change in the position of a bone in your foot or a lump of extra bone (bone spur) causes rubbing when wearing shoes. Where the shoes repeatedly rub, irritation causes dead skin to build up and result in corns or calluses. These will eventually disappear if the shoes are altered so that they no longer rub the area. **Do not** trim or use chemicals to remove or dissolve calluses and corns. Have your doctor or a foot specialist treat them for you.

Hammertoes—If the muscles in the feet become weakened and the tendons shortened, the toes may buckle under and form hammertoes. This may be an inherited problem, a result of neuropathy, or a result of wearing shoes that are too short. Shoes with a large toe area are important to prevent corns from forming on the tops of hammertoes. Sometimes surgery is necessary to straighten the toes.

Bunions—An enlargement of the joint at the base of the big toe is called a bunion. It is usually inherited. Wearing shoes with a wide toe area is helpful to prevent irritation of the skin surrounding the bunion. Sometimes surgery is necessary to remove the extra bone.

If You Have Foot Problems

Foot Infection or Sore:
1. Stay off your feet.
2. Maintain good blood glucose control.
3. Consult your physician. An antibiotic may be prescribed. Sometimes a cast, surgery, or hospitalization is necessary.

Foot Deformity
1. Have a physician or foot specialist prescribe special shoes to protect your feet.
2. Sometimes surgery is necessary to correct the problem.

Nerve or Blood Vessel Disease
1. Wear only shoes that fit properly.
2. Inspect your feet daily for cuts, sores, redness or other signs of infection.
3. Protect your feet from injury.
4. Maintain good blood glucose control.
5. Do not smoke.

Corns, Calluses, and Problem Toenails
1. Do not use over-the-counter remedies to care for these conditions.
2. If you have difficulty trimming your toenails have your physician or a foot specialist trim them for you.
3. If these problems persist see a physician or foot specialist.

Risk Factors for Diabetic Foot Problems

The American Diabetes Association has identified several risk factors for diabetic foot problems. You can determine if any of these risk factors apply to you:

1. Age greater than 40.
2. Cigarette smoking.
3. Having had diabetes for more than 10 years.
4. Decreased blood supply or loss of feeling in the feet and hands.
5. Changes in foot shape (bunions, hammertoes, or bumps).
6. History of foot infections or amputation.

You can't change how old you are or how many years you have had diabetes, but several of these risk factors may be affected by choices you make.

Smoking: The nicotine in tobacco causes your blood vessels to spasm and narrow, which decreases the blood flow to your feet. Your circulation will be greatly decreased if you have diabetes and are a smoker.

Decreased circulation or sensitivity: By following your diabetes management plan and testing often to make sure your blood glucose is under good control, you may delay or avoid the complications related to nerve and blood vessel damage. If you don't know how to keep your blood glucose under good control, ask your health care team for help (see Chapter 4). If your doctor has told you that you have decreased circulation or loss of sensation in your feet it is especially important to check your feet daily for problems. You may be referred to a specialist who will evaluate your foot problems and give more involved advice about caring for your feet.

If your doctor has told you that you have decreased circulation or loss of sensation in your feet it is especially important to check your feet daily for problems. You may also be referred to a specialist who will evaluate your foot problems and give more involved advice about caring for your feet.

Changes in foot shape: Shoes can cause pressure areas on your feet that you may not feel. Corns, calluses, and infections under the skin may develop from the pressure of shoes that do not fit well. If you have deformities of your feet, you are more likely to develop pressure sores.

History of foot infections or amputations: You have a greater risk of having foot problems if you've already had a foot infection or amputation. It is very important to prevent injury to your feet and to reduce your other risk factors, especially by avoiding high blood glucose levels. The body's ability to resist and fight infections can be reduced when blood glucose levels are high. The white blood cells, which normally attack germs and help to fight infection, do not work as well when there is a high level of blood glucose.

Foot problems are not an automatic result of having diabetes. PREVENTION is the Key!

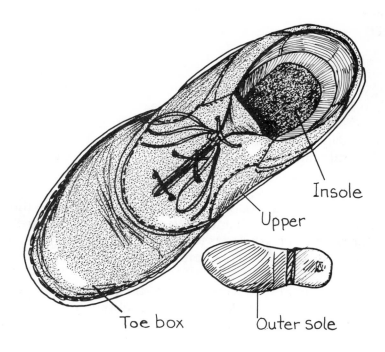

Insole

Upper

Toe box

Outer sole

Footwear

The type of shoes you wear is very important. Shoes that fit well can help prevent corns, calluses, and blisters.

Characteristics of Proper Shoes:

1. The **upper** should be made of soft leather which will mold to your feet and allow them to breathe.
2. The **insole** and inner lining should be soft without rough areas which may irritate your skin.
3. The **outer sole** should be made of a rigid material. This encourages a rocking motion when walking and helps to prevent extra pressure on the ball of your foot.
4. The shoe should be about 1/2 inch longer than your longest toe when standing.
5. The **toebox** (toe area) should be wide and shaped like your foot. Many women's styles have a narrow toebox and contribute to corns, calluses, and deformities. A good way to make sure your shoe is wide enough is to draw an outline of your foot while standing and another outline of your shoe. By comparing the two outlines, it will be easy to determine if the shoe is wide enough and long enough for your foot.
6. It is especially important to wear well-fitting shoes and thick, soft cotton or wool blend socks (not nylon stockings) when you will be on your feet for long periods. Wearing socks which cushion your feet can help protect them from corns, calluses, and blisters. Never wear shoes without socks.
7. Tight stockings or those with bands to hold them up may reduce blood flow to the feet. Socks with seams or creases may irritate your skin.

Footcare

Make footcare a part of your daily routine. Washing your feet daily will decrease the amount of bacteria on your feet and help to prevent infection. Wash your feet as part of your daily bathing routine or use a basin if you are unable to take a shower or tub bath. Use warm water, not hot, and test it with your wrist or elbow before entering. A thermometer can be purchased for testing water and used to make sure it is in a safe range of within a few degrees of 100 degrees Fahrenheit.

Use a washcloth and mild soap to gently wash your feet and the area between your toes. Rinse well and pat feet dry with a soft towel, gently drying the area between your toes to prevent fungal infections. Soaking your feet is not necessary and may cause more dryness.

Sometimes the joints in your toes become stiff and affect the way you walk. This may be the cause of pressure and rubbing on small areas of your feet which could lead to infection. Rolling a pop bottle with your toes is a good way to prevent or delay stiffness in the joints of your toes.

Rub corns and calluses GENTLY with a pumice stone to remove the build-up of dead skin. If your feet have lost sensitivity, be especially careful not to rub too hard, which could break the skin and cause an infection. Corns and calluses can become infected easily if not treated properly.

Do not use harsh commercial wart-removing products which often have chemicals that can burn your skin. Do not cut your corns and calluses, because that can cause injuries which may be very difficult to heal.

Callus formation should be avoided because calluses can become hardened and cause pressure on the healthy tissue underneath. This can lead to infection under the callus that you may not be able to see or feel. Buying new well-fitting shoes or having a foot specialist fit a shoe insert can help prevent the formation of calluses.

Dryness of the skin can lead to cracks in the skin which can become infected. To prevent this, apply a small amount of cold cream or vaseline every day. If you use vaseline, apply it when your skin is moist. Rub the lotion into the dry areas of your feet. Do not put lotion between your toes as this may contribute to the development of a fungal infection.

Careful trimming of your toenails is important. After soaking only your toenails for 10 to 15 minutes in warm water, your nails should be soft enough to trim. This is the only time soaking your feet is recommended, unless suggested by your physician. Make sure the water is warm (100 degrees F), not hot. Cut your nails straight across using a toenail clipper. File the sharp toenail edges to prevent irritation of the other toes. Sometimes toenails can become too thick to cut by yourself. If this is true for you, see a foot specialist or your physician for help with nail care.

If you are unable to trim your toenails, ask your health care team for help.

Foot Care for Athletes

If you exercise regularly and/or participate in sports, you must be aware of how this activity may affect your feet. The following guidelines will help:

- If you are having foot problems, avoid sports such as basketball and tennis, and exercise such as jogging, because they cause added stress on your feet.

- Inspect your feet after participating in activities which cause stress on your feet.

- Wearing two pairs of socks may provide an extra cushion for your feet and help avoid blisters and calluses.

- Follow the shoe selection guidelines in this chapter. A good quality shoe designed for the sport is very important.

- Special shoe inserts or insoles may help to decrease the pressure many activities exert on the bottoms of the feet.

- A light dusting of cornstarch between the toes can help prevent excessive perspiration.

- See your doctor promptly if any sign of foot injury occurs.

Footstress

Footstress refers to things that could cause injury to your feet, such as wearing open toe or open heel shoes, going barefoot, or walking too far. The main purpose of shoes is to prevent injury to your feet. Wearing safe shoes provides protection from sharp objects which you may not see or feel.

Shake out your shoes before putting them on, to prevent injury from hidden objects. Look at your feet daily for signs of irritation or injury, using a mirror if you have difficulty seeing the bottoms of your feet. Feel them for areas of warmth. Pay special attention to the bony areas of your feet. Redness and hotspots indicate irritation of the tissue over the bone. Try to find out what is causing the irritation.

Shortening your stride when walking can help prevent repeated force on bony areas of your feet.

If you have a loss of feeling in your feet you may not be able to tell when you've walked too far, too fast, or too long. Sore, tired feet are a signal to slow the pace, shorten your stride, or stop and rest. Shortening your stride is especially helpful in preventing repeated force on bony areas of your feet. The effect of continued pressure on your feet, especially when walking on hard surfaces, can cause irritation of the skin and underlying tissue. You may not be able to feel the problem, so checking your feet for hotspots or blisters is the best way to know when to rest or quit for the day. If you were to continue to irritate the sore tissue, a serious infection may develop. By checking your feet every day, you will know which shoes are safest for you and how far you can walk without injury to your feet.

Change your shoes midday and evening to avoid continuous pressure on the same areas of your feet. If you are breaking in new shoes, wear them for one hour the first day and look at your feet closely. If there aren't any areas of redness, wear them for two hours on the second day. If you notice redness or hotspots, don't wear the shoes until the irritation has healed. Gradually increase the amount of time that you wear the new shoes, or return them if you can't wear them safely.

There are other measures which are important to consider:

- Avoid extremes of heat and cold.
- Never use hot water bottles or electrical heating pads.
- Wear warm socks if your feet are cold—not battery-operated feet warmers.
- Sandals are recommended for beachwear since the the hot sand or pavement may burn the bottoms of your feet. They also provide some protection from sharp objects hidden in the sand.
- Call your physician if you notice any sign of infection such as tenderness, swelling, redness, warmth, or drainage. An infection or injury that is healing slowly should be evaluated by your doctor without delay.

Your feet should be examined by your doctor at every visit. Taking off your shoes and socks will help your doctor remember to check your feet.

What You Can Do

1. Maintain normal levels of blood glucose and blood fats.
2. Reduce your risk factors for foot problems if possible.
3. Wear well-made protective shoes.
4. Make foot care and inspection part of your daily routine.
5. Call your physician if you detect a problem.
6. Make sure your physician examines your feet at every visit.

What Your Health Care Providers Can Do

1. Help you maintain normal levels of blood glucose and blood fats and reduce other risk factors for foot problems.
2. Advise you in selecting shoes that will be safe for you to wear.
3. Teach you how to care for your feet and prevent minor problems from becoming serious.
4. Examine your feet at every visit and ask you about any foot problems you have had, as well as any foot or leg pain when you sit, stand, or walk.
5. Check the blood flow to your feet and test your ability to feel light touch or other sensations in your feet and legs. If you have poor blood flow or insensitive areas, advise you how to avoid injury and what to look for during daily checking of the affected areas.

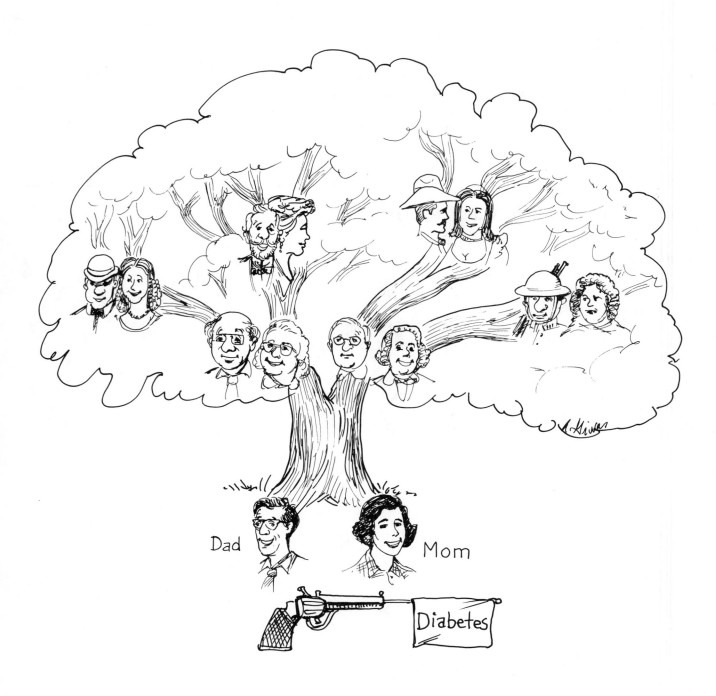

Dad

Mom

Diabetes

Chapter 24
Why Diabetes?
The Genetic Trigger and
How It Is Pulled

Jose Barbosa, M.D. and Priscilla Hollander, M.D.

In Chapter 1 we discussed what diabetes is and what goes wrong in the body to cause insulin-dependent (Type I) or non-insulin-dependent (Type II) diabetes. But before you were told **WHAT** causes diabetes, you probably wondered **WHY** it happened to you. This is a normal feeling, and it is a question that scientists are getting closer to being able to answer. Genetics, or the study of how we inherit characteristics from our parents, is the field of science that is closest to explaining why some people develop diabetes. This chapter will explain what is known about the genetics of Type I and Type II diabetes.

(Sometimes the question "Why me?" has more to do with feelings than with a need for information. If you are finding it hard to accept that you have diabetes, or if you are just feeling really mad about the disease, Chapter 6 may help you understand and deal with your feelings. It may also help you reach an agreement with yourself to learn as much as you can about diabetes and how to control it. That is when the information in this chapter—and the rest of the manual—can be most helpful.)

Why does the body stop making insulin in Type I diabetes?

We have already explained (Chapters 1 and 8) that in Type I diabetes there is a complete lack of insulin because of the death of the cells in the pancreas that produce it. But why these cells die is one of the mysteries of diabetes. Most scientists think that two factors play a role, one genetic and the other environmental.

Our understanding of the genetics of Type I diabetes has been helped by the discovery of a group of genes called HLA and located on the sixth human chromosome. Genes are chemical messages passed from one generation to the next to control characteristics. Studies of families with one or more children with diabetes have shown that there is a gene in the HLA group of these families that is not present in families with no history of Type I diabetes. Each person carries two number 6 chromosomes, one from the father and one from the mother. The diabetes gene can be present in both, one, or neither chromosome. Usually, diabetes will develop only when there is a double dose of this gene.

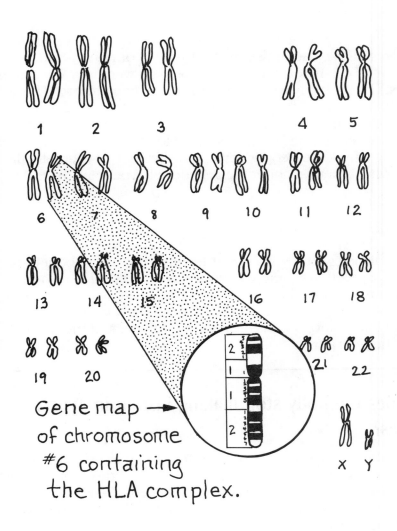

Gene map →
of chromosome
#6 containing
the HLA complex.

We are also making progress in understanding the environmental factors by which the diabetes genes can cause the disease. It seems that the genes give faulty instructions to the white blood cells responsible for defense against viral infections. This results in a number of abnormally behaving white blood cells. One way they behave abnormally is by making substances called **antibodies**, which instead of acting normally and attacking cells foreign to the body, actually damage the insulin-making cells. A second way they may help cause diabetes is by attacking insulin-making cells infected by viruses and in the process doing more harm than good.

Much research is currently being focused on these problems and there are justified hopes that better understanding of these abnormal genes and white blood cells will result in prevention or even cure of Type I diabetes.

It may help you to understand the complex interactions described above if you think of the diabetic gene as a loaded gun waiting for someone to pull the trigger. One of the environmental factors—the virus—can then be thought of as the actual culprit that shoots the gun.

Not all people who have the gene for Type I diabetes actually get the disease, however. Some people may have a resistance to the triggering virus, or there may be other factors that are not yet understood. The best way to estimate how many of the people who carry a Type I diabetes gene might be expected to develop the disease is to study identical twins. Identical twins have the same genetic makeup. So if one identical twin develops Type I diabetes, we know that the other twin also carries the gene for Type I diabetes. Studies have found that if one identical twin develops Type I diabetes, there is a 50 percent chance that the other twin also will develop Type I diabetes.

Scientists now have a fairly good understanding of how Type I diabetes is inherited. It is believed that for a person to be prone to develop Type I diabetes, he or she must receive a diabetic gene from each of his or her parents. If only one diabetic gene is present, the person will not be susceptible to diabetes, and he or she will not even know the gene is present. If this person happens to marry another person who also has a diabetic gene, then their children will receive a double dose of diabetic genes and will be likely to develop the disease. This is why Type I diabetes so often skips generations. A single gene may be passed along by many family members before it meets another diabetic gene, allowing the Type I diabetes to appear.

It is thought that a genetic factor and an environmental factor combine to cause Type I diabetes.

Geneticists have determined that if you have Type I diabetes, the risk for diabetes in your children is 5 percent or less (only 5 out of 100 children will develop diabetes). In general, the risk for brothers and sisters of children with Type I diabetes is less than 10 percent. The risk for children of diabetic fathers seems to be higher than for children of diabetic mothers. Becoming pregnant at an older age also may increase the risk that a woman with diabetes will have a child that will develop diabetes. If both parents have Type I diabetes, the risk would then be higher, possibly 20 to 40 percent. In general, these risks would rarely justify a decision not to have a family. Current research efforts will probably result in predictive tests to use in relatives of people with diabetes.

Why does Type II diabetes occur later in life?

Type II diabetes is also a genetic disease, but we do not yet understand how the genes work to produce it. No gene such as the Type I diabetes HLA gene has been found in people with Type II diabetes. In Type II diabetes, obesity seems to be the factor that sets off the genetic trigger. (Remember, a virus is thought to be the culprit in Type I diabetes.) A person who carries the gene for Type II diabetes can usually avoid the disease by keeping a close to normal body weight. Type II diabetes usually occurs later in life because of the effect of excess body weight. It takes many years for the obesity to wear down the effectiveness of the body's insulin, and then to release the genetic trigger.

Type II diabetes is inherited more easily than Type I diabetes.

One thing that is known about the genetics of Type II diabetes is that it is inherited more easily than Type I diabetes. This greater genetic tendency for Type II diabetes can be easily shown using the identical twin example from the Type I discussion. If one identical twin develops Type II diabetes, the chances are almost 100 percent that the other twin will develop Type II diabetes at some time in life.

Many families have more than one person in each generation who has diabetes. People without diabetes who are members of such families have a much higher risk of developing Type II diabetes than do people without such a family background. So if you have Type II diabetes, it is not only important for you to attain a more ideal weight, it is also important for other members of your family to avoid obesity and be checked regularly for diabetes, especially after the age of 40.

Genetic Counseling

If you have questions about your family's genetic possibilities regarding diabetes, you may want to consult a genetic counselor. However, this can be very expensive, and because very little is known about why diabetes occurs, it seldom yields useful information. This is especially true in the case of Type I diabetes, because there is no way known to prevent it, so there is little value in knowing a person's chances of developing the disease.

Genetic research is just one of the areas of diabetes research that are beginning to show great promise for making possible a future free of the effects of this disease. In the next chapter we will look at other types of research that are underway.

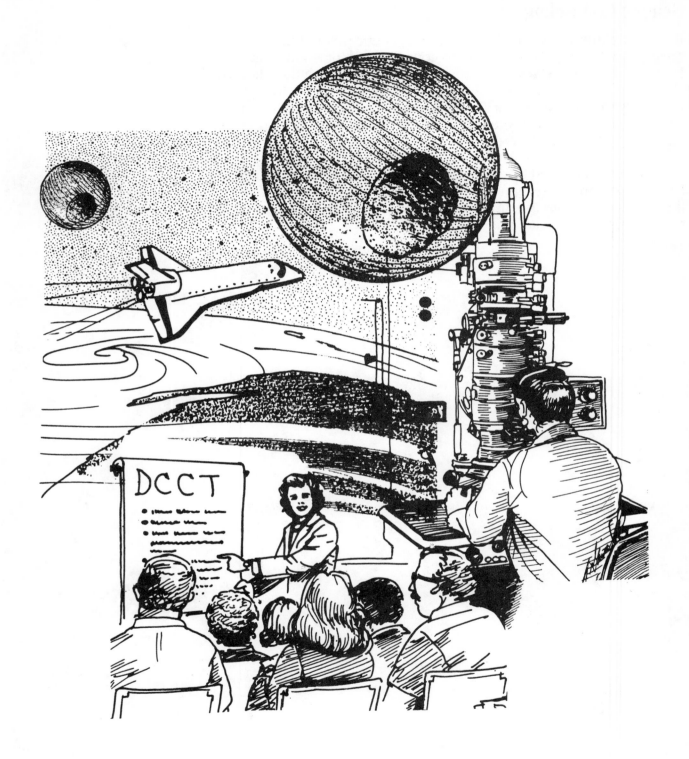

Chapter 25
Diabetes Research: Hope for Today and the Future

LeAnn McNeil, R.N., M.S.; Richard Bergenstal, M.D.; and
Donnell D. Etzwiler, M.D.

At the mention of diabetes research, most people think of the search
for a cure. This is very important and does have a very high priority in
diabetes research. However, it is helpful to remember that research can
provide present benefits which can help people with diabetes live
better until a cure (or cures) is found.

Two Basic Types of Research

There are two main types of health research: basic and clinical. Basic
research brings to mind images of scientists working in sophisticated
laboratories, making discoveries and testing new theories. This
research is called "basic" because it starts from the basic level of
pursuing ideas of how the human body normally functions. A recent
example of basic diabetes research is the discovery of ways to splice
genes (recombinant DNA technology) to make human insulin
(Chapter 9). The development of this process to produce insulin led
the way for the production of many hormones and drugs using the
recombinant DNA technology.

Clinical research is the evaluation of techniques, medications, and
products when used by people. After basic researchers developed the
technique for making human insulin and tested it extensively in
animals, the U.S. Food and Drug Administration then reviewed the
studies carefully. Approval was given for clinical research to find out if
the new human insulin was safe and effective when used by people
with diabetes. The International Diabetes Center was one of the first
centers chosen to evaluate human insulin.

The results of the clinical testing of human insulin showed that it is
indeed safe and useful in the treatment of diabetes. Human insulin is
now available in pharmacies, thanks to the combined efforts of basic
and clinical researchers, groups who provided funds, and research
participants.

Basic Diabetes Research

There are several areas of basic research which are important in the field of diabetes. Much of the initial work starts in animal studies. The most important example of this was the isolation of insulin by Banting and Best, who used dogs in their research (Chapter 1).

Besides animal studies there are different kinds of basic research done using advances in a field called **pathology**. This is the study of changes in the human body as a result of diseases. The development of very powerful electron microscopes has made it possible for researchers to see what actually happens in and around the cells of the body.

For instance, the cells of a section of the pancreas can be viewed through a microscope, which reveals the complexity of the substances and processes it controls. Using different chemical stains has shown that there is much more than just insulin produced by the pancreas. It was discovered that insulin begins as part of a larger molecule called **proinsulin** (Chapter 9). Other hormones have been discovered in the pancreas, including **glucagon**, which you read about in Chapter 8. There are also hormones called pancreatic polypeptide and somatostatin, which were unknown until just recently. It is probable that all these pancreatic hormones interact to maintain normal blood glucose levels. Currently if the pancreas is not producing enough insulin the treatment is to give just insulin injections. But maybe in the future a better method will be found, such as using proinsulin or somatostatin in combination with or in place of insulin injections.

Through basic research we have learned that diabetes is a complicated process, and there are many things remaining to be explained. A major area in basic diabetes research involves explaining the action of insulin receptors, the places on the cell wall where insulin attaches and allows glucose to enter the cell. This is an especially exciting area for people with non-insulin-dependent diabetes (Type II). Is there a way to increase the number of receptors or to help them work more effectively? We know that losing weight increases the number and effectiveness of insulin receptors, but further studies are revealing even more about these very important areas on cells.

Antibodies are another interesting area of investigation. Antibodies are proteins made by the immune system, whose job it is to find and destroy germs or other foreign substances. For unknown reasons the antibodies sometimes begin attacking the beta cells that make insulin. A test to detect this has been developed in which a blood sample is taken from a person with newly diagnosed insulin-dependent (Type I) diabetes. The blood is placed in a dish containing beta cells taken from an animal. Then a chemical dye is added, which glows if there is an antibody which is attaching to and possibly destroying the beta cells.

Electron microscope

We now know that these antibodies attacking the beta cells may be present for quite a while before diabetes actually develops. The fact that the immune system has been shown to be an important factor in causing Type I diabetes, as well as there being a test to show if an immune reaction is going on, have led to an area of research called **immune suppression** (preventing the immune reaction). Medications have been developed that prevent the immune system from producing antibodies that may destroy the insulin-producing cells. One such medication you may have heard of is called **cyclosporin**; it and similar medications are still experimental, but in the near future they might be used successfully to prevent or slow the development of Type I diabetes.

Besides discovering new information about diabetes, basic research also involves the development of tools and techniques that can be used to control diabetes. This of course led to the very fine blood glucose monitoring systems that are recognized as being far superior to urine glucose testing.

The success of blood glucose monitoring has led to the search for even better ways to monitor the blood glucose level. It is known that if the glucose level is high in your bloodstream it also tends to be high in the lens of your eyes. This led to the thought that perhaps a light could be shone through the front of the eye, which would reflect back a certain amount of light according to how much glucose is present. A method such as this would remove the need to draw a drop of blood for testing.

Another challenge is to go beyond the idea of performing a single self blood glucose test at a time, in favor of a system that continually reads the blood glucose. This would be particularly helpful for individuals prone to rapid and unexpected swings in blood glucose that result in dangerously high or low levels. It would be ideal if such a device could have an alarm that would notify the person when the blood glucose level went past a safe level.

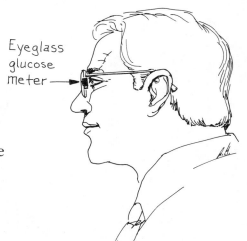

Eyeglass glucose meter →

But even more exciting would be to connect a continuous blood glucose sensing device to some type of insulin pump (Chapter 8) that could be worn externally or implanted in the body. The sensor would constantly monitor a person's blood glucose level and then instruct the insulin pump to deliver the appropriate amount of insulin. In effect, this combined system would act as an artificial pancreas. This would be a very rewarding result of the great efforts in basic and clinical research that have gone into the development of blood glucose monitoring systems and insulin pumps.

Clinical Diabetes Research

Once a drug, technique, or tool has been developed by basic researchers and has been reviewed and found safe by the Food and Drug Administration or other government body, it then must be tested in a select group of volunteers. Animal testing allows this step to be taken with as little risk to the human volunteers as possible. If the new development does improve the health of the people for whom it was intended, the challenge then becomes to make it available to all the people it could help. This often takes many years, so it is important that diabetes health professionals and people with diabetes learn as much as possible about new methods of treatment.

An example of an area of ongoing investigation by clinical researchers is the use of human insulin to improve diabetes care. Approximately 60 million dollars were devoted to the development of human insulin. One reason for this investment was because it was estimated that by the year 2000 there will be so many more people needing insulin injections that there would be a very large demand for limited amounts of insulin available from animal sources. The development of the recombinant DNA technique for creating human insulin appears to have answered this problem.

After clinical researchers found that human insulin was safe and effective and it became commercially available, work began on determining the proper indications for using this new insulin in controlling diabetes. That work is still underway, and the results are beginning to reveal ways in which human insulin can be used most appropriately.

A major effort in clinical research was begun in 1982. At that time the National Institutes of Health (NIH) decided to conduct a research project to try to determine the effects of strict blood glucose control in preventing or delaying chronic complications of diabetes. The name of this study is the **Diabetes Control and Complications Trial (DCCT)**. NIH selected 21 centers, including Park Nicollet Medical Center/ International Diabetes Center, to begin recruiting volunteers for the DCCT. It is hoped that the results of this study will be a confirmation of the widely held belief that maintaining blood glucose levels within the normal range will prevent or slow the development of long-term complications.

Clinical researchers evaluate ways to improve diabetes care.

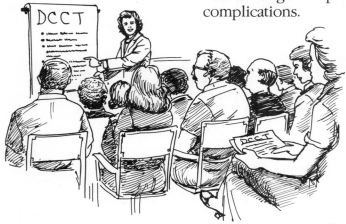

The diabetes research that shows the greatest promise of being a cure for insulin-dependent diabetes involves transplantation of part or all of the pancreas. Transplanting an entire pancreas into a person with insulin-dependent diabetes has been successful in some cases, but unfortunately the person's new pancreas can be affected by the same process that led to the disease in the first place, or it may be recognized as foreign by the body and rejected, so repeated transplants may be necessary.

Another complication of pancreas transplants involves the fact that the pancreas has functions other than producing insulin. For instance, the pancreas supplies digestive enzyme to the intestine to help break down food after eating. The pancreas of a person with diabetes is still functioning in this regard. When a pancreas transplant is performed, the person's own pancreas is not removed, a second pancreas is surgically implanted. As a result, the flow of digestive fluids from the second pancreas must be blocked to prevent an excess of digestive action. This is just one example of the very delicate and difficult procedures in a pancreas transplant operation.

An alternate approach to transplanting the entire pancreas which is being tested clinically is to transplant healthy beta cells into a person with insulin-dependent diabetes rather than transplanting a whole pancreas or large sections of a pancreas. The challenge is first to separate the tiny beta cells from the rest of the pancreas, then find a way of placing them inside the person's body so they can begin making insulin, and finally to prevent the immune system from destroying the new beta cells. The separation process is being investigated in many ways, including taking advantage of the zero gravity conditions made possible in the space shuttle program.

Transplanting healthy beta cells is one method being tested that may lead to a cure for Type I diabetes.

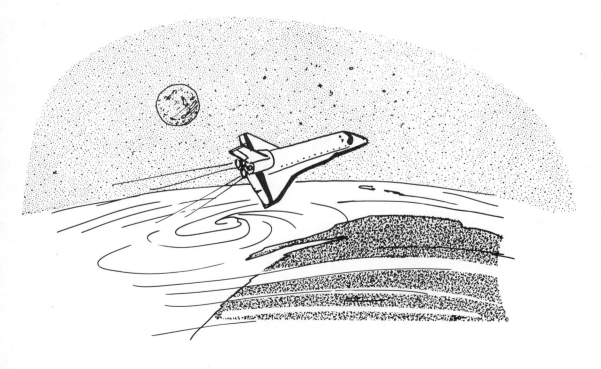

Once the beta cells have been isolated it is necessary to either physically protect them from being destroyed by the immune system or modify the beta cells in some way so they will not be rejected by the person's body. Research is being performed in both areas. Early studies have involved placing a group of beta cells inside a protective container or shell. The shell has tiny holes which allow glucose to seep in and stimulate the release of the necessary amount of insulin. The holes allow insulin to seep out but are small enough to prevent antibodies from entering. It is thought that beta cells protected by this type of shell could be injected into the person or placed under the skin at regular intervals to provide an internal supply of insulin.

The procedure of implanting beta cells that have been protected against attack by antibodies has been talked about as a cure for diabetes, but it may not help people with non-insulin-dependent (Type II) diabetes, who are already producing enough insulin. It will be several more years before we know if this indeed will be a cure for insulin-dependent (Type I) diabetes.

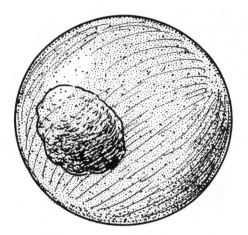

Encapsulated
Beta cells

What Can You Do?

Many people with diabetes and their families want to become involved in diabetes research. There are several ways to do this. The most active way is to become a research volunteer. Your local affiliate of the American Diabetes Association, the Juvenile Diabetes Foundation, the International Diabetes Center or a diabetes center in your area will refer you to a scientist or physician needing volunteers for diabetes research.

A second way to get involved is to become active in persuading Congress to appropriate more money for diabetes research. Research is like any other commodity—it must be paid for. The best way to make sure the exciting progress in diabetes research will continue is to contact your representatives in Congress. Legislators must make very hard decisions about how to distribute money for health research. A large part of this decision-making process depends on input from the people they represent. If they hear from people they represent who have diabetes, they will be more likely to vote for funds for diabetes research. You can contact your Congressmen and Senators, either by writing, calling, or visiting them.

Contact your legislators to urge continued support for diabetes research.

A third way to become involved in diabetes research is to contribute money to be used for that purpose. Again, all of the diabetes groups mentioned above and listed in the Appendix can tell you how to contribute. Contributions from individuals are very important in maintaining funds for all types of diabetes research.

In all these ways we can help to assure that the "light at the end of the tunnel" mentioned in Chapter 1 keeps growing brighter and brighter until the day arrives when diabetes has indeed been cured!

Chapter 26
Adding Flexibility to Your Meal Planning

Marion Franz, R.D., M.S. and Nancy Cooper, R.D., B.S.

One of the keys to your success in living well with diabetes will be your ability to add flexibility to your meals. The more you learn about nutrition and the exchange lists, the more you can experiment with different foods and types of meals without upsetting your blood glucose control. This knowledge will also help you add flexibility and interest to meal planning, as well as being able to stay within your meal plan when you are eating away from home.

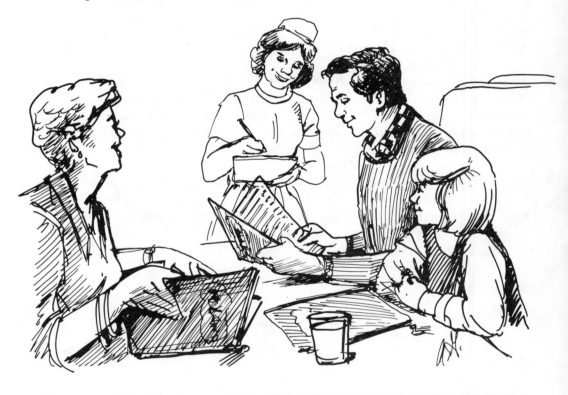

Eating Away from Home

When eating at a restaurant, cafeteria or someone else's home, bring your common sense with you. You can follow your meal plan and enjoy yourself at the same time. The following guidelines may be of help:

- **Know your meal plan.** Know how many exchanges you have for each meal and make selections appropriately.

- **Continue to watch portion sizes.** If portion sizes are too large for your meal plan, ask for a "doggie bag" or leave the food. It's more important to keep your diabetes under control than to clean your plate!

- **Ask how foods have been prepared.** How foods are cooked affects their exchange value. For example, deep fat fried foods such as chicken and shrimp contain an additional bread exchange as well as one or two additional fat exchanges per serving. Meat weight listed on a menu refers to the portion size before cooking. It will lose about a fourth of its size in cooking. For example, a steak listed on the menu as an eight-ounce steak is approximately six—not eight—meat exchanges.

- **Request that condiments** such as salad dressings, gravy, sauces, etc., be served separately so you can control the amounts.

- **Know which food groups can be exchanged for other food groups.**
  For example:
  1 fruit = 1 bread; and 1 bread = 1 fruit
  1 nonfat milk = 1 bread plus 1 lean meat

- **Know how to adjust your meal times.** People with Type I diabetes must remember to eat on schedule. If a meal is delayed by one hour, have a fruit or bread exchange from your meal plan at the scheduled meal time. If the meal is delayed for longer than one and a half hours, move a snack to the meal time and have the meal at snack time. For example, if you will be eating dinner out at 8:30 and your dinner hour is usually 6:00, have the same exchanges as your evening snack at 6:00 and then eat dinner at 8:30. This is especially important if you are taking only one injection of an intermediate-acting insulin in the morning.

  For individuals with Type II diabetes that is controlled by meal planning alone, timing of meals is not as essential. When eating away from home, however, it is important to continue to watch your portion sizes. Eat half of the portion and take the rest home for lunch the next day in a "doggie bag," or split the portion with a friend.

- **Know how to adjust your insulin injection times.** If you normally take insulin before dinner as well as in the morning, you have two options. 1) You can take your insulin at the usual time, have your snack and then eat dinner later. 2) If dinner is not delayed more than one and a half hours, you can wait, take your insulin before the meal, and then have the snack before bedtime. However, delaying the second injection too long may cause an overlap of insulin action the next morning. Making these changes will probably affect your blood glucose tests, because you may be testing closer to the larger meal than you normally do. But because you will know why your glucose level is higher, you won't need to make any changes in your insulin dosage.

- Use diet and low calorie products when available. Some restaurants now have diet syrup, jams and jellies. These items may not appear on the menu but may be available if you request them.

- Oops! Lastly, if you feel you have indeed "blown it," remember the one thing you can do is exercise! Granted, it takes a lot of exercise to burn many calories, but dancing, bicycling, or a brisk walk can help.

In summary, when dining away from home it is helpful to do some planning. Plan where you will eat, what you will eat, and how much you will eat:

Where: It helps if you are familiar with the menu of the restaurant. The more choices on the menu the more apt you are to find choices appropriate for you.

What: Decide ahead of time what you are going to order. By doing this you won't be as tempted by inappropriate food choices. Be the "trend setter"—order first, so you won't be tempted as you listen to what others are ordering!

How Much: Being able to judge portion sizes by "eyeballing" will help you decide how much to take home and save for another meal.

By planning, understanding your meal plan, and correctly judging portion sizes, you will find you can enjoy dining away from home while keeping your diabetes in control.

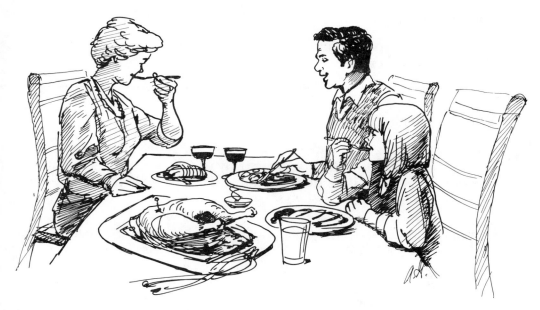

Holidays

By following some simple guidelines, people with Type I diabetes can make changes in the meal plan to adapt to holiday eating schedules. For example, if the family chooses to have the holiday meal at 2 or 3 p.m. and you are scheduled to eat at 12 noon and 6 p.m., what can you do to enjoy the holiday festivities with your family and friends? Begin by having the exchanges of your afternoon snack at 12 noon. Then, at 2 or 3 p.m., have the exchanges of your lunch meal plan. If you are really being honest about it, this holiday meal will probably use up part of your dinner meal plan as well. Do save a portion of the evening meal plan exchanges to eat at the regular dinner hour.

Making the above changes will probably throw your blood glucose tests off for the day because you may be testing closer to meal times than you normally do. But knowing what has affected the blood glucose tests, no changes need to be made in the insulin program. The principle to keep in mind is that dividing your meal plan into different size meals and snacks won't get you in trouble as long as the total for the day (preferably for each four to six hour period) remains the same. For individuals taking insulin, delaying meals **WILL** cause problems! One of the factors that determine how much insulin is needed in a day is the total number of calories eaten, and this should remain constant. Remember that making these changes should be reserved for **very special** occasions.

The same principle applies to days when you need to have your larger meal at noon instead of in the evening. For that day, exchange your noon and evening meal plans.

Meal planning by the person with diabetes depends on a certain amount of self-control as well as adequate information. With this combination, you too can enjoy an active social life and even "have a ball!"

Foods Can Be Sweetened without Using Sugar

There are two types of alternatives to sugar: non-nutritive sweeteners and nutritive sweeteners.

Non-Nutritive Sweeteners

Non-nutritive sweeteners are usually very sweet. Although some of these products contain calories, they are usually used in such small quantities that they cause very little increase in caloric intake. Two examples are saccharin and aspartame.

Non-nutritive sweeteners contain few or no calories.

Saccharin: Although saccharin has been used for about 80 years in the United States, in 1977 it was designated by the FDA as a possible cancer-causing agent. A study showed that when rats were fed large amounts of saccharin, a small percentage of their offspring developed bladder cancer. However, studies of more than 6,000 persons with diabetes have reported no association between saccharin use and the occurrence of bladder cancer. Six studies involving more than 5,000 bladder cancer patients and which adjusted for other known risk factors (smoking, etc.) could find no association between a risk of developing bladder cancer and the use of artificial sweeteners. Although these studies do not "prove" that saccharin is safe for humans, they do offer assurance that saccharin is not a major health threat. The policy of the American Diabetes Association is that, in light of current evidence, the use of saccharin is safe for people with diabetes.

Aspartame is marketed as a tabletop sweetener called Equal. Under the brand name NutraSweet, aspartame is used in a variety of food one-tenth calorie in the amount necessary to produce the same sweetness as one teaspoon of sugar.

Aspartame is marketed as a tabletop sweetener called Equal®. Under the brand name NutraSweet™, aspartame is used in a variety of food products. The use of aspartame is limited due to its instability in heat. With cooking or baking, it loses its sweetness. The taste is similar to sugar, without the bitter or metallic aftertaste that occurs when saccharin is used as a sugar substitute.

As with saccharin, questions have also arisen about the safety of aspartame (Equal or NutraSweet). Before aspartame was approved by the Food and Drug Administration (FDA) for use in foods, it underwent more than 100 scientific studies. FDA has said that "few compounds have withstood such detailed testing and repeated close scrutiny."

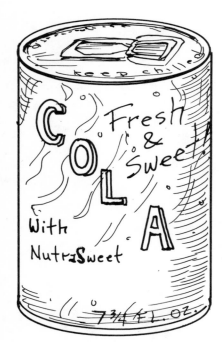

The concern about aspartame has mostly focused on the fact that it "breaks down" to a simple alcohol called methanol when digested. It has been suggested that this is harmful to the person consuming it, but what is never mentioned is that many common foods produce methanol when digested. For comparison, if all the sugar an average American consumes in a day were replaced by aspartame (which would be virtually impossible to do) it would produce the same amount of methanol—54 milligrams—produced by 8 ounces of fruit or vegetable juice or 2 ounces of gin.

It has also been suggested that one of the parts of aspartame, "phenylalanine," can cause changes in the brain and affect behavior, especially in children. However, extensive studies have found no evidence that it causes harm, even at levels of aspartame consumption six times greater than what 99 percent of the general public is estimated to consume. The phenylalanine in aspartame is used by the body just as is the phenylalanine in foods such as meat, dairy products, vegetables, and fruits. Again, if all the sugar in an average diet were replaced by aspartame it would provide 280 milligrams of phenylalanine, which is the same amount provided by 6 ounces of milk or 3 ounces of beef.

The only documented harm from aspartame can occur to people with a very rare inherited disease called phenylketonuria, or PKU. This is why a warning to people with PKU appears on all foods containing Equal or NutraSweet.

Nutritive Sweeteners

Nutritive sweeteners have 4 calories per gram, the same number of calories per gram as sucrose (table sugar). Fructose, sorbitol and other sugar alcohols fall into this category. Sugar alcohols are artificial products made from sugars whose names end in "ose." Fructose and sorbitol have been used in Western Europe as alternatives to glucose-containing sweeteners such as sucrose. Although they may be more slowly digested and absorbed, they end up in the body as glucose and therefore must be counted in the diabetic meal plan.

Nutritive sweeteners contain 4 calories per gram—the same as sugar.

Fructose: Fructose is a commercial sugar that is considerably sweeter than sucrose, although its sweetness actually depends on how it is used in cooking. If used in products that are cold and acidic in nature, it is sweeter. If used in products that require heat, such as baking, it is usually not sweeter than sucrose. It is suitable for baking, canning, and freezing.

In people with well-controlled diabetes, foods containing fructose cause a more modest increase in blood glucose levels than do foods containing sucrose. However, use of fructose is not recommended for people in poor control of their diabetes, because with an insulin deficiency, fructose is readily changed to glucose. It is also equal to sucrose in caloric value, so it must be counted by obese people as part of total caloric intake.

Sorbitol: Sorbitol is the most commonly used sugar alcohol. It is readily converted to fructose and is similarly used by the body. One of the major problems with sorbitol is its laxative effect. Also, many food products sweetened with sorbitol end up with more calories than the product they are replacing, because of added fat used to dissolve the sorbitol.

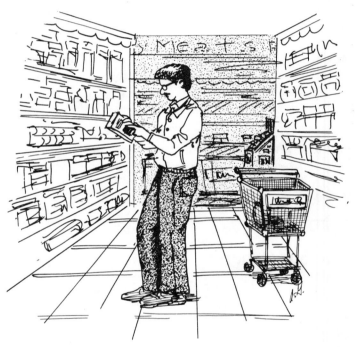

Using Food Labels in Meal Planning

Some general guidelines can be used in making decisions about which foods are appropriate to use in your meal plan and how to use them correctly. Labels on foods can help you decide. To make the best use of the information included on labels, first look at the list of ingredients.

Some ingredients are of concern because they are similar to sugar. Words ending in "ose" are generally a form of sugar. Sugar used in cooking and at the table is sucrose; other sugars are dextrose, fructose, levulose, lactose, and glucose.

A phrase that often appears on labels is "nutritive sweetener." This identifies a sweetener that contains calories. Examples of nutritive sweeteners are: invert sugar, corn syrup, dextrin, molasses, sorghum, honey, maple or brown sugar, sorbitol, mannitol, and xylitol. If the label contains the phrase "non-nutritive sweetener," it indicates that the sweetener contains few or no calories. Examples are saccharin and aspartame (Equal or NutraSweet).

After you have checked the ingredients list, look to see if nutritional labeling is provided. This information can help you fit the product into your meal plan. Companies are not required to provide nutritional labeling. However, it is required on any food product for which special nutritive claims are made (such as low sugar, low salt, low calorie, etc.) or to which extra nutrients are added.

A food product with nutritional labeling must follow a standard format. The label must state the serving size and the number of servings per container. It also must state number of calories; grams of carbohydrate, protein, and fat; milligrams of sodium, and the percentage of important vitamins and minerals per serving.

Knowing the number of calories per serving can be helpful in deciding how to fit a product into your meal plan. If a food contains less than 20 calories per serving, it may be used either at mealtime or snacktime and need not be counted in the meal plan (it is a "free food"). However, free foods, if they contain calories, should be limited to one per meal or not more than three or four per day.

Dietetic products are products in which some ingredient has been restricted or changed and a substitution has been made. "Dietetic," "diet," and "dietary" are terms that mean the same thing when used on labels. They do not necessarily mean the product is low in calories or useful for people with diabetes. If used, they must be counted in the meal plan as other products are, since they are generally not free foods. Dietetic products must comply with the nutritional labeling code because of their nutritional claims.

Dietetic products that might be useful are: artificial sweeteners, diet pops, and fruits canned without added sugar. Dietetic products that may be useful as free foods include: dietetic syrups, diet jams or jellies, diet hard candies and sugar-free gum. However, always check the caloric content to be sure these products do not contain more calories than you expect.

Nutritional labeling must be provided on any product for which special nutritive claims are made.

Dietetic products to be wary of include: dietetic ice cream, cookies, candy bars, and cakes. Many of these products are actually higher in calories than the products they are replacing. They are frequently made with sorbitol, which contains 4 calories per gram just as any other carbohydrate. But the fat content of these products is usually greater than in regular food products. Products containing large amounts of sorbitol can cause diarrhea. Other considerations in the use of dietetic foods may be cost and quality of the product as well as the number of calories.

By looking at the nutritional information on the label, you can estimate how many exchanges are in a serving of a food, which will help you include it in your meal plan. You must pay particular attention to the grams of carbohydrate, protein, and fat, but the grams do not need to be exactly equal to the exchanges in your meal plan. Variations of a few calories or grams of protein, carbohydrate, or fat are not significant in most meal plans.

The following table may be used to convert the information on a label to the exchange system.

Amounts of Nutrients in Food Exchanges

Exchange	Calories	Carbohydrate	Protein	Fat
1 starch/bread	80	15 gm	3 gm	—
1 lean meat	55	—	7 gm	3 gm
1 medium fat meat	75	—	7 gm	5 gm
1 high fat meat	100	—	7 gm	8 gm
1 vegetable	25	5 gm	2 gm	—
1 fruit	60	15 gm	—	—
1 milk (skim)	90	12 gm	8 gm	trace
1 fat	45	—	—	5 gm

Steps for Converting Nutritional Labeling to Exchanges

The following label is from a 10 oz. box of frozen pizza:

Nutritional Information Per Serving

Serving size...1/2 pizza (5 oz.)
Servings per container 2
Calories 350
Protein .... 17 gm
Carbohydrate .... 33 gm
Fat.. 16 gm

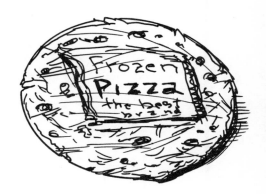

To make it easier to convert label information to the exchange system, follow these steps:

1. Check the label for the information you need to convert to the exchange system. You need:

Serving size ....1/2 pizza
Calories 350
Carbohydrates...33 gm
Protein ....17 gm
Fat...16 gm

2. Check for serving size. Is this a reasonable size for your use?

3. Compare the label information with the carbohydrate, protein, fat, and calories on the exchange table. First, convert the grams of carbohydrate in your serving size to exchanges. In this case, 33 grams of carbohydrate would be 2 starch/bread exchanges:

	Carbohydrate	Protein	Fat
1/2 pizza	33 gm	17 gm	16 gm
2 starch/bread exchanges	30 gm	6 gm	—

4. Next, subtract the grams of protein you used in converting the carbohydrate to exchanges. Then convert the remaining grams of protein to meat exchanges. Use the medium fat meat exchange values.

	Carbohydrate	Protein	Fat
1/2 pizza	33 gm	17 gm	16 gm
2 starch/bread exchanges	30 gm	– 6 gm	—
		11 gm	16 gm
2 medium fat meat exchanges		14 gm	10 gm

5. Next, subtract the grams of fat in the meat exchanges from the fat contained in the serving size. Then convert the remaining grams of fat to fat exchanges.

	Carbohydrate	Protein	Fat
1/2 pizza	33 gm	17 gm	16 gm
2 starch/bread exchanges	30 gm	– 6 gm	—
		11 gm	16 gm
2 medium fat meat exchanges		14 gm	–10 gm
			6 gm
1 fat exchange			5 gm

6. If you eat 1/2 of this 10-oz. pizza, you use the following exchanges from your meal plan:
2 starch/bread, 2 medium fat meat, 1 fat

7. Final check:

	Carbohydrate	Protein	Fat	Calories
1/2 pizza	33 gm	17 gm	16 gm	350

Exchanges:
2 starch/bread,
  2 medium fat meat,
  1 fat
	30 gm	20 gm	15 gm	355

8. If difference between the grams per serving and the grams accounted for by the exchange system is less than half of an exchange, you do not need to count those extra grams.

Summary

The more information you have about food and nutrition the more flexibility you will be able to introduce into meal planning. Keep in mind the overall goals of nutrition:

- Healthy food choices,
- Normal blood glucose levels, and
- Normal blood fat levels.

With increased food knowledge and skills you can meet these challenges while eating tasty and enjoyable meals!

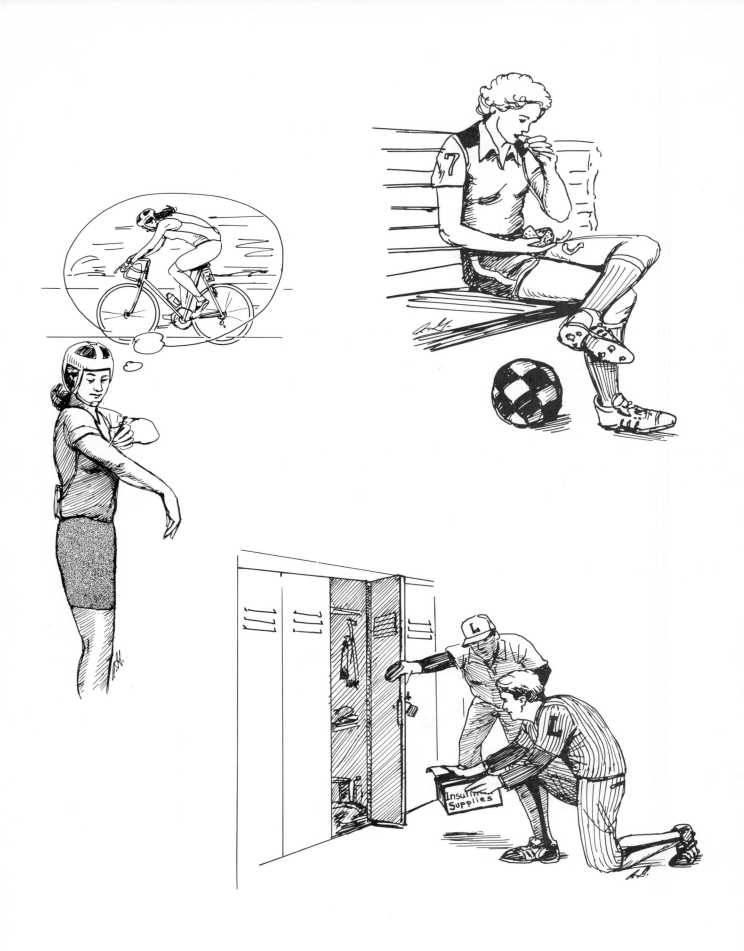

Chapter 27
Making Individual Adjustments for Sports and Exercise

Marion Franz, R.D., M.S.

Sports and exercise are an important part of a healthy lifestyle. Children and adults with diabetes who wish to participate in sports and/or exercise need to be able to continually juggle insulin, food, and their activity in order to perform to the best of their ability and training level.

The availability of blood glucose monitoring (BGM) has expanded the opportunity for people with diabetes to enjoy sports and exercise. BGM has made it possible to make routine adjustments to maintain the delicate balance of food, insulin, and activity. It has allowed individuals to learn about their own response to different activities and has helped many to safely challenge the limits of their athletic abilities.

General information about diabetes and exercise was discussed in Chapter 3. This chapter will suggest wise food choices for sports and exercise and will offer guidelines for adjusting insulin dosages. Of course, every individual is different, and any strenuous athletic activity or change in your health care plan should first be discussed with your health care team.

What are appropriate food choices for exercise, training, and sports competition?

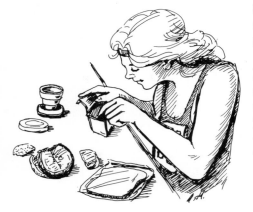

Carbohydrate and fat are the major fuel sources for exercise. During the first 20 to 30 minutes of aerobic exercise the body uses glycogen (carbohydrate stored in the liver and muscles) as its main fuel source. The body can burn carbohydrate more efficiently than fat, but there is a limited amount of stored carbohydrate. While this supply lasts, the exercising person uses a mixture of mostly glycogen, glucose, and some fat for energy.

If moderately strenuous exercise is continued for more than an hour, carbohydrate stores will run low, so fat use must increase. This adds to the exerciser's fatigue, because the body uses more energy to burn fat. By the end of an endurance competition or exercise session longer than two hours, almost all of the energy will be coming from fat. Training increases the body's ability to use fat and therefore makes the limited supply of glycogen last longer. This, along with the training effect on the heart and lungs, increases the individual's endurance.

Because regular exercise requires frequent replenishing of stored carbohydrate, there is a need for more carbohydrate in the diet. This should come mostly from "naturally occurring" sugars, starches, and fiber-containing foods rather than refined sugar foods, which supply only calories without other nutrients. There is no need for an increase in fat or protein intake. In fact, excessive protein intake can make it harder for the body to use its most efficient fuel, carbohydrate. Foods high in fat contain large amounts of calories, so they will contribute to excessive body fat, which is both unhealthy and an unnecessary burden for athletes.

In general, the percentages of carbohydrate, protein, and fat needed by an active person are similar to those recommended for everyone else:

50-60% carbohydrate
15-20% protein
25-30% fat

The difference is that an active person will need more calories to maintain weight. Total caloric needs will depend on the type and duration of activity (see chart on page 59). Most of the additional calories should come from carbohydrate foods, meaning that the active person will be eating closer to 60 percent carbohydrate and 25 percent fat. If weight loss is desired, daily caloric intake can be reduced slightly. The easiest way to do this is by eating less of high calorie fat-containing foods. Chapters 3 and 10 discuss weight loss and exercise.

Nutrient Guidelines

The most important nutrient needed during regular exercise is not often thought of as a nutrient: water. Large amounts of water can be lost during exercise, and if not replaced the body can become dehydrated and unable to cool itself. The result can be a very dangerous condition called heat stroke, in which body temperature can rise so high that the brain or other body systems are damaged.

Dehydration is especially likely in hot humid weather, but large amounts of body water can be lost in any weather. Thirst is not a good indication of how much fluid to drink, because thirst will be satisfied long before the body's fluid needs are met. The following guidelines will help you maintain adequate body fluid during exercise and sports of long duration:

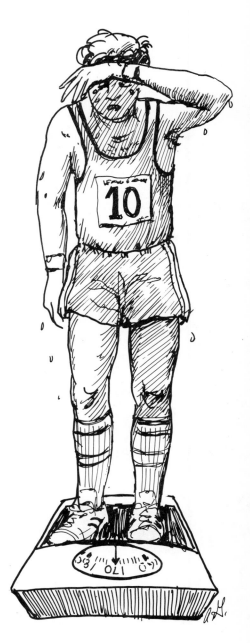

- Drink eight 8-ounce glasses of fluid the day before an athletic event or exercise session lasting several hours.
- Drink three or four glasses of fluid about two hours before the event.
- Drink one or two glasses of water 5 minutes before beginning the event.
- In hot and/or humid weather, drink about 8 ounces of water every 20 minutes during the event.
- If you are exercising regularly for long periods or in hot humid weather, weigh yourself before each session to make sure you have replaced fluid weight loss. Do not rely on thirst. You need to drink approximately two cups of water to replace each pound of body weight lost during exercise. Water is absorbed into the system faster than juices and special "sport drinks" that contain sugar, glucose, sodium, potassium, and other ingredients. This is why water is the best drink for quick fluid replacement. Cool water will be absorbed the fastest.

Individuals with diabetes may require a source of carbohydrate during exercise of long duration, such as a long run or athletic event lasting several hours. Blood glucose monitoring will help you find out how much extra carbohydrate you need during different types of activity. Fruit juices or other glucose-containing beverages can be a good source of carbohydrate and fluid, but they should be diluted with about twice the normal amount of water so they can be absorbed more quickly to supply the body's needs. Try to consume some carbohydrate (10-15 grams) every hour during a long run or athletic event. Don't wait for symptoms of hypoglycemia such as tiredness, loss of coordination, and loss of concentration. Obviously, you want your senses in top condition when competing in sports.

Snacks Before Exercise

Contrary to the popular idea that a source of "quick energy" such as a candy bar is helpful when eaten before exercise, it is best to avoid high sugar foods before exercise. High concentrations of sweets, such as candy and pop, are absorbed into the blood very rapidly, causing blood glucose to rise very quickly and then to drop abnormally low.

Quick energy is already stored in the liver and muscles as glycogen, and is available as fuel for exercise as long as there is enough insulin available. To prevent an insulin reaction when glycogen stores become low, it is helpful to eat slowly-absorbed carbohydrate foods before exercising. The following pre-exercise snack suggestions are either complex carbohydrates or fruits containing "natural sugars" as well as vitamins and minerals.

Pre-Exercise Snacks

Food	Amount	Carbohydrate (grams)	Exchanges
Breads			
Bagel	1	28	2 starch/bread
Bread sticks	3	14	1 starch/bread
Crackers			
Graham	2	11	1 starch/bread
Rusk	2	15	1 starch/bread
Rye Wafers	3	16	1 starch/bread
Rye-Krisp	1 triple	15	1 starch/bread
Saltines	6	14	1 starch/bread
Triscuits	4	13	1 starch/bread
English Muffin	1 whole	28	2 starch/bread
Muffin	1	17	1 starch/bread
Pretzels	6 three-ring	14	1 starch/bread
Soup (not cream)	1 cup	15	1 starch/bread
Yogurt (plain)	1 cup	16	1 milk
(fruit flavored)	1 cup	43	1 milk, 2 fruit
Fruits			
Apple	1 medium	22	1½ fruit
Banana	1 small (6 in.)	22	1½ fruit
Dates	2 medium	15	1 fruit
Dried fruit	1/2 cup	20	1½ fruit
Grapes	22 medium	16	1 fruit
Orange	1 medium (3 in.)	18	1 fruit
Pineapple	1 slice (1/2 cup)	12	1 fruit
Raisins	2 Tbsp.	15	1 fruit
Fruit juice	1/2 cup	15	1 fruit

During breaks in athletic events lasting several hours, watery fruits such as oranges, apples, peaches, plums, and pears can help prevent low blood glucose without providing too much sugar. They are approximately 85 percent water, so they provide fluid as well.

Meals the Night Before Competition or Long Endurance Events

Eat a high carbohydrate meal the night before an event to increase the amount of glycogen stored in muscles. The following foods are suggested:

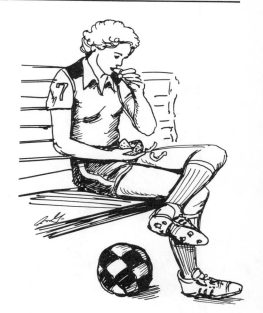

spaghetti	banana	bread
rice	pineapple	muffins
potatoes	fruit juices	crackers
squash	dried fruits	roll
noodles		

Avoid foods that contain large amounts of fat in addition to the desired carbohydrate. Pizza and ice cream are examples. Also consider the following to minimize fat:

- Replace butter, margarine, or peanut butter with dietetic jam on toast, muffins, and bagels.
- Replace whole or 2% milk with skim milk.
- Replace doughnuts with English muffins or bagels.
- Replace cheese with low fat crackers.
- Replace eggs with pancakes and a fruit topping.
- Replace meat sauce on spaghetti with tomato sauce.
- Replace red meats with protein sources such as broiled chicken or fish.

Meals the Day of Athletic Events

On the day of competition eat a light breakfast and lunch. Toast, juice or fruit, and cereal with skim milk are good breakfast selections. A turkey sandwich, skim milk, and fruit make a good lunch.

A lighter pre-event meal should be eaten one to two hours before the starting time. This meal should contain mostly carbohydrate and some protein, but a minimal amount of fat. The menu could include lean meat, such as poultry without the skin or fish; potatoes without gravy; vegetables; bread with no butter; salad without dressing; fruit; and skim milk.

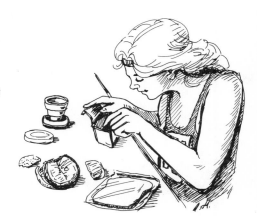

Practice to Help Prevent Problems

Of course, the above suggestions will not automatically result in an athletic event or exercise session free of problems. Use blood glucose monitoring to find out what works for you in different situations and under different conditions. Just as practicing athletic skills and building endurance lead to better performance, learning your food needs and response to exercise will be a major part of reaching your athletic potential. Building up gradually to competitive activity levels while learning how to keep your blood glucose in the normal range will help prevent unpleasant surprises in sports and exercise.

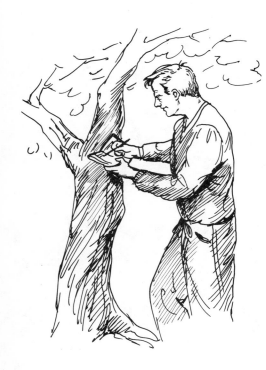

An exercise diary is a good tool to use to make decisions about food, insulin, and activity. Write down your usual records such as injection times and amounts and blood glucose testing results, but add comments about what activity you did, how hard you exercised, for how long, how you felt, and any changes in your usual daily routine or variations from your meal plan. Also keep track of insulin reactions and how much food was needed to treat them.

If you have decided to begin jogging (or other type of exercise or sport) and have obtained your doctor's approval, you will first need to purchase a pair of shoes that are appropriate for the activity. Be sure they fit correctly, are well constructed to cushion and support your foot (not dime-store tennis shoes) and do not cause blisters. Wearing cushiony athletic socks will help prevent friction sores. Break in the shoes slowly and inspect and care for your feet carefully (see Chapter 23) after each exercise session. It is very important for people with diabetes to prevent or treat promptly any minor foot irritations because they can easily become infected and cause major problems.

Next, you will need to find out how to prevent an insulin reaction during the jog. Start by testing your blood glucose at the time of day you plan to jog. Follow the "General Guidelines for Making Food Adjustments for Exercise" table on page 56 according to your blood glucose test result. Eat the suggested amount of food and then begin your jog (or other type of exercise or sport). Every 15 to 20 minutes during the exercise, stop and test your blood glucose. If it is falling near 80 mg/dl or less, eat the amount of glucose food you would use to treat an insulin reaction. If it is above 180 mg/dl, you probably ate too much food before exercising.

Continue to test your blood glucose every two hours for the next 12 hours to find out how the exercise has affected your pattern of blood glucose levels. Exercise can continue to lower blood glucose for 12 to 24 hours after you stop exercising. Your body will be changing glucose to glycogen to replace the muscle and liver glycogen that was used during the activity.

It is a good idea to do the above test several times to make sure you know how your body usually reacts to exercise. Repeat the test whenever you make a major change in the intensity or duration of the activity, or whenever you begin a new sport or exercise. DO NOT attempt to compete in any sport until you have gradually worked up to the intensity and duration of activity required by the event. ALWAYS carry a source of fast-acting glucose food with you when you exercise or compete. A roll of chewable sugar-containing candy is easy to carry; about 6 or 7 LifeSavers contain 10 grams of carbohydrate.

As you become better trained you may find you need less injected insulin. This is because training improves the body's ability to use insulin. Your daily insulin dosage may have to be decreased if your blood glucose levels are frequently too low. General guidelines are provided at the end of this chapter.

It is wise to do everything possible to prevent an insulin reaction during sports and exercise, but it is also necessary to be prepared in case one occurs. Use the following guidelines to design your insulin reaction plan:

If you feel symptoms of an insulin reaction:
1. STOP your activity immediately—DON'T WAIT.
2. THINK—Use your brain to decide on action. Test blood glucose if possible.
3. EAT the amount of glucose-containing food that experience has taught you is enough to recover.
4. REST—let your body absorb the glucose.
5. RESUME your activity only when a blood glucose test is above 80 mg/dl and you are sure you can continue without further problems.

Informing your exercise partners or teammates and coach:
1. Tell them about your diabetes and the possibility of an insulin reaction.
2. Explain how they can help you, making them feel comfortable with rather than fearful of your situation.
3. Show them where you keep your supply of glucose foods and emphasize its importance so they do not snack on the foods.
4. Arrange an "insulin reaction signal" with your coach so you can remove yourself from the action to treat it.
5. Don't use your diabetes as an excuse for poor performance, and don't play on anyone's sympathy with your diabetes.

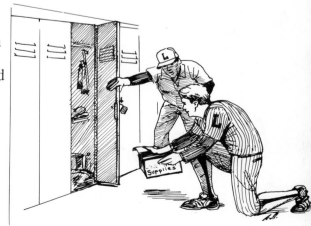

What your coaches, teammates, or exercise partners should be able to do:
1. Recognize the signal you give when you need to treat an insulin reaction.
2. Detect the signs preceding a reaction.
3. Supply glucose foods to you.
4. Know emergency telephone numbers.
5. Help you decide if you have recovered from a reaction.
6. Be supportive but not too protective.
7. Allow you to handle your diabetes as you choose.

What insulin adjustments are necessary for sports and exercise?

If you exercise or participate in sports on a regular basis, your insulin dosage may be reduced or your injection schedule changed to allow for the glucose-lowering effect of exercise. The following table includes some guidelines that can be used as starting points in making changes in the insulin schedule. Frequent blood glucose monitoring will give you and your doctor the additional information needed to adapt your insulin schedule to your sports or exercise schedule.

General Guidelines for Adapting Insulin and Food Schedules for Endurance Exercise

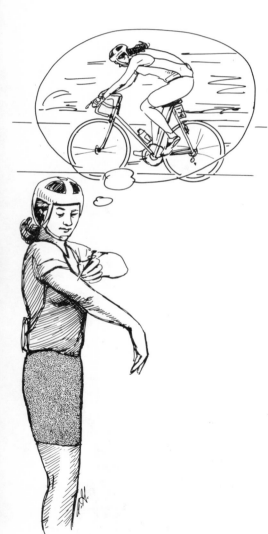

1. If you don't exercise regularly, increase food before exercise but do not change your insulin.
2. If your daily exercise includes aerobic exercise for more than 60 minutes, you may be able to reduce by 10 percent the dose of the insulin that will be acting during the time you are exercising. For activities of very long duration, try reducing by 15-30 percent the dose of the insulin acting during the activity. It is very important to do frequent blood glucose monitoring to help you and your health care team determine the effects of a change in your insulin dosage. (See page 57 for guidelines for adjusting insulin for extended exercise.)
3. If you exercise in the early morning, test your blood glucose level and eat a fruit and/or a bread exchange before the exercise. After you finish exercising, retest your blood glucose, take your morning insulin, and have your regular breakfast.
4. Inject insulin into your stomach or buttocks if you will be exercising your legs or arms within an hour after doing the injection. Be aware that exercising immediately after injecting insulin into an area of the body mainly involved in the exercise, as well as heat and increases in body temperature associated with exercise, may increase the rate of insulin absorption.
5. Eat a light carbohydrate meal about two hours before long duration exercise. Another small carbohydrate meal may be needed immediately before a long endurance event.

6. Consume only water during exercise or events lasting 1 hour or less if blood glucose levels remain in the normal range. Carry a fast-acting glucose in case of an insulin reaction.

7. Consume water and liquid carbohydrate during exercise or events lasting longer than 1 hour, and be especially aware of possible symptoms of low blood glucose.

8. On precompetition days you may want to eat more carbohydrate and decrease training to increase glycogen stores. Your insulin dosage may need to be increased slightly during this period.

9. On the day of a long-distance competitive event, reduce insulin dosage as you think necessary—perhaps 10-30 percent of your usual dosage.

10. Above all, although it is helpful to have basic guidelines to follow, remember that you are an individual. All athletes have variations in their response to training and physical stress. Adjustments that work well for one individual with diabetes may not work for you! You must constantly be aware of the signals your body is giving you; all good athletes become experts at interpreting these signals.

By learning how your body responds to the physical stress of training and competition, you can reach your full athletic potential.

With the proper preparation and attention to your body's needs as you exercise and/or compete, you can enjoy the thrill of becoming physically fit and athletically active to the best of your ability and desire.

The author wishes to thank Dan Hall, a marathon runner who has insulin-dependent diabetes, for reviewing this chapter.

Section V

Children
and
Diabetes

Chapter for Children
Normal Growth and
Development
Tips for Feeding Children

Information for Children with Diabetes,
Their Families, Relatives and Friends

Chapter 28
Taking Care of Me

(To be read by or to a child with diabetes)

Barbara Balik, R.N., M.S.

Note to Parents
This chapter was written for two reasons:

1. To explain diabetes in basic terms to your child.
2. To help you to talk to your child about all sorts of things, including diabetes.

This chapter is meant to be read with your child. As you read, you will come across frequent questions. Use the questions as an opportunity to see your child's view of life and diabetes. Don't expect to answer all the questions. Discuss topics honestly with your child. Keep a list of questions you and your child can ask your health care team. If your child asks a question about diabetes, ask what she/he thinks first. There are lots of thoughts behind children's questions. If you don't know, say so. It's OK not to know everything.

What children can manage by themselves varies. See Chapter 29 for general information. Remember, your child needs your support and involvement even as he or she gains greater independence. How to stay involved while letting go is a tricky balance. One way is to work at listening to and communicating with your child. It's a skill that takes time to learn. Communication is important for all families, but diabetes requires all family members to communicate especially well. There are more reasons to talk—about insulin, food, blood glucose, "Did you test?". If there are problems with communication, talking about diabetes becomes a source of constant friction. Diabetes can become the focus of an entire family. We hope your family will focus on health and love and fun and communication. In that environment, diabetes will be managed best. Children who grow up feeling good about themselves will be more likely to succeed at self-management and live life well.

Parents of children with diabetes have an enormous job. You manage the diabetes daily, with many decisions to be made. As we tell children, you sometimes have to ask grown-ups for help. Parents need to know which "grown-ups" they can turn to when they need help with diabetes, with feelings, and with communication concerns. Resources to help you may include:

- Friends
- Relatives
- Church
- Professional family counselors
- Health care providers
- Community resources
- Diabetes centers
- American Diabetes Association
- Juvenile Diabetes Foundation

Use the resources you need to help with a large task. Children need to know about diabetes so they can help themselves, so they can be involved.

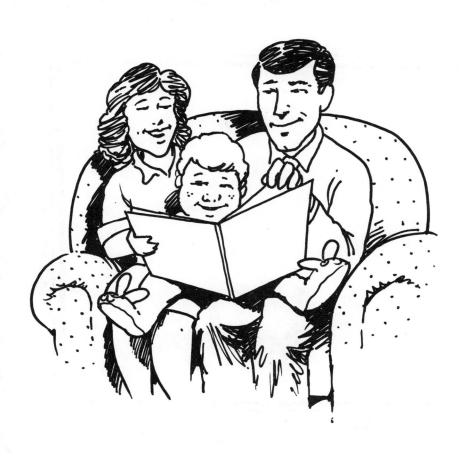

TAKING CARE OF ME

My name is Chris and I have diabetes. I got diabetes about 3 years ago. My grandma had diabetes but I didn't think kids got it. I didn't know I had diabetes at first. My Mom thought I was acting tired all the time. I was drinking lots of water and I had to go to the bathroom all the time. A couple of nights, I even wet the bed. My doctor said those were signs of diabetes.

How did it feel when you got diabetes? Write the signs you had or draw a picture of how it felt.

I wanted to know why I got diabetes and how long would it last? Do you want to know what I learned at my diabetes clinic and my special diabetes class?

First: I didn't do anything to make me get diabetes.

Second: There was nothing I or anyone else could have done to keep me from getting diabetes.

Third: Right now, no one knows how to make diabetes go away.

But I still didn't know what diabetes is or why I got it. Why do you think you got diabetes? Write down or draw what you think.

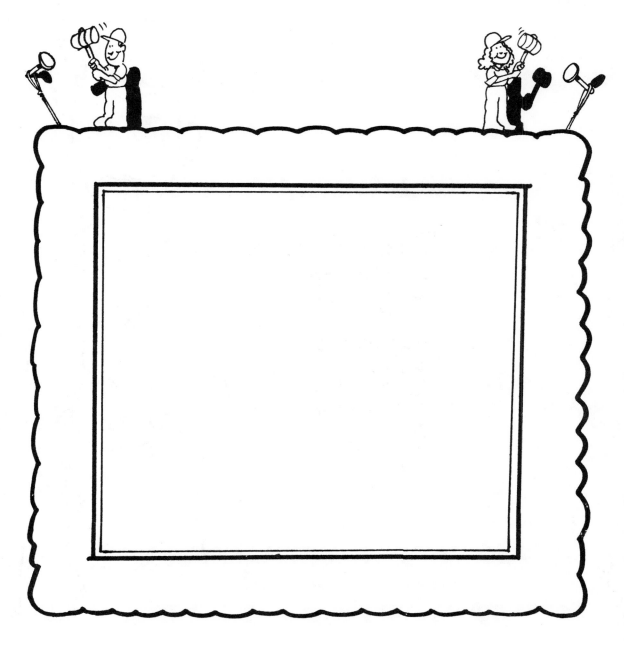

Here is what I learned from the people who help take care of my diabetes:

Inside my body are lots of things. There's my stomach and my lungs. Can you name or draw things inside your body?

One of the things inside my body is my pancreas. Can you find your pancreas in the drawing? A pancreas does lots of things to help my body. One part of a pancreas makes insulin. Insulin helps your body use the food you eat. Diabetes means your body doesn't make enough insulin.

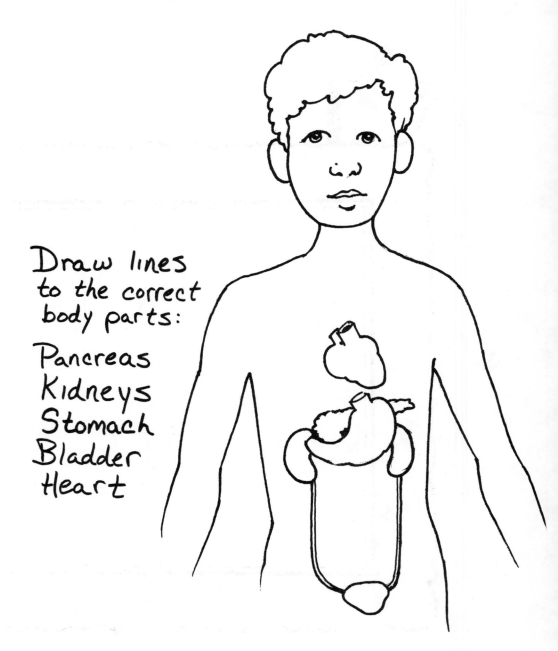

Draw lines
to the correct
body parts:

Pancreas
Kidneys
Stomach
Bladder
Heart

What happens if your body doesn't have enough insulin?
  Do you turn green? No!
  Do you fly like a bird? No!
  Do you grow four extra hands? No!

So a person with diabetes doesn't look different.

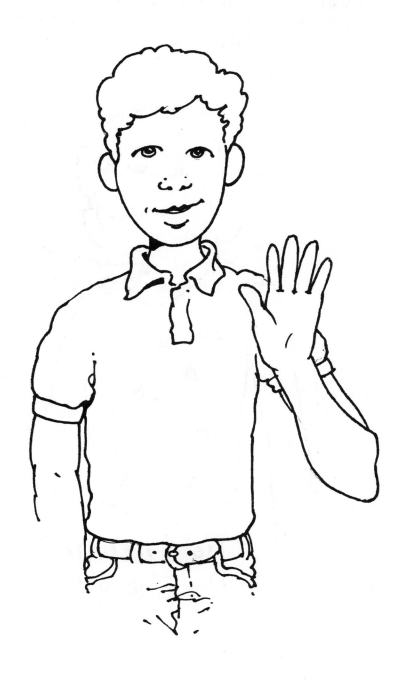

What does happen is that when there's not enough insulin, your body can't use the food you eat. Food makes us strong and helps us grow and gives us energy to play. The food changes to a kind of sugar called glucose. Your body needs insulin to help use this sugar for energy. If you have diabetes you don't have enough insulin, so your body can't use the sugar. Too much sugar stays in your blood and urine. That is why my friend Ann thought you got diabetes because you ate too much sugar. She was wrong! You get diabetes because you don't have insulin to help food make you strong and help you grow. Instead, you feel tired and go to the bathroom a lot and all those other signs of diabetes.

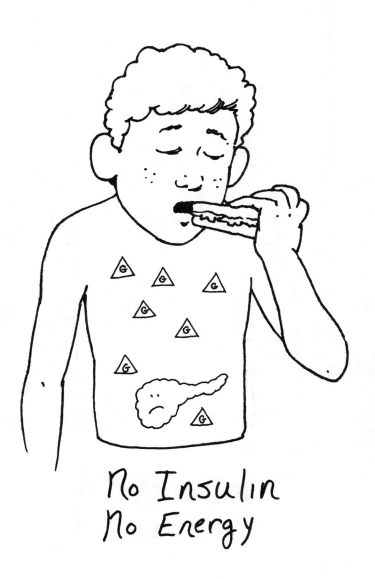

No Insulin
No Energy

So part of my pancreas stopped working and I wanted to know why.

Dietitians and nurses and doctors aren't sure why kids get diabetes. Here are some of the reasons they think people get diabetes:

You are born with differences in your pancreas that later make the pancreas stop making insulin.

You get sick and sometimes that makes your pancreas not work.

But most of all, they don't know, so remember:
There was nothing I or my mom or dad could have done to keep me from getting diabetes.
I didn't do anything to make me get diabetes.

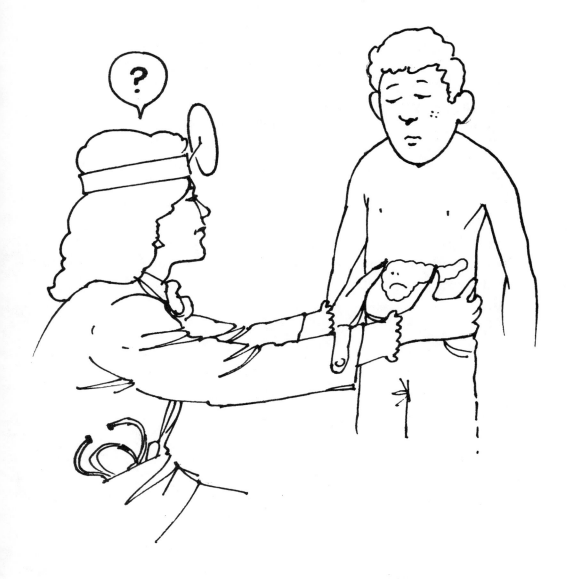

So now do you know what diabetes is and why you got it? Let's practice:

Find some of the things inside your body.
Where is the pancreas?

What is one of the things a pancreas does?
    Makes insulin.

What is insulin?
    It is something that helps your body use the food you eat.

What is diabetes?
    Diabetes means your body doesn't make enough insulin.

So what happens when you get diabetes?
    Your body can't use the food you eat.
    You might feel tired and go to the bathroom a lot and drink more.

Why do people get diabetes?
    Is it because they eat too much sugar? No!
    Is it because they did something wrong? No!
    Is it differences in your pancreas you might have been born with? Yes!
    Is it that sometimes grown-ups don't know why? Yes!

Even if part of my pancreas doesn't work, the rest of my body works just great! Can you find all the parts of your body that work just great?

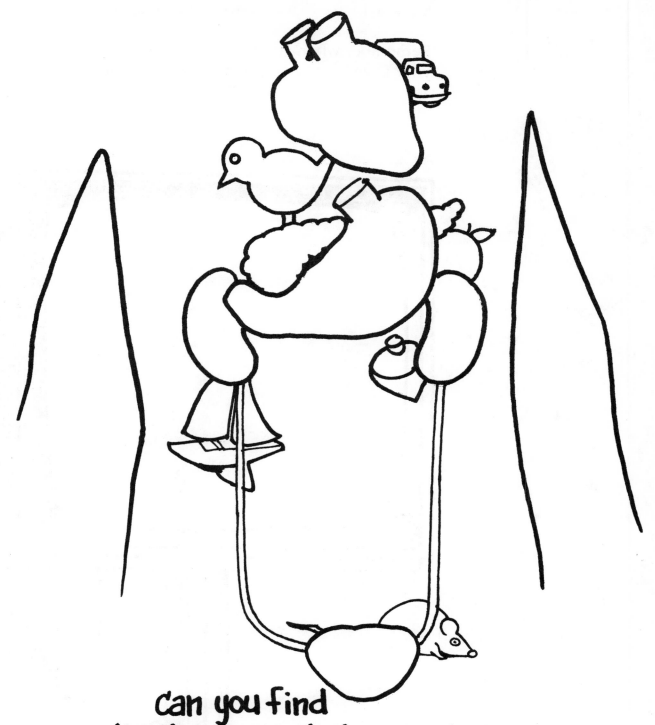

Can you find
the things that do not belong
in this picture?

So now I have diabetes, what happens now?

Remember when you first got diabetes? What happened to you? Draw a picture or write a story about what happened.

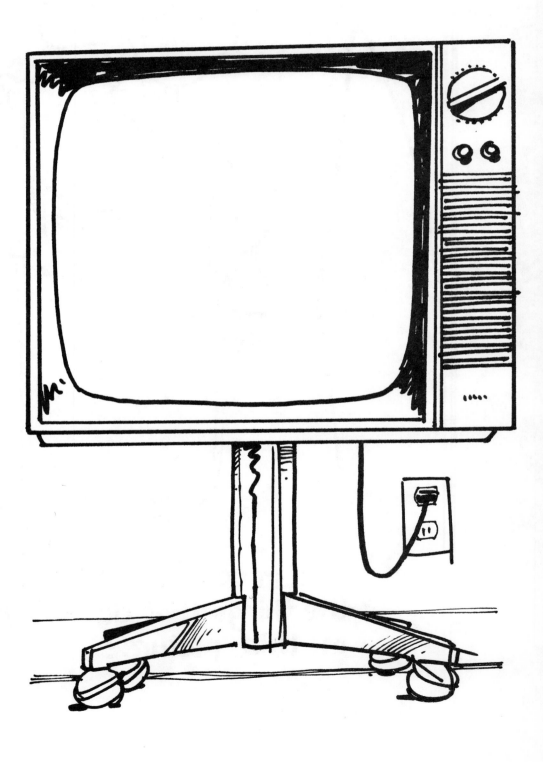

Some kids get sick, like my friend Jamie. She went to the hospital and stayed four days.

Some kids are not very sick when they get diabetes, like me. My mom and dad took me to the clinic. The doctor knew I had diabetes when they checked my blood and urine for glucose. Then my mom and dad and I talked to a dietitian and a doctor and a nurse and a family counselor to learn how to take care of my diabetes. Mom and Dad called the clinic a lot. They had bunches of questions. We can always call the clinic with questions.

My mom and dad also looked worried and tired. They were worried about learning all about diabetes and helping me take care of my diabetes.

What did your mom and dad look like?

Do you know what I learned at the clinic? Lots of things. They told us that since my pancreas doesn't make insulin, we have to learn to do some of the things my pancreas used to do.

First thing I had to learn was to give myself a shot. When I heard that, I said, "A shot!! NO WAY!!" But the nurse helped me and Mom and Dad to learn. It wasn't that hard and I felt proud that I could do it!

I learned that insulin won't work if you take it in a pill so it has to be a shot.

Next I learned to check my blood for sugar. You need to know what your blood sugar is to know if you are getting enough insulin and food. Checking your blood sugar gives you information. Blood sugars are not good or bad. They just let us know what's going on inside our bodies.

Let's pretend:
A kid just checked his blood sugar and it's 350.
What does he think?
What does his mom or dad say?
What would you think?

I'm real good at checking my blood sugar. I can do it as well as my mom and dad or my nurse or doctor can!

The dietitian helped us learn about food. I thought I already knew enough about food but we learned a whole lot more! My Mom said because I had diabetes, the whole family was going to eat so much better. She said it was a chance for us to eat smart. We learned to balance my food and insulin and activity (like swimming, running, riding my bike, or just playing). I learned that I had to eat at the same time for breakfast, lunch, dinner and snacks because I had taken my insulin. It was already working and ready for my food.

Draw a picture or write three of your favorite foods.

1. _____

2. _____

3. _____

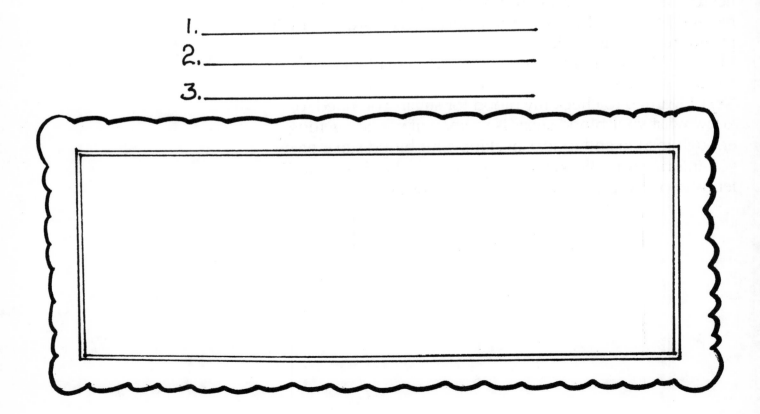

I wanted to know why I couldn't eat all I wanted of foods like candy bars and ice cream sundaes or pie. The dietitian said that foods with lots of sugar make your blood sugar go way up. Then I don't have enough insulin. She said even people without diabetes need to eat smart. Eating smart means eating lots of different kinds of foods—foods that help your body grow and fix itself.

Can you draw foods that are smart foods for your body?

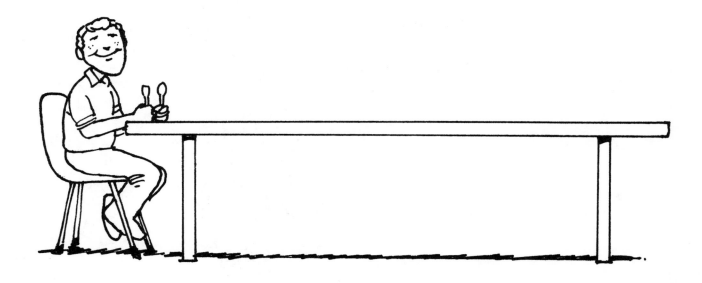

If I'm active and play, my body uses insulin better. The people at the clinic call it exercise—I call it fun. What do you like to do for fun?

For a healthy body, exercise is real important. Sometimes it is hard to balance my food and insulin and activity. Sometimes my blood sugar is high and sometimes it is low and sometimes it is in the middle. If my blood sugar is too low that's called a reaction. I get reactions if:
- I didn't eat all my meal or snack.
- I ate my meal or snack late. Remember, my insulin is already working and ready for the food.
- I played real hard. Sometimes when I play real hard, I need an extra snack. Remember, exercise helps my body use the insulin better.

So a reaction means not enough blood sugar. How do I know if I don't have enough blood sugar?
There are some signs. I may feel:

- sweaty

- dizzy

- shaky

- sleepy

- grouchy

- have a headache

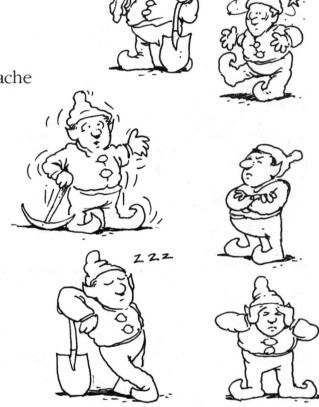

Sometimes I feel one of these things, other times I feel a lot of them. Sometimes I don't feel any of them, but my mom and dad notice I am acting different.

What do I do to make a reaction stop?

I eat something right away. That makes my blood sugar go up. Then in 10 or 15 minutes, the signs of a reaction go away.

Here's a list of some foods that help with a reaction:

1 small box of raisins
1 Fruit Roll-up
½ cup fruit juice
6 or 7 Lifesavers
4 or 5 pieces of dried fruit

Can you guess why you always need to carry some food with you for a reaction? What do you carry with you for a reaction?

I also learned about too much blood sugar. Too much blood sugar happens if:

I don't take enough insulin.

I'm sick.

I watch TV or just sit around all the time.

I eat extra food or I don't eat smart food.

I forget my insulin shot.

I get real worried or scared or excited about something.

Feelings can make your blood sugar go up.

When I have too much blood sugar, I:

May not feel any different.

Or I may drink a lot.

Or go to the bathroom a lot.

Or have a stomach ache.

I try to check my blood sugar 3 or 4 times a day before I eat. Then I write the blood sugar and how much insulin I took in my record book. I try to remember to write if something different happened that day, like a long bike ride or I was sick.

My mom and dad and I look at the record book once or twice a week and talk about if we need to change anything like my food or insulin or exercise to help my blood sugar.

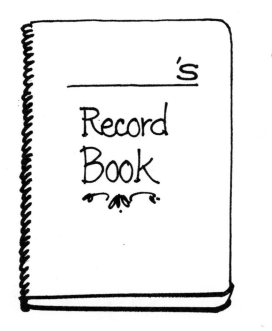

_____'s

Record Book

Can you write your name?

Sometimes, we need to call the clinic to get help. We work on things together. Then every 3 or 4 months we go to the clinic. They check my height and weight and we talk about diabetes. My mom and dad and I learn more about diabetes. Sometimes it's boring to go to the clinic and sometimes it's fun.

What do you do when you go to the clinic?

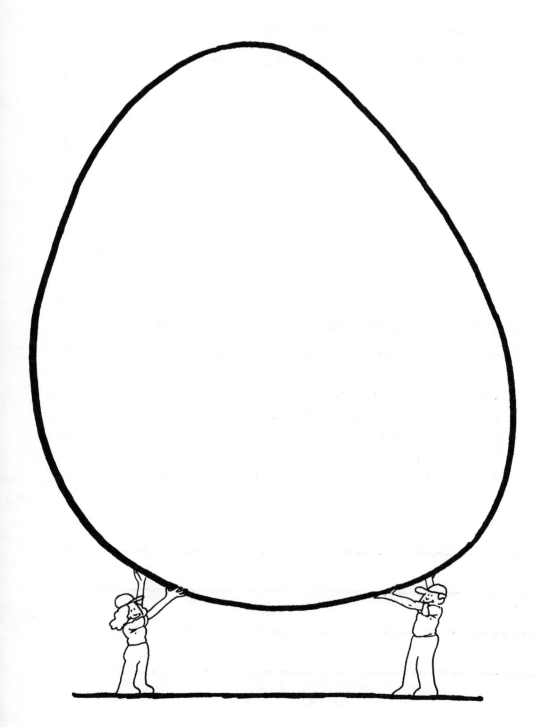

I used to need help:
    getting dressed
    tying my shoes
    riding my bike
But now I can do them by myself. I just need some help sometimes like getting a tight shirt over my head. What things can you do yourself?

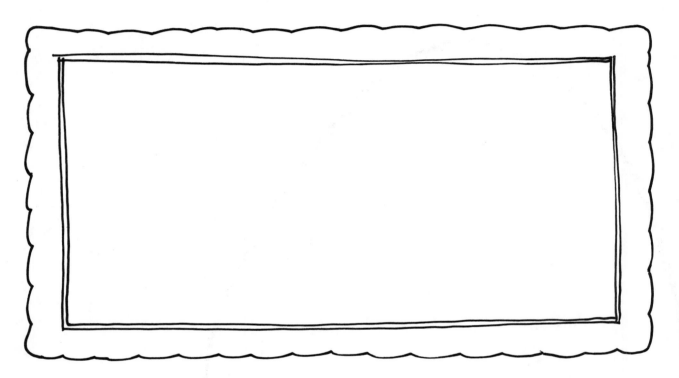

There are new things I do because I have diabetes. I check my blood sugar. My mom and dad help me sometimes.
I get a shot twice a day. I do my legs and Mom or Dad does my arm. Next year I'll do my shots all by myself.
What things do you do because you have diabetes?

1. _____

2. _____

3. _____

4. _____

Sometimes I don't want to do things like clean my room or take a bath or test my blood. But some things you just have to do. That's when I tell my mom and dad or friend about my feelings. Sometimes I:

Feel angry—like when my brother scribbled in my favorite book. What makes you feel angry?

Sometimes I feel afraid—like sometimes when I am by myself in the dark. What makes you afraid?

Mostly I feel happy—like on my birthday. What makes you feel happy?

I have feelings about my diabetes too. Sometimes it doesn't seem fair that I got diabetes. Sometimes I want to pretend I don't have diabetes—but I know I do! It helps to talk about my feelings.

What do you want to do with this space?

Sometimes I need a grown-up to help me.

A grown-up needs to drive a car.

A grown-up needs to help fix some things.

A grown-up sometimes needs to help check my blood sugar or give me my insulin.

A grown-up needs to help if I have a reaction that won't go away.

Grown-up help is nice to have when you need it.

I'm in charge of some things.

Getting my shot on time.

Eating what I'm supposed to.

Telling my friends I have diabetes.

Making sure my teachers know I have diabetes.

Taking something to eat with me in case I have a reaction.

Asking grown-ups if I need help.

What do you tell your friends about diabetes?

When I get bigger, I will be in charge of more things.

So that's what I learned about diabetes.

I can do lots of things.

I can take care of diabetes, like give my insulin shots, eat smart, test my blood sugar, and get lots of exercise.

Then, I can do all the things I want to do!

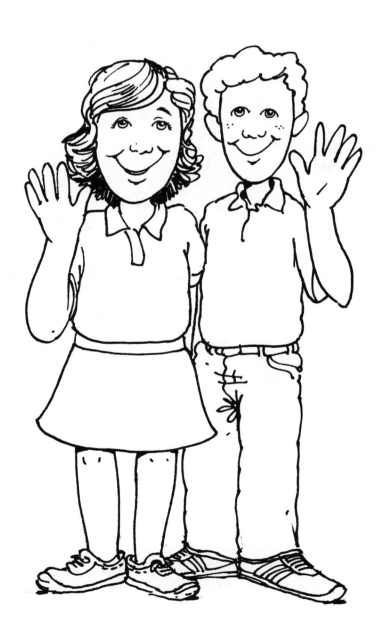

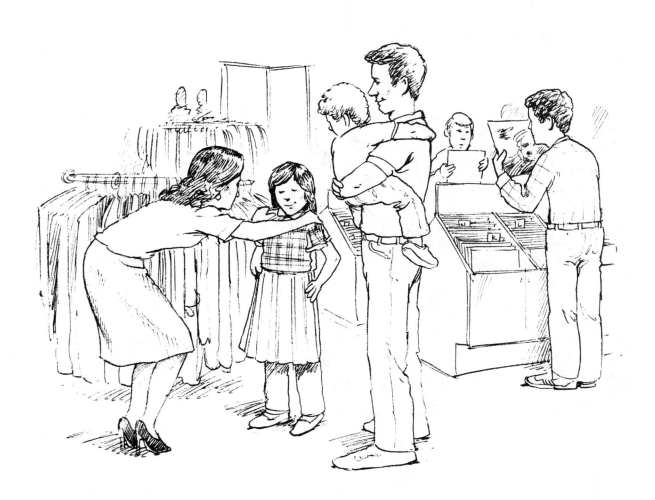

Chapter 29
Children: What Every Parent Should Know about Normal Growth and Development

Patricia M. Moynihan, R.N., M.P.H.

When Johnny developed diabetes at the age of 2, he became the terror of the household. But because of his diabetes, his mother excused his actions and blamed everything on the disease. The rest of the family was told they would have to put up with Johnny's behavior and give him whatever he wanted so that he would not get overexcited. When Johnny was 5, he was still an undisciplined terror "because of his diabetes." His father gave up trying to reason with him and his brothers and sister stayed away from him as much as possible so they wouldn't get blamed for causing his tantrums. Now Johnny is a teenager, and even his mother has given up hope, forcing herself to realize that "diabetes was just too much for poor Johnny to handle." There is a great deal of tension within the family and they never really talk to each other anymore. Johnny's diabetes is in very poor control and he spends most of his time in his room; he never really made any friends because his diabetes prevented him from playing with the other kids and participating in activities at school.

A ridiculous and unnecessary situation? Certainly, but unfortunately it happens all too often because families don't keep in mind that a boy or girl with diabetes is more alike other children than different. When a child has diabetes, there is a very common tendency for everyone to focus on the disease—on how to control the diabetes—and to forget to look at the broader picture. Our expectations of the child must take into consideration the broader issues of growth and development. Children are changing physically, intellectually, and emotionally, and what works to help control diabetes when they are 6 may not work when they are 10.

For this reason, it may be helpful for you, as parents of a child with diabetes, to understand some basic ideas about the growth and development stages that every child goes through. This chapter will help you become better able to anticipate changes, encourage independence in your child at the right times, and avoid feeling guilty that his or her behavior is not always what you think it should be.

We will discuss normal childhood development by dividing the age span of the child into three stages: the preschool ages from 2 to 5, the school ages from 6 to 12, and the adolescent ages from 13 to 19. Within each stage the physical, intellectual, and social needs of the child will be explored together with some ideas about expectations based on these needs.

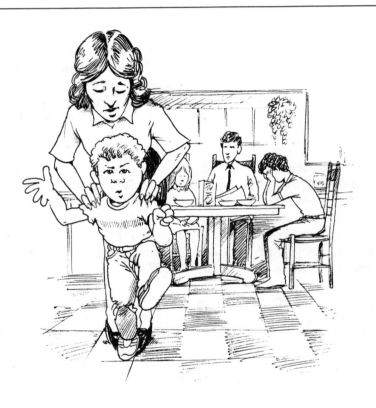

What does your preschooler understand about diabetes?

Peter's worst time of the day was in the morning when it came time for his shot. He would scream and hide and eventually upset the entire family before breakfast could begin. His parents tried a different approach every day, searching for the way to satisfy and quiet Peter. What they didn't know was that by changing their approach each day—a different family member giving the shot, sometimes before and sometimes after breakfast—they were acting as their own worst enemies. Peter needed one routine, done firmly and matter of factly, in order to understand and accept that this was the way he could count on things happening each day. Shortly after a consistent structure was developed for the family's mornings, everyone, including Peter, stopped reacting to each other's frustrations and breakfast once again became a calm and enjoyable family gathering.

Physical growth in childhood occurs at different rates. There are times of accelerated growth and change, and times of slower growth and change. For the preschooler, physical growth begins to slow compared to growth in the first two years of life. It is important for parents to monitor their child's growth (height and weight), and to have it checked by their doctor at least twice a year. The child's growth can be plotted on a growth chart to compare it to other children of the same age and sex. Children with diabetes should grow like other children if their diabetes is in reasonable control. If a child's growth does start to slow, his or her caloric requirements, food intake, and insulin dosage should be examined. Short-term delays in growth can be reversed if discovered early and the appropriate changes in food intake and insulin are made. If a delay continues for six months or more, it can have a lasting effect on the child's overall growth and development.

The preschooler's slowed physical growth usually has an effect on appetite and food intake. This is a time when your child may become very "picky," with strong food likes and dislikes. Substitutions in the meal plan can be made if you understand the food exchange system (see Chapter 2). Fluids that have carbohydrate in them can also be used to meet caloric requirements. Fortunately, this period of fussy eating usually passes with increasing age. Natural hunger helps the appetite of the child, assuring that overall food intake is sufficient. The attention span of children this age is short—15 to 20 minutes—so long drawn-out meals are usually not productive. Shortened meal times with small snacks throughout the day are usually more successful.

The preschooler's bladder and bowel control improves and toilet training is usually mastered. Urination is more frequent when blood glucoses are high, so increased difficulty with toilet training may tip you off to a problem with your child's diabetes control. It is important not to make your child feel guilty when he or she has an accident during these times. Illness normally increases children's dependence and causes changes in behavior. Illness is also a time of higher blood glucose, so toilet accidents may be more frequent during these periods.

Urine testing for glucose and ketones may be part of your child's regular management or to supplement blood glucose testing. In either case, it is important to allow the child to participate in this care so he or she begins to understand and not be fearful of it.

Muscle strength and coordination improves in preschoolers. The child becomes more active and begins to play harder, so food and insulin needs may change during this time.

Children whose diabetes is in good control should grow and develop just like other children.

Those who care for a preschooler with diabetes must be aware of his or her signs of an insulin reaction.

The preschooler's intellectual and social development affects how the child will behave and what adults should expect of him or her. A 4-year-old basically sees the world through his or her own eyes and feelings. He or she cannot separate his or her feelings from the feelings of others. Your child understands diabetes on the basis of the day-to-day behaviors that are asked of or done to him or her. He or she also understands diabetes from the hospitalization that may have been necessary at diagnosis or during illness. A preschooler cannot truly understand the need for insulin shots or the threat of becoming ill.

The preschooler begins to develop a sense of time and an understanding that things and events happen in a sequence. Routines throughout the day are important to your child because they give him or her a sense of predictability and control of the world. Children need routines in their day so that they know what they can count on. The morning routine of insulin injection, blood glucose testing, and eating will be more successful if done in a short time and if the time, place, equipment and people are usually the same rather than if always changing and chaotic.

The ability of a child this age to tell others of an insulin reaction is unpredictable. Many 3- to 4-year-olds cannot identify their own signs of a reaction, so it is important that those who care for the child know how to identify one and how to treat it. After a child has had a reaction and is feeling better, it is important to explain in simple terms what happened and why. This will help lessen fear of reactions and will begin to help your child make an association between his or her shakiness and ill feelings and not eating enough food.

Finally, preschool is a time to prepare yourself and your child for the separation that will occur when school starts. Any parent may be anxious about this separation, but parents of a child with diabetes may be even more anxious about entrusting someone else with the responsibilities for their child's daily care. A successful separation requires two things: being able to trust your child's ability to take care of himself or herself, and good planning with specific school personnel about the basic management of your child's diabetes.

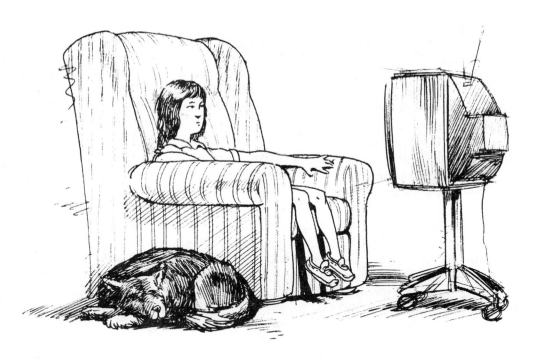

How will your child cope during the school years?

"Penny is an inactive girl who would rather watch TV or read than play," her parents told the counselor and school nurse at the fall school conference. What they didn't mention was that her inactivity was due in large part to their fear and overprotectiveness in trying to prevent insulin reactions. They did not want Penny to participate in any rigorous activity at school and did not allow her to play active games with her friends at home. What Penny's parents needed to learn—painful and frightening as it may be at first—was that Penny and her school needed to be and could be trusted to handle reactions. Preventing her from participating in exercise activities was hurting her more than helping her in the long run.

As your child grows, the world in which he or she lives and the number of people he or she has contact with also grow. These physical and emotional changes are accompanied by changing needs for diabetes care.

The physical growth of a school-age child is slow but steady. Caloric requirements reflect this and should show slow increases over the years. To match this, insulin requirements will also slowly increase. Food requirements will begin to increase significantly when the physical growth spurt of adolescence begins, but this is not until ages 10 or 11 for girls and 11 to 12 for boys. Before this time, appetite may naturally be low, and children with increasingly active lives tend to forget to eat. You may need to remind your child to eat consistent meals and snacks. Children can become bored with the same food ideas, and they usually begin to prefer more variety and convenience in their food selections. Regular discussions with a dietitian can be very informative and helpful during these years.

Basic physical coordination in both large and small muscles improve tremendously during the early school years. Your child's interest and ability in physical activity should increase. Sports and athletic events for both boys and girls should be encouraged if the child shows interest. Having diabetes is not a reason to avoid activity. In fact, exercise can be very helpful both physically (muscle development and a lowering effect on the blood glucose) and emotionally (feeling a part of the group and learning how to participate and compete in groups). The exercise needs to be planned and balanced with food, but this is relatively easy to do.

Dental development at this age will include the eruption of the permanent teeth. Because the child with diabetes is eating frequently (meals and snacks), he or she may need to brush more often. Dental cavities occur frequently in many children this age. Diabetes does not cause an increased risk for dental cavities as long as blood glucose control is reasonable. But if blood glucose is high for prolonged periods of time, the risk can increase.

Most preteens can do injections and testing and will feel more independent if they do so.

Because the small muscles and fine motor coordination are developing during these years, and your child's need for independence is increasing, it is a good time to teach him or her how to do insulin injections and test blood glucose and urine ketones. Children this age can add numbers, compare colors, and print and write increasingly better. They also want and need to control more situations. This is the prime time to teach a child about diabetes management. Children vary in their readiness to take over these responsibilities, as do parents, but most children by the age of 12 can do injections and testing (with recording) and will feel more independent and ready to start their teen years if encouraged to do so.

The world of school is a big step for all children and their parents. Children with diabetes make this transition and progress through the school years as well as any other child, but there are a few additional steps that the family must take. You must tell the school that your child has diabetes, and you must inform the school personnel (teacher, coach, bus driver, cook) how best to help your child take care of himself or herself. At the beginning of each school year, it is important that you and your child have a conference with the school. The purpose of this is to update the school on changes in the diabetes management, review the upcoming school schedule, and plan accordingly.

It is neither necessary nor realistic to tell the school everything you know about diabetes. But there are basic topics that need to be discussed regularly. These include:

1. Your child's usual symptoms of an insulin reaction.

2. The foods that should be readily available to treat reactions. You should make these foods available to the school and check the supply several times throughout the school year.

3. Times when your child may be likely to experience a reaction, such as during unplanned physical activity, when snacks are missed, and during times of emotional stress.

4. Reactions can be prevented by simply planning ahead. Teachers and coaches most commonly fear that a child with diabetes will have a reaction and the teacher will not know what to do. Reassure the teacher that most reactions can be prevented, and that your child is capable of treating most of his or her reactions (if this is true).

5. If your child does blood glucose testing during the school day, review the method with the school and discuss the amount of supervision required. You need to provide all necessary supplies and check the supply regularly. School personnel may not be expected to interpret the results of the testing, but they should be told when to notify you about unusual results.

6. Discuss with school personnel a reasonable length of time and place for your child to test and eat snacks. This time should not be used by your child as a way to avoid other activities. The less these routines disturb the child's school day, the better.

7. Discuss your child's use of the school lunch system, especially any food alternatives that will be necessary to meet his or her meal plan. The child with diabetes can eat the school lunch, but school lunches are typically higher in carbohydrate and fat and need to be planned for. Substitutes for desserts may have to be brought from home. Many schools publish or otherwise provide the weekly menu to parents in advance so they can plan accordingly. Your child may prefer to bring a lunch to school. Either option can work well, but the lunches must be planned.

8. Planning for parties and special school events will help your child to participate and not feel left out because of food restrictions. You can suggest kinds of party snacks your child may have, or you may want to provide them for special occasions.

9. Tell the school personnel what kind of information you need to know about your child's handling of diabetes (such as the occurrence and severity of reactions). Ongoing communication between you and the school will make everyone feel more comfortable.

The Following Information Should Be Given
To School Personnel When Conference is Held
at the Beginning of the School Term

General Advice The child with diabetes should be carefully observed in class, particularly before lunch. It is best not to schedule physical education just before lunch; and if possible the child should not be assigned to a late lunch period. Many children require nourishment before strenuous exercise. Teachers and nurses should have sugar available at all times. The child with diabetes should also carry a sugar supply and be permitted to treat a reaction when it occurs.

Diabetic coma, a serious complication of the disease, results from uncontrolled diabetes. This does NOT come on suddenly and generally need not be a concern to school personnel.

Child's Name   Date

Parent's Name   Address   Phone

Alternative person to call in an emergency   Relationship   Phone

Physician's Name   Address   Phone

Signs and symptoms the child usually exhibits preceding insulin reaction _____

Time of day reaction most likely to occur _____

Most effective treatment (sweets most readily accepted) _____

Kind of morning or afternoon snack _____

Suggested "Treats" for in-school parties _____

**SUBSTITUTE AND/OR SPECIAL TEACHER SHOULD HAVE ACCESS
TO THE ABOVE INFORMATION**

Prepared by the American Diabetes Association, Committee on Diabetes in Youth
Endorsed by the National Education Association, Department of School Nurses

Parents frequently are concerned that their child may be more prone to illness and infection because of diabetes. All children are at increased risk of illness when they start school each year, because of greater exposure to other children with infections. Children with diabetes are not at increased risk as long as their blood glucose control is good. If blood glucose is high for prolonged periods of time, this can increase the risk of illness. It is important to remember that during any illness, blood glucose tends to increase and insulin requirements go up. Monitoring of the blood glucose and urine ketones is very important during these times (see Chapter 8).

During the school years, your child will develop and mature in how he or she understands diabetes and how he or she feels about having it. Socially, the school-aged child grows increasingly independent and the circle of friends with whom he or she plays also increases. The child tends to judge himself or herself in comparison to these friends. Your child may learn that there are no other children with diabetes in his or her class or school and this can make him or her feel different. The truth is that your child is different because of diabetes, but he or she must learn that all children are different and have things that set them apart. This is a time for you to talk with your child about these feelings of being different, and to discuss how being different can be as much of a strength as a weakness.

School experiences should not be limited by diabetes.

Children this age are better able to deal with present reality than with the abstract future. Their understanding of diabetes can increase, but it is still not oriented to the future. The school-age child deals in the here and now and can gain some understanding of what causes reactions and how to prevent them. He or she is ready for a deeper explanation of what diabetes is and means, but he or she is not ready to understand diabetes in the same way you do. Long-range complications and their prevention have little meaning to your child at this age.

The experiences of the school years—the successes and the failures—will affect how your child enters adolescence. Each year, as your child matures and as interests and social contacts increase, there are new opportunities for growth. These should not be limited by diabetes.

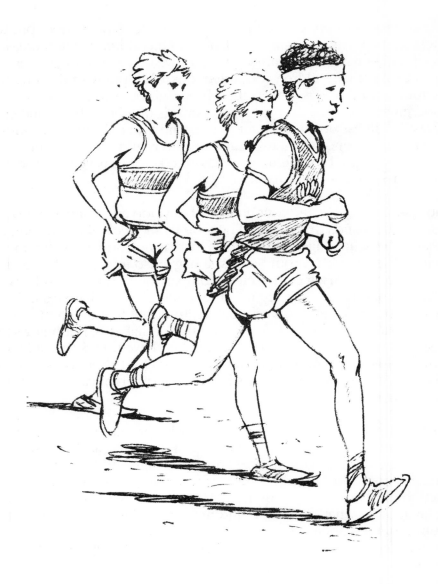

How can your teenager best be guided to adulthood?

When Dan was told by his doctor and parents that he has diabetes, he thought it was the most unfair and cruel thing imaginable. He had worked hard in school, had always respected his parents and teachers, and was looking forward to running on the varsity cross-country team. Was this how he was being rewarded for all his hard work and energy? Why should he bother to do anything now, least of all follow the diabetes tasks that were now being "shoved down his throat?"

What Dan learned in his first year with diabetes was that he had built all the resources he would need to control diabetes and do all the things he had planned. His self-discipline and motivation would carry over to allow him to take control of his diabetes, enjoy his teen years, and become a productive and responsible adult.

Increased physical growth and maturity and the onset of puberty mark the entry to adolescence. It is often distinguished more by the physical and emotional changes that begin to occupy the child's mind than by the chronological years. The rate of physical growth is faster during adolescence than at any other time in a child's life, except for a newborn's growth in the first six months.

This rapid growth will affect your child's sleep patterns, eating, and activity. Food intake must increase as growth increases. There may be a marked increase in caloric requirements to fuel the physical growth and development. Insulin requirements reflect this increase. Increases in insulin dosage during adolescence are normal and to be expected. The insulin needs do not change suddenly, however. There is usually a slow but steady increase in blood glucose testing results. One injection of insulin in the morning cannot usually keep up with the physical and hormonal changes, and your child may be started on two or more injections per day. Again, this is normal and not a sign that the diabetes is worsening. It is simply a change in the needs of the body, which are best matched by increasing the dosage and frequency at which insulin is given.

Increases in insulin dosage can be expected during the growth spurt of adolescence.

As growth slows in the mid to late teens, insulin requirements need to be reevaluated. When growth is complete, insulin dosage may even be decreased. Insulin can stimulate the appetite, so if not reevaluated at this time, obesity can become a concern.

Physical growth and development, including the development of sexual characteristics, should progress in the teenager with diabetes and have the same end results as in any other teenager. There is no evidence that young adults with diabetes will necessarily be short-statured or underdeveloped physically, as long as their diabetes is kept in reasonable control.

Poor blood glucose control for prolonged periods (six months or greater) can alter growth and development in the adolescent years. High blood glucose interferes with the hormones that stimulate growth and development. Weight is usually affected first, followed by height. This is a reversible situation if caught early and if changes are made in food and insulin to improve control. If it is not identified, or if it is identified but no change is made in food intake and insulin, there can be a lasting effect on body size and stature.

Having a "successful" period of growth and development is usually very important to the teenager, and it can be a strong reason for him or her to take care of diabetes. It is important that your teen understands the relationship between the two.

Intellectually, the adolescent's ability to think and reason becomes more adult-like. He or she begins to be able to think logically and understand the consequences of his or her own behavior and that of others. Your child now has the ability to look not only at the past and present, but also at the future. Interest and concern for the future will extend from your child to the world around him or her. It is important that you understand that although your teenager has the ability to do these things, he or she does not do them automatically nor consistently. It is very common for a teenager to fluctuate between thinking like an adult and thinking like a child.

Your teenager is trying out new abilities but still needs the security of the childlike ways of seeing the world. He or she is naturally stimulated to test new abilities. This is part of the reason the teenager, though seeking independence, still is dependent on parents and others for guidance and reassurance. You need to continue to have rules and expectations of your teenager. These can provide the guidance and reassurance that is needed and wanted, although seldom asked for.

Out of your rules and expectations comes a sense of values that are important for your teenager and your whole family to understand. Because the teenager can now understand that there are several consequences to any specific behavior and many different opinions on a subject, he or she is likely to question values and what they stand for. He or she may even question the value you place on his/her health and diabetes control.

The teen years are a time of experimentation to discover what is real and what is not. As the teenager experiments, values and their strength or lack of strength are tested. This experimentation may include experimentation with diabetes. The questions "How serious is my diabetes?" and "Does it really matter if I take care of myself?" surface and are looked at and explored with new insights.

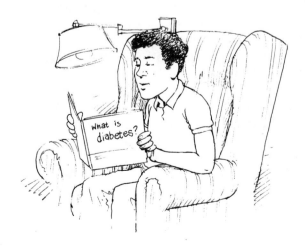

Because your teenager is now capable of understanding the future, his or her feelings about diabetes may change. He or she may begin to understand that it is a serious, chronic disease that does not go away. This realization may be too much to handle all at once, so he or she may choose to deny that the diabetes exists. This denial of diabetes actually serves a purpose by allowing time for the teenager to get comfortable with the reality he or she knows will follow. But denial can become destructive when it is prolonged. Even though the teenager is denying diabetes, it is important that parents and family do not. You need to continue to voice an interest in diabetes management and support the value that your teenager's health is important. Not all teenagers go through a period of denial of their disease, but if they do, it is important that you understand its purpose and remember that it usually passes. When it does, your teenager will have a clearer understanding and better acceptance of his or her diabetes.

Your teenager needs the contact and support of the family throughout this period, but he or she also needs the contact and support of peers. The need to belong to a group of peers is perhaps stronger now than at any other time in life. Within the peer group, your child continues to try out roles and values. He or she comes to understand that people accept him or her with diabetes just as they accept others with their unique differences.

Teenagers move in groups from school to extracurricular activities to evening parties and to other social activities. It is important that your teenager participate in all these things if he or she chooses. But he or she must realize that with this right to participate comes the responsibility for self-management of diabetes. Insulin and syringes and testing equipment must go along on overnights and into the wilderness. The opportunity for the teenager to make self-management decisions, and your willingness to trust him or her to act responsibly, are very important in helping your son or daughter develop a sense of self-trust and independence.

New interests and opportunities face the teenager. A driver's license is something seen as a sign of independence. It is important that teenagers understand that there are no restrictions to their getting a driver's license, but at the time of application they must state that they have diabetes. A medical form also must be completed on a regular basis by the physician, who will evaluate if your child's diabetes is under reasonable control. Its purpose is to protect the safety of the driver and others. Traffic accidents can occur during severe insulin reactions. All people with diabetes who drive should have food in the car for easy access if needed.

The amount of attention your family places on diabetes will affect the growing up process; each family can work together to discover what is the right amount of attention.

Employment opportunities are open to the teenager with diabetes if he or she takes care of the diabetes and is honest with the employer. States vary on restrictions, if any, regarding employment of people with diabetes. Generally, the only occupations in which people with Type I diabetes cannot work are those that involve commercial transportation, such as commercial flying and interstate trucking. The armed services also do not employ people with Type I diabetes.

Finally, you and your teenager must deal with the issue of intimate relationships and the development of sexual identity. Teenagers with diabetes naturally have the same fears, questions, and curiosities as any other teenager. They all usually go through the stages of friendship, dating, romantic love, and sexual love as they mature. Within the privacy of these relationships, they continue to find out who they are and how others feel and think about themselves. Teenagers with diabetes are usually no more or less fearful than anyone else in this discovery. They may have very practical and real questions about pregnancy and impotence, and these questions need to be discussed with the diabetes health care team. Most of all, the teenager needs to know that his or her fears and questions are normal, and that he or she is like other teenagers.

It is important to remember that "growing up" is a process that takes more than just time to complete. Your child with diabetes will move through this process at a different rate than your other children—not becuase of diabetes, but simply because each child is different. The amount of attention your family places on diabetes will affect the growing up process. Each family must determine what is the right amount of atttention. Listen to your child and family; they will give you cues. And include your health care team in the decision process; they can provide suggestions based on experience and an impartial but concerned interest.

The final outcome is what parenting is all about!

Chapter 30
Tips for Feeding a Child Who Has Diabetes

Marion Franz, R.D., M.S. and Broatch Haig, R.D., B.S.

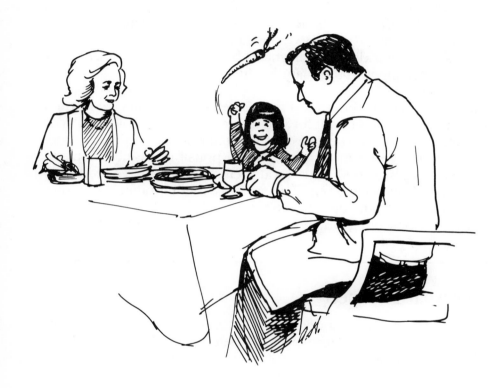

Remember that old saying, "Do you eat to live or live to eat?" We all must eat to live, but diabetes focuses our attention on how central food is to our very existence! Children and their unpredictability complicate the food situation, increasing parents' anxiety. Consistent and informed parents who have realistic expectations and a close working relationship with the health care team are most successful at working through the tough times.

Parents of children who have diabetes worry about how to feed the finicky eater, what to do when their child doesn't eat the entire meal or snacks, how to live by meal plan recommendations—and still avoid power struggles. How do parents deal with this on a meal-by-meal and a day-to-day basis? This chapter will discuss eating habits of children and adolescents, common eating problems, and tips for making permanent changes in eating habits—especially for a child who has diabetes.

To begin with, it is important to realize that the nutritional and exercise recommendations for anyone with diabetes are part of a healthy lifestyle. To expect a child to make major changes when the rest of the family continues eating in inappropriate ways is certain to cause problems. The whole family benefits from eating changes that can help prevent heart problems, stroke, cancer, high blood pressure, Type II diabetes, and many other major health hazzards. Parents should not feel guilty or feel they are depriving other family members, especially if there are no longer as many "sweets" and high fat snacks and foods around the home. If parents feel anxious or sad themselves, kids will pick it up. Even the lean teenager needs to learn good eating and exercise habits. We know of one family who celebrated the anniversary of their diabetes diagnosis because they were thankful for the positive changes in their family's lifestyle.

Children learn their eating habits from their parents and brothers and sisters.

Children are born without food prejudices. Eating habits are learned. So as parents it is important for you to set a good example with your own eating habits. You serve as an essential role model. This is true whether or not you want to accept the responsibility. Since Moms most often plan meals around Dad's food preferences, fathers need to be involved in food decisions and be aware of the importance of their nutritional role modeling. Children quickly learn which foods are desirable by observing which foods their parents and brothers and sisters relish most.

Know what to expect

As parents you need to understand what are normal eating patterns for children. Knowing what to expect can help you anticipate problems and find creative and workable solutions for eating problems you may face with your child who has diabetes.

Children's appetites change frequently for no apparent reason. Children go through whimsical phases of alternately liking and disliking certain foods. They may want the same food for a long period of time and then abruptly refuse it. Try not to overreact—assume that the food fancy will soon pass.

Children grow extremely rapidly during their first year of life, after which the rate of physical growth slows considerably. Children's appetites also wax and wane with growth rates. Periods of rapid growth will usually be accompanied by increases in appetite. Sometimes the increased appetite and weight will preceed the growth spurt. Don't immediately assume it is the beginning of obesity—watch carefully and wait awhile before curbing portions.

Youngsters usually have larger appetites during the summer when they are physically more active. Not only do appetites vary by season, but there are daily variations as well.

Children are good judges of the **amount** of food they need, but it is up to parents to provide the **kinds** of foods that children need. If at all possible, leave young active children at home while grocery shopping. Wise food purchases are most often the result of factual nutrition information, planned menus, and unhurried selection. If only appropriate, nutritious foods are in the cupboards and refrigerator, good eating habits are encouraged. Other family members not following a meal plan can snack on what they wish away from home.

Families whose menus are varied and interesting introduce the pleasure of variety. Children who taste new foods each time they are served learn to know and enjoy many different foods. But don't be disappointed when foods are not a hit the first time around. It is important to introduce only one new item at a meal, perhaps along with a favorite food. Offer unfamiliar foods when children are hungry and in good health—never when ill, cross, or tired. Serve very small portions of new foods and be sure to compliment children—even when only one bite is eaten.

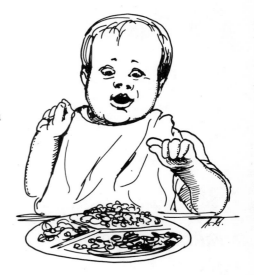

Children do not eat foods in the same order as adults. Youngsters often eat one food at a time, which is perfectly acceptable. Children tend to prefer mild-flavored, lightly seasoned, and crunchy foods. Stringy, lumpy, sticky, and very dry foods are usually rejected. Brightly colored foods served attractively whet everyone's appetite—even young people. Try to look at meals as children see them. A large plate with a mass of food can be overwhelming to those little eyes. Scale your portions down to their size.

All children thrive on regularity and routine in daily activities. They need to have meals served at approximately the same times. When meals are served at irregular times, hungry, irritable children are usually the result. A regular meal schedule for the whole family is a benefit as you plan meals for a child with diabetes.

Children find sitting difficult. They need excuses to move and stretch. Small tasks, such as carrying plates to the kitchen, can be useful for the child as well as for parents! Children become restless during long waits. Serve food as soon as the child is seated. When children are done eating, excuse them from the table.

Children, just like adults, have "off" days when they are irritable and don't feel like eating. Accept this as gracefully as possible!

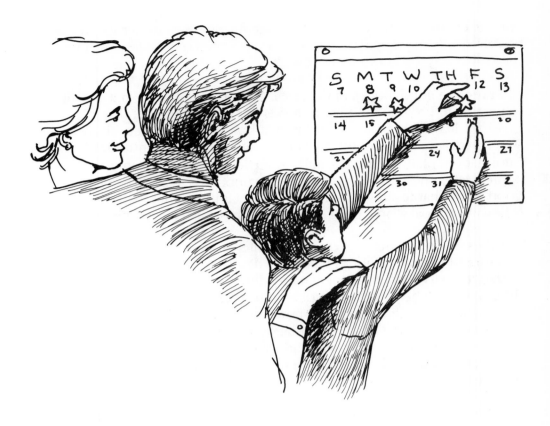

What can parents do?

Knowing what to expect is the first step, but there are other things parents can do to make nutritional management of diabetes easier. Meal time atmosphere has a significant influence on how the whole family enjoys a meal. If meal times are a tense battleground, children often rebel by refusing to eat anything. This sets up a vicious cycle. Children who feel they are under constant scrutiny at the table lose their appetite in a hurry. Don't lay on guilt. Don't lecture on school grades or other behaviors during meals. A relaxed atmosphere at meals helps children eat better. If you are very tired and rushed, prepare a fun, friendly meal of cereal, milk, and fruit rather than a three-course frantic and grumpy dinner. Prepare for a mess at meals. Children who are nagged about neatness may refuse to eat.

If rejecting food gets attention, it may become a routine; a game to play with parents whenever extra attention is desired. Food dislikes may then become permanent.

Continue planning and serving nutritious and attractive meals. Serve a wide variety of foods. Whenever possible, allow children to have two menu options. Families who share meal preparation tasks find that children who are given simple cooking tasks are better eaters. They will eat foods they prepare and most often are fair about tasting meals others prepare.

Meal time atmosphere influences how the whole family enjoys a meal—and often how well a child eats.

Establish a rule that all foods must be tasted before having a second serving of preferred foods or returning to play. This can increase food acceptance over time. Encouraging children to play outside and be physically active perks up appetites. There are more overweight children as a result of underactivity than overeating.

Snacks should be at least one and one half hours before mealtime. If children don't eat well at meals, snacks may be too large or have been eaten too close to mealtime. A pattern of too much food for the child's appetite is a signal that the meal plan needs reevaluation.

Feeding Problems

In the real world, feeding problems develop in all children. These problems seem to be magnified when a child has diabetes, because eating is such an important part of the management plan. When an eating behavior becomes a problem, what can parents do? First, make sure you are serving meals on a regular schedule; providing table, chair and utensils that are the right size for the child; serving snacks and meal portions of appropriate size; and setting a good example by the foods you are eating.

The next step is to use behavior modification. To begin changing an established behavior, clearly define what behavior is expected and reward that behavior. Common sense tells us that when an act is followed by a reward it tends to occur more frequently. Ignore or at least do not overreact to undesirable behavior. Although it may be difficult to do, avoid criticizing. Criticism is a common means of trying to change a child's behavior, but it is a form of attention, and attention of any kind often acts like a reward, leading to more of the behavior. Criticism can also arouse anger and a desire to get even.

Criticism and talking about a child's dislikes in his or her presence are not effective means of behavior modification.

Verbal praise from parents or brothers and sisters for eating good meals can encourage and reinforce a child's eating behavior. On the negative side, attention given to undesirable behavior, such as talking about the child's dislikes in his or her presence or by frequently correcting undesirable traits or table manners, teaches the child to use these behaviors to get attention.

A "star chart" can be used effectively as a reward plan for children. If the behavior you want to change is to have the child finish dinner, a star on a chart can be an immediate award for finishing the meal. It usually works best if stars are used for only one meal—breakfast, lunch, or dinner. The habit of finishing a meal or changing any behavior tends to carry over to other meals or similar situations. The task for which stars are given should be simple and easily achievable. When a certain number of stars have been received, they can then be exchanged for a reward—playing a game, going to a movie, or buying something special.

Resist interference from grandparents, other relatives, and neighbors. The more people involved, the larger and more complex problems become. Also, the problem child need not and should not know of the parents' concern. Food is a great battleground, and the less the child views it as a weapon, the better.

Remember that progress takes time. It takes children a while to make the connection that eating right makes them feel better. Sometimes children need to experience a reaction to realize that finishing meals is important. You can't always prevent a child's insulin reaction, but the best way to guard against one is to keep meals on schedule, stick to the meal plan, don't let your child skip snacks or meals, and if needed, provide extra food to compensate for extra exercise.

It takes children awhile to associate eating right with feeling good.

Do not play games or employ trickery to encourage eating. Inform the child—after about 30 minutes at the table—that there will be no more food until the next planned snack or meal is served. Let the child decide whether to eat or go without. If the child still shows no interst, remove the food without further comment. Follow through with your plan or you defeat the purpose. If a reaction occurs, treat it appropriately, but without a lot of fuss or attention, or "I told you so." Remember, it is not uncommon for children to rebel when forced to eat. Rejecting food is a way to assert independence.

In a situation where appetite just isn't what it usually is and not a behavior problem, the child should eat as much of the planned meal as possible. Take note of what is left to be eaten and offer an equivalent amount of food an hour or so later. This is especially important if blood glucoses have been in the normal range. When the overweight sedentary child is hungry for an extra snack, is it hunger or boredom? Test the child's blood glucose and if it is not low, create a physical activity diversion.

Since appetite will wax and wane with growth rate, it is important to keep the child's meal plan updated. If the meal plan is reviewed at every three-month check-up, it will be easier to keep current with the child's growth and appetite. It is especially important to have the child's meal plan updated in the spring and fall, since these are times that are natural breaks in the child's routine. A child may have a large appetite during the summer when physically more active and then need less food or a rearranged food schedule when school begins in the fall.

Children should not feel continually hungry or "stuffed." If this is the case, the meal plan needs adjusting. The child with diabetes needs the same amount of food as the child without diabetes. To grow normally, children need adequate nutrition. Consistent timing and spacing of meals and snacks is what is essential for the child with diabetes.

Remember that although vegetables are nutritionally excellent foods, they are low in carbohydrate and calories and do not have much effect on blood glucose levels. Introduce them gradually to the child with diabetes, just as you would to any child. Don't force the child to eat entire servings of vegetables. Try adding them to stews, soups, and breads.

It is important that children continue to be offered food choices. "You have a fruit exchange—what would you like?" Allowing selection from two offered choices leaves the child feeling some control over which foods are eaten.

Keeping a food diary can sometimes be helpful for older children. However, the child should not be made to feel that the family is "checking up" or trying to make him or her guilty. It is easy for the family to be critical of the eating habits of the individual with diabetes. The family has to be careful not to be judgmental.

Stock your refrigerator and cupboards with appropriate food choices—everyone finds it easier to avoid temptation when "treat" foods are not facing them at every turn. Great snacks are fruit, small cubes of cheese, yogurt, half a sandwich, nuts, unsalted popcorn, or cut-up raw vegetables. Dried fruit can also be a good snack. (One-fourth cup of dried fruit is one fruit exchange.) Crackers and cereal are other good snack choices. Avoid high fat and high salt snack foods such as weiners, bologna, chips, etc. Variety in snack choices is important. Be creative and make snacks fun when time and talent permit. How about fresh apple slices spread with peanut butter and decorated with an animal cracker, or pear-half bunnies with cottage cheese?

Because snacks are essential in diabetes management, you may need to use some snacks because of their convenience even if there are more ideal ones. For example, granola bars are convenient because they are wrapped individually and can be carried in a purse or pocket. One regular granola bar equals one bread and one fat exchange. Check labels for number of calories.

Treats such as ice cream, cake, and cookies can be used occasionally as bread exchanges, but try to save them for special occasions. The best time to use these foods is with a meal or before exercise.

Sugar-free hard candies can be used for treats. Chocolate dietetic candies are high in fat and calories and are not good choices. Just because the label states "dietetic" does not mean it is a good choice for people with diabetes. "Dietetic" food products such as chocolate candies, cakes, ice cream, and cookies usually contain more calories than the foods they are replacing and are not recommended.

Diet pops (or any pop for that matter) can be a significant source of caffeine for children. Caffeine is a special concern in children because of their body size and weight. A child drinking 12 ounces of pop has a caffeine intake comparable to an adult drinking 4 cups of instant coffee. Restlessness, irritability, sleeplessness, and nervousness are reported in children and teenagers consuming large amounts of caffeine beverages and foods.

The Importance of Education

It is essential that the child with diabetes and parents be well informed about diabetes management. Education increases the parents' confidence in the decisions they must make. Correct information is a vital support for good consistent parenting skills. It will also help determine priorities. Appropriate decisions need to be made to safely handle birthday parties, holidays, camping, vacation, travel, etc.

Education also helps in knowing what are realistic expectations of children at various ages. See Chapter 29 for more information on normal growth and development. For example, with very young children you can't expect as close control of blood glucose as you can in older children. But even for the very young child it is important to have a meal plan and to begin to establish appropriate eating habits. If a child develops diabetes at age 2 or 3 but is not introduced to an appropriate meal plan until age 6 or 7, it will be difficult for the child to understand why this is necessary. It is easier to start changing and improving eating habits as soon as diabetes is diagnosed. But be realistic in your expectations. Realize that many changes will be gradual.

Education in nutritional management of diabetes is important as well. Injected insulin continues to act throughout the day, unlike insulin produced naturally in response to eating. Consistency of food intake is important because of the predictable action of injected insulin.

You can generally divide food intake into smaller snacks or meals if necessary, without causing low blood glucose, but don't delay meals. It is important to take insulin injections at the same time each day, which makes it important to eat at set times. If meals must be delayed—such as when eating out in restaurants or when traveling—a fruit, bread, or milk exchange should be eaten at the usual meal time to prevent low blood glucose. This should allow the meal to be delayed by about one hour.

The amount of insulin needed by each child is individual and there is no "magical" insulin dosage. Nor does an increased dosage signal that diabetes is worsening. Higher blood glucose levels aren't a sign that the child is "bad," nor are they always preventable or a result of "cheating."

Raising any child requires good judgment and firm but loving discipline. When a child has diabetes, it is easy to want to give in to his or her every desire to make up for having diabetes. Food is easy to use for a treat or reward! You need to treat food and meals as part of a very normal and accepted routine. Backing positive eating habits with a supportive family that treats diabetes matter of factly is the best way to give the child confidence and pride!

Realize that it is normal for children to "sneak" forbidden foods. Encourage the child to exercise to burn off extra calories from irresistible binges.

Knowing which substitutions you can make in the meal plan is helpful to give the child more flexibility. Since calories are approximately similar in most fruit, bread, skim milk, and meat choices, they can be used interchangeably. Consistency in the number of servings from these groups is important at meals and snacks. Try to keep the calories as consistent as you can. However, don't worry about using up or skipping fat exchanges. Fat exchanges have a way of being used even when you are trying to be careful of them!

Skim milk is recommended for everyone—starting with children at age 2. If your family now drinks whole milk, gradually change to 2%, 1%, and then skim. It takes time to get used to the taste of skim milk, so it is a good habit to learn at a young age.

Cut back on salt in cooking and at the table. This is another good habit to establish at a young age.

Sharing your recipes and snack ideas with other families can help with common challenges. Try to avoid sharing dessert recipes, even if they are sugar-free or so-called "dietetic" desserts.

Children can learn about nutrition, exchanges, and their meal plan by playing different games. "Exchange cards" are available as games, which can be a fun way to learn new eating habits.

What about holidays with special treats?

Halloween poses special problems for the child with diabetes. Try some creative problem-solving with your child. Some families have tried the following:

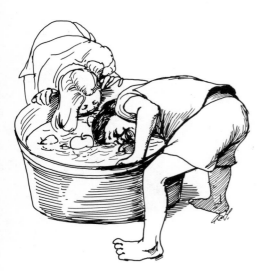

- Giving candy to children who are in the hospital, praising the child for being generous and suggesting a special occasion—play, sports event, or museum trip for him or her.
- Collect money for UNICEF and become pen pals with children in other countries.
- Divide collected candy with friends, brothers, and sisters.
- Take treats to school for other kids. It is a good feeling to be the giver of special treats.
- If children must have some candy, plan strenuous physical activity to teach balancing moderate increases in calories with exercise.

Easter baskets can be another problem. Try using other small gifts, such as coloring books, books, jewelry, etc., rather than candy in the Easter basket. Sugar-free gum and hard candy can also be used, but not dietetic chocolates. Ask grandparents to bring treats other than foods—such things as books, small toys, jewelry, records, and puzzles can be enjoyed by kids just as much as sweet treats.

Adolescents

Adolescents are in a precarious balance between striving for independence from the family and needing to depend on the family for basic physical and emotional needs. Adolescents are not free from the family nor do they desire total freedom. At the same time, they are attempting to become self-reliant and independent and to have more privacy.

An adolescent's friends are important—what they do sets the norm, and what they think (or what the adolescent thinks they think) is important. Being different is difficult for teenagers. Being on a diabetic meal plan suggests they are different. They do not want to seem odd, sick, or to be singled out for attention.

Adolescents have wide emotional swings. Nutritional changes to manage diabetes usually imply long-term or difficult lifetime changes. Persistence is needed. It is easier to do this when life seems rosy, but food modifications may take too much energy when anger, despair, or boredom get in the way. Food can be used to attempt to reduce tension or to make people happy. It can seem to reduce anxiety, alleviate depression, reduce boredom, and instill peace.

Changes need to be made gradually. Diabetes education helps to provide facts adolescents need to know and may want to know to better understand diabetes. Once you're confident they really understand the necessity of a meal plan and know their allowance of food, assure them of your confidence in their judgment and your love and support. Then let go. Expect that there will be times when they do not totally follow the meal plan. All the nagging in the world will not change this.

Teens do not need to know every nutrition detail, but instead need skills to help them change eating behavior. As an example, teens need to know how to refuse family or peer pressure to eat inappropriate but tempting foods. They also need the opportunity to practice and to experience success in a safe situation. They will not always succeed— nor do we. Threats of chronic complications are more likely to encourage them to ignore the rules and enjoy life "while they can!"

Assertiveness skills are helpful for teens, sometimes just to tell parents to "bug off." Better to say it than eat the world just to show us. A polite refusal has two parts: 1) a thank you for the offer or a compliment to the person making the offer, and 2) a refusal plus the reason for refusing ("Thanks Mrs. Smith, that cake looks wonderful, but I'm already full"). If people continue to be insistent, continue to refuse politely. No one needs to eat because someone else thinks they should!

Involve teenagers in problem-solving. Help them learn how to analyze and solve dietary problems. Start by brainstorming. Come up with as many solutions as possible to a problem that has been identified. Role-playing situations with adolescents in groups is helpful. Once all the ideas are exhausted, select a solution and plan how to use and evaluate it.

Don't give up hope if teenagers seem to rebel against the "diet" for awhile. High blood glucose causes fatigue and emotional lows. Most teens will gradually equate feeling good with normal blood glucose and will choose to stick to a consistent well-designed meal plan. Teenagers need to know it is their choice to make appropriate changes. "You really do have a choice and it is up to you. You can feel bad or you can try to control your diet. Either way we love you."

Summary

Children's eating habits become magnified when diabetes enters the picture. How well your family copes with this situation depends on attitude and ability: An attitude of willingness to make changes as necessary to make eating part of a healthy lifestyle for the child with diabetes as well as the rest of the family; and the ability to make substitutions within the child's meal plan to control diabetes while keeping meals and snacks fun and enjoyable. Look for all the help you can get—from cookbooks, other parents, a dietitian, etc. The tables on the following pages may be helpful in solving a child's eating problems.

Good enjoyable nutrition is a major part of a healthy and fulfilling lifestyle that will benefit your child for the rest of his or her life!

Suggestions For
Solving Children's Eating Problems

Ages 2 to 5

Eating Problems	Why?	If a child has diabetes
"Roller coaster" appetite. Desire for food changes day to day.	• May be changes in physical growth. • Amount of physical activity varies from day to day.	• Monitor blood glucose in order to adjust insulin needs to appetite changes. • Offer choices between two foods. • More snacks, smaller meals. • Understand child's response to food while encouraging sound food habits. • Offer half portions, praise, offer other half portion.
"Food jags" — eating only certain foods for a period.	• Child may be trying to establish independence or to attract attention.	• Ask child to take a "no thank you bite." • Don't overreact, offer a substitute. • Go along with it; can be helpful if it aids in food consistency for a period of time. • Establish a variety of foods to choose from early in life. • Understand that "food jags" are a normal part of a child's development. Express optimism that it will change later.

Ages 2 to 5

Eating Problems	Why?	If a child has diabetes
Child refuses vegetables and foods with a sharp taste.	• Children have an acute sense of taste and smell and usually prefer mildly or non-seasoned foods.	• Children enjoy foods that are crunchy, chewy, crackly and smooth. They dislike foods that are lumpy, mushy, slimy or stringy. Plan accordingly. • Serve vegetables raw with low calorie dip. • Cook strongly flavored vegetables with more water and for a shorter time to decrease strong flavors. (Use cooking water in soup.) • Serve vegetables in taco shells or pita bread. • Introduce new vegetables gradually in small amounts. • Vegetables are low in carbohydrate and calories so do not have much effect on blood glucose. Tastes will change — don't worry too much about them.
Child can't finish meal.	• Children have small stomachs and need to eat often.	• Plan five to six small meals. Make sure snacks contribute to nutrition. • Smaller meals and snacks are helpful for diabetes management. • Can divide foods up into more frequent feedings, but meals or snacks should not be skipped or delayed. • Look at meal plan if routinely too much food; perhaps food needs to be reduced for a time.
Child doesn't like certain foods.	• Children assert independence by rejecting things they don't like.	• Serve food cut in fun shapes. • Children often imitate what they see parents, brothers and sisters and teachers do. Extremely important to set a good example. • Assume tastes will change. Offer food again at meal with other favorite food.

Ages 2 to 5

Eating Problems	Why?	If a child has diabetes
Child refuses new foods.	• Children are curious but distrustful of the unknown.	• Introduce only one new food at a time. Offer a very small amount at the beginning of a meal. Finish meal plan with foods child already is familiar with and likes. • Don't offer new foods when child isn't feeling well. • Study how foods are grown, color pictures, grow new foods in own small garden. • Plan meals with new foods to try each month.
Child refuses to eat.	• Child may be asserting independence or may actually not feel like eating for some reason.	• Simply remove the food without making any bribes or punishment. Don't let food become a weapon against parents. • Monitor blood glucose levels or watch for symptoms of hypoglycemia — treat accordingly.
Dawdling or playing with foods.	• May be trying to attract attention or may not be hungry.	• Wait a reasonable time and then remove food. Watch for symptoms of hypoglycemia. • Offer help if needed. • Offer more at next snack or meal. • Make sure child is getting enough exercise. Limit TV watching time.
Wants to feed self.	• Eating is a way to be independent.	• Offer as many choices as possible that child can handle — finger foods such as raw vegetables, strips of fruit, bite-size sandwiches, etc. • Offer food in utensils and dishes that are easy for child to handle. • Encourage independence for child with diabetes.

Ages 6 to 12

Eating Problems	Why?	If a child has diabetes
Wants to eat what other kids may be eating — junk foods, etc.	• Need for peer acceptance; child needs to feel that she/he belongs and is accepted by classmates and friends.	• Help child learn that uncontrolled blood glucose equals not feeling good. • Help child realize that all children have differences. • Know that most children will try forbidden foods — don't forbid, work toward the positives of other ways of eating. • Make special treats just for "you" and whole family gets to share it too.
Typically eats four to five times a day.	• Growing children need to eat more frequently.	• May prefer to prepare own snacks after school. • Encourage independence. • Works great for child with diabetes, encourage consistency.
Accepts more foods but still may reject vegetables and casseroles.	• Food likes and dislikes change rapidly during middle years.	• Children should be encouraged to try new foods, help in food preparation and menu planning. • Keep offering food with positive expectations for change.
Child affected or influenced by television.	• Children look to parents, teachers, and other media as authorities on many things, including foods.	• Parents buy the groceries, parents make the choices. • Parents need to set a good example; not just right after diagnosis, but always. • Make a house rule not to have sugared cereals — not because of diabetes but for the well-being of the whole family.

Adolescents: Ages 13 to 20

Eating Problems	Why?	If a teen has diabetes.
Teen resists others' attempts to encourage good eating habits.	• Environment important; teen will often eat anything that is available.	• Deal with weight control and fitness, not diabetes (positive vs. illness). • Cartoons on the refrigerator can help. • Post charts and graphs that support positive change.
Sabotaging statements from family and/or friends about the kinds or amounts of foods to eat.	• Friends are major influence on teens.	• Discuss thoughts that create problems and those that foster progress. • Identify family member or friends who will be supportive or who might help if asked. • Don't threaten with diabetic complications.
Emotional problems related to food.	• Our society (ads, TV, books, movies, etc.) is filled with confusing information about food and eating.	• Discuss thoughts that create problems and those that foster progress. • Identify emotions associated with inappropriate eating and those that help the teen stick to his or her dietary goals.
Poor food habits.	• Teen may exert independence by displaying poor food habits.	• Support teen's values, such as physical appearance. Good nutritional habits support being the most attractive we can be. • Discuss whether eating can really make us popular.
Snacking common.	• Teens like and sometimes need to eat frequently — always on the go.	• Can be helpful if good snacks. • Assure yourself that he/she understands the meal plan. • Expect teen to act maturely. Let go!
Trouble complying with meal plan.	• Teens have hard time focusing on one issue for any length of time.	• Look for gradual improvement. • Consider professional help if necesssary. • Compromise with your expectations for a time. • Support all compliance efforts. • Applaud self-care measures. • Encourage testing to monitor control.

INDEX

—A—

Albumin—268
Alcohol—38-40 (table), 178, 215, 222, 240
Aldose reductase inhibitors—176, 281
Alpha cells—5, 145
American Diabetes Association (ADA)—3, 30, 288, 307, 312
American Dietetic Association—30
Amino acids—22-23
Antibodies—297, 302-03, 306
Arthritis—176
Aspartame—312-13
Atherosclerosis—27, 181, 250

—B—

Banting, Frederick—5, 302
Bell's palsy—277
Berson, Saul—6
Best, Charles—5. 302
Beta cells—5, 153, 302-03, 305-06
Bladder infections—221
Blood glucose (sugar)—5, 8-10, 14, 19, 23, 25-26, 35, 38, 54, 56, 70-71, 97, 117, 119-20, 123, 135, 140, 160, 172, 173-177, 182, 186, 189, 193, 194, 199, 220, 223, 227, 228, 240, 242, 244, 263, 269, 280, 304, 306, 361, 365, 374, 376
Blood glucose monitoring—26, 35, 56, 57, 69, 72-74, 93-95 (how to do), 123, 139-40, 160-62, 190, 192, 215, 228, 303, 309, 311, 321, 323, 326, 328, 358, 360-61
Blood pressure, high (hypertension)—29, 55, 177, 179, 180, 190, 194, 197, 210-12, 215, 230, 250, 252, 254, 262, 269, 270
Blood pressure, low—278
Blood vessel disease—14, 175-76, 178, 185, 189, 190, 210-12, 238, 243, 250, 252, 253, 284, 285
Body weight
   desirable—164, 197
   loss of—54, 62, 165, 197, 198, 199-204
   measurement of body fat—197
Brain (see also stroke)—11, 275, 323
Bread—31, 42
Breast feeding (nursing)—206

—C—

Caffeine—376

Calories—21, 22, 24, 27, 30, 31-34, 38, 39, 54, 60-61 (table: Using Up Calories with Activity), 162-65, 195, 198, 229, 359

Carbohydrate—8, 15, 21, 22, 24-26, 30, 31-34, 39, 58, 148, 167-68, 322, 325, 357

Cardiovascular disease (see heart disease)

Cataracts—212, 258

Children

    chapter for—334-53

    growth and development—15, 135, 163, 174, 354-68

    eating habits—369-79

Cholesterol—21, 23, 27-28, 149, 159, 177, 189, 190, 194, 195

Chromosomes—296

Complications of diabetes

    Sudden or short-term (see also hypoglycemia and hyperglycemia, infections, and vision)—15, 173-74

    Intermediate (see also pregnancy and growth and development)—15, 174

    Long-term (see also specific body areas)—4, 6, 15, 149, 175-82, 185, 190, 193, 209-15, 304, 363, 379

Congress—4, 307

Contraception (birth control)—228, 235, 243-47

C-peptide—153

Crapo, Phyllis—25

Creatinine—268

Cyclosporin—303

—D—

Dehydration—10, 62, 147, 323

Dental care—219-20, 360

Diabetes

    Control of—3, 14-16, 19-20, 56, 81, 97, 117, 119-20, 135, 140, 171, 175, 182, 186, 189, 193, 194, 206, 209, 211, 230, 235, 236, 241, 280, 304, 314, 357, 366, 367

    History of—4-7

    Search for cure—3, 299, 302-03, 305

    Types of (table)—13

      Gestational—13-14, 232

      Insulin-dependent (Type I)—12-14, 133-51

        "brittle"—133, 137, 143

        causes of—13, 295-98

        complications—14, 171-82

        diagnosis—14, 134

        exercise in—56-59, 320-29

        "honeymoon period"—137

        "juvenile"—12, 133

        meal plan for—139, 159-68, 309, 311

        prevalence—4, 133

        symptoms—134

        treatment—14, 134-51

      Non-insulin-dependent (Type II)—12-15, 166, 179, 185-215

        "adult-onset"—12, 185

(*Diabetes, continued*)

causes of—21, 186, 188, 194, 298
complications—14, 209-15
diagnosis—14, 188, 189
exercise in—55, 60-62
meal plan for—194-204, 309
"nonketosis-prone"—185
prevalence—4, 186
"stable"—185
symptoms—13, 14, 189
treatment—13, 15, 183, 187-93

Diabetes Control and Complications Trial (DCCT)—182, 304
Diabetes pills (oral hypoglycemic agents)—15, 20, 40, 60, 85, 185, 191, 205-08
Dialysis—270
Diet (see meal plan)
Dietary Guidelines for Americans—21
Dietetic foods—310, 312-16, 376, 378
Dietitian, registered (R.D.)—159, 197, 359
Diets, fad—204
Digestion—8-9, 22-23, 277-78
Driving—142, 367
Drugs ("street" or illegal)—224-25

—E—

Eating habits, changing—199-204
Education—150, 376-77, 379
Electromyogram (EMG)—181, 279
Emotional adjustment—101-15, 363, 367
Employment—368
Exchange lists—30 (table)-33, 35, 42-51, 316-19
Exercise—35, 53-67, 136, 139, 141, 142, 162, 165, 198, 204, 253, 291, 310, 320-29, 360

Food adjustments for—57, 58 (table), 162
Heart rate during—64-65 (table)
Insulin adjustments for—59, 328-29

Eye problems—4, 14, 55, 173, 179, 190, 212, 256-65 (prevention tips), 277

—F—

Fat (lipids)—8, 11, 15, 19, 21-24, 27-29, 33, 48, 177, 189, 194, 210, 253, 285, 322
body fat (see body weight)
monounsaturated—28
Omega-three—28
saturated—27, 28, 159
unsaturated or polyunsaturated—28

Feelings about diabetes—101-15, 363
Feet, foot care—55, 214, 282-93 (prevention tips), 326
Fiber—25-26 (table)
Fitness, World Health Organization definition—53
Flu shot—174
Food labels, how to use—314-19
"Free" foods—33, 49, 203, 315
Fructose—313-14
Fruit—32, 46, 325

—G—

—H—

—I—

—K—

—L—

—M—

—N—

—O—

—P—

—R—

Rebounding (Somogyi effect)—143-44
Recombinant DNA—154, 301, 304
Renal threshold—72, 75, 189
Research—3, 4-7, 182, 300-07
Restaurants—169, 201, 308-10
Retinopathy—212, 260 (photos), 261-62
Rewarding good behavior—123, 203

—S—

Saccharin—312
Salt (sodium)—29, 159, 196, 270
Sanger, Frederick—6
School personnel—358, 360-62
Self blood glucose monitoring (see blood glucose monitoring)
Sexual concerns
    for men—237-40
    for women—241-47
    for adolescents—368
Shoes—67, 289, 326
Smoking—178, 215, 222-23, 240, 253, 288
Snacks
    before exercise—58
    for children—375-76
Somatostatin—302
Sorbitol—176, 314
Space shuttle—305
Sports—291, 320-29, 360
Star chart—373
Starch—25
Steiner, Donald—7
Stress—124-25, 133-34, 136, 139
Stress hormones—141, 143, 145, 166
Stress management—124-26
Stroke—4, 14, 211, 243
Sugar—25, 313-14, 322, 324
Sulfonylurea agents (see also diabetes pills)—208
Support system—112-13, 128

—T—

Toilet training—357
Transplantation—271-72, 305
Triglycerides—23, 27, 149, 177, 189, 190, 194

—U—

Urea (BUN or blood urea nitrogen test)—268
Uremia—267-68
Urinary tract infection—221, 269, 273
Urination, problems with—221, 278
Urine glucose testing—69-70, 75-76 (table comparing to blood glucose testing), 96, 192, 357
Urine ketone testing (see also ketones)—77-78, 96 (how to), 147-48

—V—

Vegetables—32, 45, 203, 375
Viruses—174, 297
Vision, blurry—173, 258
Vitrectomy—263

—W—

Water—10, 62, 147, 323
White blood cells—288, 297

—Y—

Yalow, Rosalyn—6

APPENDIX

If you found this book helpful and would like more information on this and other related subjects you may be interested in one or more of the following titles from our *Wellness and Nutrition Library.*

BOOKS:

The Joy of Snacks — Good Nutrition for People Who Like to Snack
(288 pages)
The Physician Within (210 pages)
Pass The Pepper Please (90 pages)
Fast Food Facts (40 pages)
Convenience Food Facts (137 pages)
Opening The Door To Good Nutrition (186 pages)
Learning To Live Well With Diabetes (392 pages)
Exchanges For All Occasions (210 pages)
A Guide To Healthy Eating (60 pages)

BOOKLETS & PAMPHLETS

Diabetes & Alcohol (4 pages)
Diabetes & Exercise (20 pages)
Emotional Adjustment To Diabetes (16 pages)
Healthy Footsteps For People With Diabetes (13 pages)
Diabetes Record Book (68 pages)
Diabetes & Brief Illness (8 pages)
Diabetes & Impotence: A Concern for Couples (6 pages)
Adding Fiber To Your Diet (10 pages)
Gestational Diabetes: Guidelines for A Safe Pregnancy and Healthy Baby
(24 pages)
Recognizing and Treating Insulin Reactions (4 pages)
Hypoglycemia (functional) (4 pages)

The *Wellness and Nutrition Library* is published by Diabetes Center, Inc. in Minneapolis, Minnesota, publishers of quality educational materials dealing with health, wellness, nutrition, diabetes and other chronic illnesses. All our books and materials are available nationwide and in Canada through leading bookstores. If you are unable to find our books at your favorite bookstore contact us directly for a free catalog:

Diabetes Center, Inc.
P.O. Box 739
Wayzata, MN 55391

Slide Series By the IDC

Guidelines for Managing Diabetes During a Brief Illness (1984) 53-slide series $74.00. Narrative Cassette $10.00
Vividly illustrated instructions and food suggestions with narration and inaudible 1000-HZ slide advance.
Exchange Lists for Meal Planning (1979) 62-slide series $69.00, Narrative Cassette $10.00
Appealing food photography by General Mills, Inc., illustrates foods in the six exchange lists and nutritive values.
Healthy FootSteps for People with Diabetes (1985) 80-slide series $90.00, Narrative Cassette $10.00
Photography and anatomical illustrations show practical and easy to follow foot care steps to have happy feet.
Diabetes and Impotence: A Concern for Couples (1985) 50-slide series $74.00, Narrative Cassette $10.00
A warm presentation of the possible complication of sexual impotence, its prevention, diagnosis and treatment.

Portions of the above slide series and cassettes can be reviewed for $5.00 each.

Other Sources of Information About Diabetes

American Diabetes Association, Inc.
2 Park Avenue
New York, NY 10016

Juvenile Diabetes Foundation
23 East 26th Street
New York, NY 10010

Both of the above organizations have branches and affiliates throughout the United States.